Biodynamic

CRANIOSACRAL THERAPY

Other books by Michael Shea

Biodynamic Craniosacral Therapy, Volume One
Biodynamic Craniosacral Therapy, Volume Two
Biodynamic Craniosacral Therapy, Volume Three
Biodynamic Craniosacral Therapy, Volume Four

Biodynamic
CRANIOSACRAL THERAPY

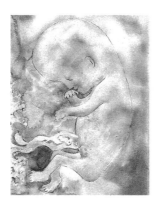

Volume Five

Michael J. Shea, PhD

With contributions from

Raymond Gasser, PhD   Carol Agneessens, MS

Christopher Muller   Ann Diamond Weinstein, PhD

Valerie Gora, LMT   Phyllis Aries

Laurie Park   Michael Kern

Alexander Berzin, PhD   Alan Lokos

Sheila Shea, MA

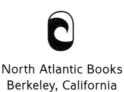

North Atlantic Books
Berkeley, California

Published by
North Atlantic Books
P.O. Box 12327
Berkeley, California 94712

Cover art by Friedrich Wolf
Cover and book design by Jan Camp
Production by Larry Van Dyke
Printed in the United States of America

All photographs in Chapter 23 used with permission from the photographers Lina Surowitz and Ivana Surowitz. Photographs in Chapter 24 used with permission from the photographer Rob Aries, except photo 24.31, which was taken by Karl Roecker. All photographs in Chapter 25 used with permission from the photographers Rob Aries, Laurie A. Hoffman, Karl Roecker, Danielle M. Polizzi. The photographs in Chapter 26 are used with the permission from the photographer Laurie Park.

Biodynamic Craniosacral Therapy, Volume Five is sponsored by the Society for the Study of Native Arts and Sciences, a nonprofit educational corporation whose goals are to develop an educational and cross-cultural perspective linking various scientific, social, and artistic fields; to nurture a holistic view of arts, sciences, humanities, and healing; and to publish and distribute literature on the relationship of mind, body, and nature.

North Atlantic Books' publications are available through most bookstores. For further information, visit our website at www.northatlanticbooks.com or call 800-733-3000.

MEDICAL DISCLAIMER: The following information is intended for general information purposes only. Individuals should always see their health care provider before administering any suggestions made in this book. Any application of the material set forth in the following pages is at the reader's discretion and is his or her sole responsibility.

New ISBN for Volume Five: 978-1-58394-547-6

Library of Congress Cataloging-in-Publication Data
Shea, Michael J., M.A.
   Biodynamic craniosacral therapy / by Michael J. Shea; with contributions from Margaret Scott … [et al.].
     p. ; cm.
   Includes bibliographical references and index.
   Summary: "a thorough description of the evolution of cranial osteopathic medicine into a new form available to many health care providers, this book presents a technique of touch therapy that is extremely gentle and subtle and gives practical exercises to be proficient in healing physical, spiritual, and emotional conditions"—provided by publisher.
   ISBN-13: 978-1-55643-591-1
   ISBN-10: 1-55643-591-6
   1. Craniosacral therapy. I. Society for the Study of Native Arts and Sciences. II. Title.
   [DNLM: 1. Complementary Therapies—methods. 2. Musculoskeletal Manipulations. 3. Mind-Body Relations (Metaphysics) 4. Sacrum. 5. Skull. WB 890 S539b 2007]
RZ399.C73S54 2007
615.8'2—dc22
                            2006031902

        1 2 3 4 5 6 7 8 9 SHERIDAN 18 17 16 15 14 13
                    Printed on recycled paper

This book is dedicated to His Holiness, the Fourteenth Dalai Lama.

May all beings be parted from clinging and aversion—
  feeling close to some and distant from others.
May they win the bliss that is especially sublime.
May they find release from the sea of unbearable sorrow.
May they never be parted from freedom's true joy.

CONTENTS

ILLUSTRATIONS

ACKNOWLEDGMENTS

This book is like a journal to me. There are more contributors to Volume Five than any of the previous volumes. It is truly a collaborative effort. My first goal was to bring forward the female voice in biodynamic practice. Carol Agneessens, who is not only a brilliant practitioner, but also an incredible teacher of the work, has written one chapter and co-authored three other chapters with me, especially in the embryology section and Appendix B as well. Ann Diamond Weinstein has contributed six chapters in the development of a body of knowledge that I believe must form the core of any approach to prenatal and pediatric therapy, especially biodynamic practice. Phyllis Aries has contributed two chapters on working with babies and moms in neonatal intensive care units. I have known Phyllis now for more than ten years and her contribution to the field of pediatric craniosacral therapy is nothing less than magnificent. Laurie Park, who also works in neonatal intensive care, has written a beautiful and emotional story about her work with babies who died in a neonatal intensive care unit. My sister, Sheila Shea, has contributed seven chapters on detoxification. It is the most thorough examination of detoxification that I know of, especially regarding constipation.

A fundamental principle of osteopathy is the balance of nutrition coming in and waste products being removed. That theme is explored throughout this volume from the first section on embryology through to the end of the book, with my sister's chapters. Finally, Valerie Gora, a certified doula, biodynamic craniosacral therapy instructor, and pregnancy massage instructor, has contributed a chapter on prenatal craniosacral therapy. All of the contributions from these women move the biodynamic paradigm into a deeper, richer, and more feminine voice. I am very grateful for their willingness to speak their voices in Volume Five.

This book is not my book but a collaboration by many people. I teach with several remarkable people. First is Sarajo Berman who has been together with me for more than ten years in the classroom. She constantly shapes my sensibility around embodiment with the depth of her knowledge and sensory skills. Catherine Vitte teaches with me and works with me, especially with the embryo presentations. Our dialogue for the past decade has sharpened and directed my understanding of the embryo and helped me to find my own embryo as it lives on in my body. Marcel Bryner is another exceptional biodynamic instructor whose sensitivity and clinical expertise is beyond mine. He has been a friend and colleague over a decade and always available to review my biodynamic thoughts and ideas with precision and clarity.

Several men have also contributed to Volume Five. Once again, Raymond Gasser, who to me is the best American embryologist, has contributed yet another interview that allows biodynamic practitioners to deepen their understanding of the embryo and how to palpate the embryo. Christopher Muller of www.booksandbones.com has graciously allowed me to transcribe a DVD that he produces called *The Protoplasm of a Slime Mold*. I have also annotated it with a focus on how the movie shows and discusses Primary Respiration and stillness. Michael Kern, one of the premier instructors and school owners of biodynamic craniosacral therapy, has generously provided a meditation on accessing a spiritual resource. Alan Lokos, the author of *Pocket Peace* (2010), one of my favorite spiritual books, has graciously contributed eighteen practices from his book in my chapter on the stages of spiritual development. Finally, Alexander Berzin has contributed a translation of an eighth-century text, specifically a chapter called Patience. I find that patience is a very important element of biodynamic practice and Shantideva, the actual author, elaborated completely and fully on the need for patience and how to be patient.

I am sitting here with my local editor, Sara Dochterman. It is likely that I could not produce these books without her help. She makes the work effortless and seamless. We had to finish the preparation for this book during Tropical Storm Isaac and I can only express my profound gratitude for her and her commitment to the well-being of the planet. Sara is a licensed social worker in clinical practice and gives up her time to midwife these books of mine. Lisa Fay, my office manager, actually holds this entire empire of mine together as I travel around the world teaching and withdraw into my office writing these books. Thank God for Lisa! Of course, I cannot actually do any of this without my wife, Cathy. As I was putting the finishing touches on Volume Five, I realized I was getting behind and my wife dropped everything she was doing and helped finish several chapters. Our marriage produces a creative energy and a collaboration that is the foundation for all of the books I produce and the teachings I give.

I am very fortunate to have had the same copyeditor for all five of these volumes. Her name is Winn Kalmon. It is through her precision and organization that this book and the others in the series retain coherence and, to me, a beauty or aesthetic that permeates the writing. This beauty comes from her editing. Wendy Taylor, my managing editor, is incredibly responsive and clear with all of my inquiries and needs in the entire publishing process. I am also very grateful to Richard Grossinger, my publisher, who holds a vision not only for the human embryo, but how the embryo is integrated into everyday life at a cellular level.

I am very grateful to Jeannie Burns, who transformed and touched up more than 150 photographs for this book and drew one of the images that I commissioned from her. She is always available and timely with her help. Finally, I am grateful to His Holiness the Dalai Lama, my teacher, because of his continued inspiration and wish that centers for the development of the heart be formed all over the world. It is through his teachings that I have come to understand that biodynamic craniosacral therapy is a protocol for compassion.

I wish to acknowledge all of the mothers, fathers, and babies shown in this book. Just by looking at the loving connection, it is possible to retrain our brains and hearts into a deeper, empathetic understanding of the human condition, and the obvious need for love and connection in this day and age. I offer praise and gratitude to all who have helped me along the way.

INTRODUCTION

We have entered the age of fear. Somewhere between September 11, 2001, in New York City, and the December 14, 2012, Newtown massacre of innocents, our culture took a step deeper into the suffering of unnecessary fear and unhappiness. This is a book about one antidote, called biodynamic craniosacral therapy.

Biodynamic craniosacral therapy is constantly evolving. This book is about an important paradigm shift in biodynamic practice. It is my experience that Primary Respiration and stillness guide this unfolding. I see the biodynamic model as having eight aspects, shown in Figure I.1. Each ring is designated with a letter. Starting in the middle with the letter A is the therapeutic intention of slowing and stilling. This, of course, specifically relates to the practitioner's ability to perceive Primary Respiration and its rhythmic, balanced interchange

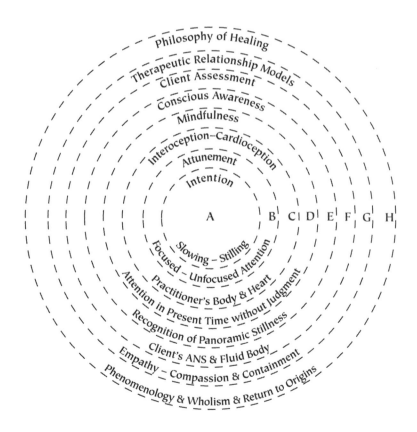

Figure I.1. The eight aspects of biodynamic practice.

with Dynamic Stillness. This perception begins in and around the practitioner and gradually is extended to include the client later in the assessment phase of a session.

Moving outward from the center, the next ring, B, is called attunement. I have written extensively about attunement, especially in Volume Four. It is the main work of a biodynamic session. Attunement is the capacity of the practitioner to move his or her attention close to the client and rhythmically away from the client in a slow tempo. This includes the simple ability to focus and unfocus one's attention. This is how nervous systems grow, develop, and stay in balance.

The next ring outward, C, is called interoception. Some literature refers to this as cardioception. The meaning of this is simple. The practitioner spends the majority of time in a session sensing his or her own body and especially the movement and activity of the heart and blood. This body awareness changes brain structure and develops resilience. Resilience is the conscious ability to return one's heart rate and mental state within a window of tolerance physiologically and a state of peacefulness. This requires the ability to notice states of arousal and work whatever skills are necessary to dissipate the arousal state as soon as possible, both mentally and cardiovascularly. Everyone comes in and out of states of arousal all day long and even during a biodynamic session. These waves come and go all day and can be normalized so that the big waves do not cause damage. I highly recommend a new book by Richard Davidson and Sharon Begley, *The Emotional Life of Your Brain* (Davidson and Begley, 2012). His research and antidotes to stress build resilience, especially with mindfulness meditation.

How does a practitioner accomplish such healthy attunement and interoception? It is through the process of mindfulness seen in the next ring, D. Mindfulness simply means that the practitioner maintains conscious attention in the present time or moment without judgment. First of all, present time refers to physical events and mental processes, such as breathing, that are only occurring on a moment-to-moment basis. A thought may be about the past, but the thought is happening in this present moment until the next thought comes along. The current breath that I am taking is occurring now, not in the past or future. Consequently, mindfulness of breathing and mindfulness of mind are essential components of biodynamic practice. This is especially true because of the relationship of breathing with Primary Respiration that I speak about in this book. Mindfulness also includes suspending any judgment or interpretation about what one is experiencing at any time. Judgment and interpretation create compression. Although compression is a normal biological dynamic, stress and trauma exacerbate compression and cause physiological problems. Biodynamic practice is about normalizing compression and allowing it to go through its reciprocal rhythmic cycle of decompression in a slow tempo.

Biodynamic practice involves two kinds of mindfulness. The first kind of mindfulness is deliberate. Deliberate mindfulness initiates the whole capacity to be in right relationship with one's mind and body. Mindfulness allows the mind and body to become synchronized. I call this orientation, as described in Volume Four, which is the first step in the biodynamic process. Gradually, the practitioner does not have to work so hard at being deliberately mindful. This leads to the second kind of mindfulness called spontaneous mindfulness. In other words, mindfulness simply becomes an alignment with a pre-existing state requiring no effort to notice or initiate. There is no effort at being mindful, but this takes a lot of practice.

Spontaneous mindfulness gradually leads to conscious awareness, seen in ring E. In biodynamic practice the practitioner becomes consciously aware and recognizes panoramic stillness. As mentioned earlier, Primary Respiration is in a rhythmic, balanced interchange with Dynamic Stillness through all the zones extending from the practitioner's midline out to the horizon. This kind of panoramic awareness usually occurs in the middle of a session, as if the zones have merged into one unified whole. If the reader is unfamiliar with the concept of the zones of awareness, please refer to my Volume Four.

The heart of biodynamic practice involves a restoration of the client's autonomic nervous system and fluid body, as seen in the next ring, F. The more mindfulness and conscious awareness generated by the practitioner, the more restorative Primary Respiration and Dynamic Stillness become for the client. Thus, client assessment involves the stability of the autonomic nervous system both in the limbic system of the brain and the heart and cardiovascular system of the practitioner's body and then the client. Assessment of the client's fluid body involves the perception of the potency of Primary Respiration to become more amplified and three-dimensional in the client's fluid body. It is vitally important that these assessments be done by the practitioner with the practitioner's own mind and body first before extending that evaluation and practice to the client.

I believe that the model of the therapeutic relationship in biodynamic craniosacral therapy is actually a protocol for compassion, seen in ring G. My previous volumes and this one discuss the neurobiology of empathy and compassion. This is based on the original research having to do with mirror neurons. It involves a four-step process in which, first, the practitioner's nervous system and vascular system merge with that of the client's, and vice versa. Second, the practitioner differentiates his or her own body-mind states. This simply means that the practitioner spends time focusing on his or her own sensory body. This creates a third element in the relationship called resonance. It is through the practitioner's ability to differentiate his or her own body sensation that the client's brain and heart unconsciously resonate with this deliberate slowing and stillness. The client's brain, heart, and body mimic what is happening with the practitioner.

As this process of empathy unfolds, a fourth step called insight is gained by the practitioner on where to move next and how to apply attention and attunement with the client. This is nothing less than compassion, which is the attempt to reduce and stabilize the client's pain and suffering. Empathy and compassion in the context of healing require a container and thus the zones and their perception become the field of healing and create containment for the transformation necessary for the client's pain and suffering.

The last aspect of the biodynamic model involves its philosophy of healing in ring H. The philosophy of phenomenology is simply the ongoing lived experience of the practitioner and also that of the client. It is highly subjective. Lived experience has to do with sensation, feeling, and perception of the totality of the human body. I have noticed over the years in practicing phenomenology and teaching it that each student and practitioner works with his or her own metaphor to describe lived experience. Thus biodynamic practice is a system of metaphors such as *fluid body, stillness, Primary Respiration, ignition,* and many other descriptions of felt, living experience. At a deep level, healing, as discussed in all of my volumes, is about sensing one's wholeness and the ability to return symbolically through Primary Respiration to one's conception as an embryo. It is here where the human body is a single-celled, undifferentiated whole. Many healing traditions have rituals designed for the patient to touch this original state of wholeness. Primary Respiration and stillness, experienced in the present moment with mindfulness, allow both practitioner and client to touch their original wholeness. Thus, Volume Five continues the exploration of these eight aspects of biodynamic practice. Please note that all the circles in Figure I.1 are drawn as dotted. This implies a continuum throughout the whole biodynamic model.

Section I of Volume Five, on biodynamic embryology, begins with an interview with Raymond Gasser, PhD. Ray is Professor Emeritus of Embryology at Louisiana State University and co-author with Erich Blechschmidt, MD, of *Biokinetics and Biodynamics of Human Differentiation,* which was updated in 2012. This section and these chapters begin to shift the biodynamic paradigm toward an understanding and a palpatory sensitivity of both biodynamics and biokinetics. In brief, biokinetics refers to local changes and metabolic fields of growth and development in the embryo and adult. Biodynamic refers to the interconnected wholeness of the local fields and the growth of the whole over time. Chapters 2, 3, and 4, co-authored with Carol Agneessens, go into detail on biokinetic and biodynamic applications in clinical practice. Chapters 5, 6, and 7 involve the various protocols that I am currently teaching, along with Carol, that resulted from this paradigm shift. It is now possible with these advanced skills to work with the blood and the heart, which, according to Jaap van der Wal in a conversation I had with him, are the active elements of the fascia. Primary Respiration moves through the vascular system and the fascial system in distinct patterns and a practitioner with thinking and feeling hands can enhance the healing benefits of Primary Respiration to the client.

Chapter 8 ends the first section with an annotated transcript of the famous biodynamic movie entitled *The Protoplasm of the Slime Mold.* Many biodynamic practitioners have seen this twenty-five-minute movie in which the protoplasm of a living slime mold found on a log in a forest is viewed under a microscope in 1954. Primary Respiration is visible in its phase changes and mentioned by the narrator. This chapter serves as a valuable interpretation and viewing guide of the movie, which is available from Christopher Muller at www.booksandbones.com.

Section II focuses on biodynamic practice. It begins with Chapter 9 on new perspectives on the therapeutic relationship, which includes a thorough review of the literature on interpersonal nervous systems and interpersonal cardiovascular systems and summarizes information also found in Volumes One through Four of this series. Chapters 10, 11, 12, and 13 detail therapeutic practices for contacting the fluid body and Primary Respiration. The biggest challenge in teaching biodynamic craniosacral therapy is helping students bypass their musculoskeletal system and to take the leap off the end of all the nerve synapses in the autonomic nervous system into the great ocean of the fluid body. The human body is 92 percent fluid and yet practitioners and clients alike hold on to that other 8 percent of tissue, especially the musculoskeletal system. These tissue systems carry the imprint of so much stress and trauma that it is exceedingly difficult to simply allow the imprint to be there and allow it to dissipate into the greater living fluid field of wholeness via Primary Respiration. These chapters are designed to help the practitioner and client liquefy the musculoskeletal system without fear through the practices of buoyancy and transparency. The fluid body is a concept. Buoyancy and transparency are the lived experience of the fluid body. Ultimately, the intention of these practices are to open the heart in a way that produces joy and happiness that is embodied.

Chapter 14 is a discussion of the Mid Tide, especially from the point of view of zone B. This zone is the immediate space around the body and this chapter details how to sense the integration of the body as it extends beyond the surface of the skin out 15–20 inches. Chapter 15, about breathing, is by Carol Agneessens. Once again, Carol has contributed a vital piece of knowledge to biodynamic practice.

Section III is on pediatric practice. It begins with Chapter 16 and a discussion of my particular history of working the children with cerebral palsy and other developmental delays. Chapters 17–22 are by Ann Diamond Weinstein, PhD. Ann has written what I consider to be a body of knowledge for pre- and perinatal psychology. These chapters comprise a primer for anyone working with pregnant moms, babies, and parents of those babies, including biodynamic craniosacral therapists. This body of knowledge is linked to the standards of practice that I proposed in Volume Three for practitioners wishing to learn pediatric craniosacral therapy. These chapters provide in-depth knowledge of the literature associated with the primary period extending from pre-conception through the first two years after birth. More information can be found on the primary period in my Volume Four. Chapter 23, on prenatal craniosacral therapy, is by Valerie Gora. It is the first clinical discussion that I am aware of for practicing biodynamically with pregnant moms.

Chapters 24 and 25 are by Phyllis Aries about her brilliant work with babies in neonatal intensive care units (NICUs). These chapters are the most thorough investigation that I have ever seen of clinical processes and techniques with small babies. Finally, Chapter 26 is by Laurie Park and entitled Singing Them to Heaven. Laurie is a music therapist who also works with babies and families in NICUs. She writes about her work, especially in assisting babies die and helping families transition through the death of their baby. Death as it turns out, is a common experience in NICUs.

Section IV is about healing principles. Michael Kern has contributed a beautiful spiritual meditation in Chapter 27 for biodynamic practitioners. Chapter 28 is about patience. It is from the sixth chapter in Shantideva's book *Engaging in Bodhisattva Behavior,* written in the eighth century CE in India. I am very grateful for permission to reprint this translation by Alexander Berzin, PhD. Patience is a virtue, as my mother used to say, and this long exposition about patience represents a cornerstone in the biodynamic work that I practice and teach. Chapter 29 includes important practices for one's own personal development and also helping clients. I am very grateful to Alan Lokos for contributing very easy practices from his book *Pocket Peace* (2010).

Finally, Section V on detoxification involves the final seven chapters in this volume; they are by my sister, Sheila Shea. To study the human embryo and human development is to study how nutrition is taken in by the body and waste products get removed. At every level of development, whether the human body is the size of a lentil as in an embryo or its adult size, the principle of nutrition and waste removal must be in balance or disease and disorders follow. Detoxification is a term that implies the removal from the body of toxic waste that derives from a contemporary lifestyle or living in a polluted city. The toxic waste must be removed from the body and Sheila elaborates on one of the principle problems, constipation, and its healing. Waste removal and detoxification are essential for proper metabolic function for the autonomic nervous system and fluid body in general. It is a theme found throughout Volume Five.

To finish Volume Five, I have included three appendixes. Appendix A is a new client brochure I recently wrote for a class I was teaching in Arizona. Appendix B is actually a poster I made for graduates of my Foundation Training in New York City several years ago with the help of Carol Agneessens. Finally, Appendix C is a complete list of all the sutures of the cranium. It serves as a ready reference for those undertaking such a study to improve their skills.

I must say in closing that this is not the Volume Five I originally conceived. It has more contributors than any other volume and in some ways I feel like I am the editor of a journal with this volume. I am hoping that it shifts the paradigm into a deeper level of biodynamic practice. It has certainly done that for me with the help of Primary Respiration and stillness.

SECTION I

. . .

Biodynamic Embryology

CHAPTER 1

The Metabolic Fields of the Embryo

*An Interview with Raymond Gasser, PhD,
January 2012*

Michael: I think a way to begin this conversation is to talk a little bit about the general characteristics of the metabolic fields to understand what these fields are and how they relate to growth and development.

Ray: The reader should understand right away that contrary to what many developmental biologists believe, differentiations begin on the outside of the cell, not on the inside in the cell nucleus. The view that many of them have about differentiations is similar in some respects to preformations, that differentiations begin in the genome located in the nucleus. They believe the appropriate signal moves out of the nucleus and cause differentiations at the appropriate time. Contrary to this concept are Professor Blechschmidt's theories that are based on differentiations starting on the outside, then transmitted to the cell membrane, through the cytoplasm and finally to the cell nucleus. The nucleus then responds in an appropriate but specific way, depending on the stimulus. It is not inside-to-outside differentiation but outside-to-inside. With this concept the nucleus is a reactive center rather than a center of genetically, preformed programs that cause differentiations.

Blechschmidt made a series of very precise reconstructions from the serial sections of human embryos. From the reconstructions he observed where structures were located at each stage of development. From his background in physics he reasoned that all movement is caused by physical force, or, in other words, physical force causes the movements. This is what biokinetics means, or simply kinetics. It is not possible to have a movement without force. This is what the biodynamic concepts of human differentiations are about. Biokinetics and biodynamics are applied to living systems and, in this case, to the living human embryo, which is composed mainly of fluid. After making the reconstructions

3

he observed the embryo wholistically as structures differentiated over time. This relates to the meaning of biodynamics or simply dynamics. He saw changes occurring on the outside (surface) of the embryo and, at the same time, changes were occurring on the inside (in the organs and cells). Developmental biologists have reported almost exclusively on differentiations occurring regionally and are mainly unaware of what is happening in a wholistic manner by observing what is happening in other regions.

As the embryo differentiates, its structures are constantly changing their shape at every level. Most developmental biologists view the shape changes as being initiated and directed by the nucleus. But, as pointed out in this book, cell membranes are very thin and flexible structures. It is easy to understand how a physical force on the outside of the cell could change the shape of the cell. The shape change then influences the nucleus to express itself in a particular way. Based on his observations he wanted to understand how the whole embryo maintained its wholeness as organs changed their position, shape, and structure over successive stages of development. He expanded on the notion of fields of activity, which he named metabolic fields in the embryo. The biodynamic model of differentiation is based on the biology of metabolic fields. These fields are three-dimensional fields consisting of an aggregate of cells changing shape in distinct patterns within a predominantly fluid matrix. Particular physical forces in the tissues operate to bring about changes in the position, shape, and structure within a given field of cells.

The embryos that were precisely reconstructed often vary remarkably from what is depicted in college embryology textbooks, where often a drawing is only a general concept of how the embryo and its internal structures are arranged. Blechschmidt's reconstructions are located in the Anatomical Institute at the University of Goettingen in Goettingen, Germany. When one observes them one is immediately struck by how much time and effort went into making them. Before the reconstructions could be made, human embryos had to be sliced into hundreds of sections depending on their size, and then each one is enlarged so that the total reconstruction was roughly a meter from top to bottom. There are over sixty models and each model took approximately three years to make.

Once Blechschmidt observed which way structures were moving and enlarging, he then examined the sections more closely under a microscope, recording the shapes of the cells and how the cell shapes changed from one stage to another. After noting where the shape changes occur, he then widened his view to determine what force could possibly cause the shape changes. He observed structures at every level of magnification, from the surface of the embryo down to the surface of the cells. To explain what he observed he used different types of arrows in the illustrations. The meaning of each type of arrow is defined in the original preface of our book that we co-authored, *Biokinetic and Biodynamic Differentiations in Human Development: Principles and Application* (Blechschmidt and Gasser, 1978, revised ed. 2012). The arrows indicate specific movements such as directions of growth, resistance to growth, and specific forces that reside in and around metabolic fields. Sometimes only an arrowhead shows the force direction and at other times the arrows are pointed toward one another or sometimes they are pointing away from one another. Some arrows have a horizontal base line. There are a variety of arrow types, but it is important to understand that each means a specific movement that takes place. Some refer to the direction of flow of nutrition, some the growth direction of the tissue, some refer to the movement of the metabolic fields, growth resistance, and so on.

What Blechschmidt then did was to observe the cell positional, shape, and structural changes. He realized that they were all synchronized with one another. They all occurred simultaneously. From these observations he divided the activity into early and late metabolic fields. For the first time one can examine the early fields using the Virtual Human Embryo DREM project of serial sections of human embryos. The section images at each stage can be viewed at http://www.virtualhumanembryo.lsuhsc.edu. Go to the section images themselves and look at the shape changes and where the cells have different shapes in different positions and different densities. Some regions become quite dense while other regions become much less dense.

Fluid movement brings about the changes. Much of what biokinetic and biodynamics are about is fluid movement. Blechschmidt stated that this fluid movement was ordered and organized. The fluid movement in turn determines the cell shapes and the organ shapes, especially in the early stages. What the monograph points out is that in the early stages the biodynamics of certain structures result from the movements and forces causing them to appear. The early structures in early metabolic fields are caused or brought about by such movements. Throughout the embryo fluid is constantly moving from one region to another. If a region changes from a very dense or fairly dense one, and subsequently becomes looser, one can safely conclude that more fluid has moved into that region. At the same time the structure and associated metabolic fields are enlarging in one direction. In the early metabolic fields the overlying epithelium is referred to as limiting tissue. The ectoderm is stretched, which is what you would expect in a growing, expanding embryo. It has a very stretched appearance under the microscope.

Some years ago I did a study on the effects of the enlarging neural tube on the structures surrounding it. The shape changes that occurred made perfect sense, as the neural tube becomes the spinal cord. Cells around the neural tube have certain shapes and positions. I examined almost every one of Blechschmidt's conclusions and verified what he observed. I have never found him to be wrong when he described shape changes and position changes. I respect his observations and I concur with them after examining sectioned human embryos at each stage over the past fifty years.

One can examine the one-cell stage embryo post-fertilization (stage 1 of the Carnegie stages) and, after about twenty-four hours the cell begins to divide into two cells. Actually the cell subdivides because there is a subdivision of the original cytoplasmic mass. The membranes move in from each side to join and then form two cells, but they are smaller. Blechschmidt believed fluid movement brings this about. The fluid presses against the cell membrane to cause it to move inward. When Blechschmidt saw a cell membrane move in a particular direction, he concluded that there is a pressure difference at that location and that if it becomes concave in its shaping process, then there is pressure on the outside pushing against the membrane, causing it to bend inward. Either this occurs or there is a reduction in the pressure on the other side of the membrane. Nevertheless, there is a difference in the pressures or forces operating that cause the structural change. These are important principles to understand in the activity of the metabolic fields.

Early metabolic fields include a variety of activities that happen during the early part of development that are described in the front section of the monograph. The late metabolic fields are described in the back section and are easier for most people to understand. The early fields address the formations of such structures as early blood vessels, early peripheral nerves, the somites, and so forth. Many of the early structures disintegrate or transdifferentiate as the embryo grows and then needs a more differentiated structure for support. The late fields provide the process for a completed or at least more differentiated complex structure and function such as how precartilage forms, then cartilage, and then muscles surrounding the cartilage segment before the cartilage become bone. They are fields that generally occur a little later than the early ones. There is some overlap, but it's generally the late metabolic fields that are more three-dimensional force fields that operate a little later and over a longer period of time. The early fields usually operate over a shorter period of time, like subdivision of the ovum, somite formation, and neural tube closure.

M: So the metabolic fields as described have a lot to do with fluid direction or organized movement of the fluids, as Blechschmidt said. It would also seem that there is a densification or one might say a viscosity related to some of the metabolic fields, just in terms of the thickness. Is that an accurate statement?

R: I am reluctant to use the word *viscosity.* The tissue becomes denser if the intercellular fluid leaves. In other words, if you observe that from one stage to the next the tissue becomes denser, then there's less intercellular fluid. Blechschmidt looked very closely at the intercellular substance, i.e., all the material that's between the cells. If the cells get closer, then the intercellular substance has less volume than it previously did. Blechschmidt followed how that happens physically—where does it go?

M: Well, I think it is a very good point and a challenge for a lot of students, because we have to study molecular biology and it's all about the inside. And here is a whole different view of embryology that has been developed about studying the outside. I think that's really significant.

R: It's actually because of this outside-to-inside differentiation, not inside-to-outside, that changes the whole point of view of how an embryo grows and develops. Developing structures are viewed as structures differentiating because of extracellular processes. This concept is completely different from the nucleus being in charge of differentiation.

   When I first encountered the term *metabolic field,* what came to mind was biochemical metabolism, as in the Krebs cycle and all the different chemical reactions occurring. But Blechschmidt looked at metabolism from the point of view as a change brought about by physical fluid forces, whether it's the accumulation of fluid or the reduction of fluid or the enlargement of a mass. It is simple and elegant science. He looked at the so-called biokinetic forces as a metabolic phenomenon. It's the activity of a cell or groups of cells in particular locations at particular times in the embryo that cause the changes. That's why he called them metabolic fields. The term *field* was used to describe such activity as seen in the embryo in the 1930s by developmental biologists and it is likely he expanded the concept used at that time.

M: You mentioned the type of arrows he used in his illustrations. I have always found that the key to the Blechschmidt drawings is understanding the meaning of the arrows.

R: Many of the drawings are from photomicrographs, but not all. When you read the text of the monograph you'll see a fair number of times where his conclusion is based on logic rather than actually seeing something change, such as fluid movement. When you observe in an area that it becomes loose or contains more fluid, then obviously something is moving into the tissue. These sorts of observations are repeated throughout development and therefore predictable. The definition of the arrows is very important and defined early in the preface of the book. If one doesn't understand the various arrow definitions, then one has no idea what's being presented and will become confused, as you probably have seen with some of your students.

M: Well, the osteopathic community really has quite an interest in the definitions of the terms you are describing and I think there are several osteopaths who have attempted more extended definitions that obviously would be very interpretive of what Blechschmidt said.

R: As I stated at the beginning, kinetics means force and movement and dynamics means force and movement over time. Kinetic movement is movement caused by force. Biodynamics is more about the forces and movements acting over a period of time. You add a third factor of time in biodynamics because this is biodynamic embryology, which means an embryo is simply growing and adding more tissue during its entire span of development. There are different kinetics acting at different times, but it's the biodynamics that occurs over a period of time. Thus kinetics occurring over a period of time becomes biodynamic.

M: I think sometimes the osteopathic community, in differentiating the term *biodynamic* from *biokinetic,* has referred to the word biodynamic as also relating to the activity within the whole, as opposed to just the parts. There is a dynamic occurring within the whole and I think in our last interview (Chapter 9, Volume Three) you had said that every field knows where every other field is and every cell knows where every other cell is in the embryo. And, as such, one could say that knowledge of the whole of the structure is biodynamic. Would you agree with that?

R: Well, that concept is not wrong. I think that it's a way of looking at perhaps the adult arrangement, the definitive arrangement rather than the developing arrangement. My definition was more looking at it in a developmental viewpoint.

M: I remember reading a book on embryology that had a tremendous influence on me. Called *Crystals, Fabrics, and Fields: Metaphors That Shape Human Embryos*, it was a Yale University PhD dissertation by a woman who studied and compared the work of three developmental biologists in the first half of the twentieth century. One of the observations of these three was that the knowledge of the whole physical embryo is conserved or carried over through each successive stage of development. So I think that goes along with what you just said but maybe as a corollary to your principle. The point is that some osteopaths studying Blechschmidt's work equate the term biodynamic with the principle of dynamic wholeness occurring over time and observed in each successive stage of development. The author called it the conservation of wholeness.

R: If it's an adult where things are in a definitive arrangement, it is biodynamic in that state. Adults change, as one gets bigger, as one grows up. Blechschmidt also talked about the development of function. Not just the development of structure, but also function. At no time during development is an organ without function, whatever the organ. An organ may change its function as it develops, but there is always a function present. Blechschmidt points out in one place in the monograph where function may reside in a tissue for a particular period of time. He uses terms such as limiting tissues and inner tissues. Limiting tissues are epithelium such as the ectoderm and endoderm. On the other hand, inner tissues are the mesenchymal tissue that develops into so many different things and thus it is undifferentiated but becomes differentiated over time by the physical forces we have been talking about.

M: In reading and reviewing all of his published work, including the one you co-authored with him, it's interesting that in each of the glossaries in the books there is a slightly different, nuanced description of the term *biodynamic,* but I like the way you describe it a lot, because it's a consideration of a process that's occurring over time.

R: That's how I see it with the background I have.

M: The process that's occurring over time is very complex with all the changes taking place.

R: Some developmental biologists talk about inducers or induction and use the term primarily as differentiation needing a chemical inductor. But the observations of Blechschmidt pertain actually to physical induction. Forces that operate in three dimensions bring about tissue change in the shape of the cells, their position, and what is going on inside them. To repeat, differentiation begins on the outside and then moves to the inside. This concept is dramatically different from many developmental biologists' concepts. They envision things inside the cytoplasm that move the cell membrane and cause the cell to take the shape that it has. Many of them consider shape change as originating in the cell nucleus.

M: You know, it's interesting that two weeks ago, there was a prestigious piece of research released. The researchers were studying a particular type of worm and it was the first time that they discovered that cell division did not occur as a result of the cell nucleus. In the description of the research, they were saying that this could likely turn cell biology upside down.

R: I really believe that cell biology is going to undergo dramatic changes. It's not that all the published findings are wrong. It's that their interpretations of what was discovered are not correct. When I lectured to students I tried to explain how differentiation begins on the outside. I would use as an example a cell that has a stellate shape at a particular stage as it lies between two organs. Then, at a later stage you observe that the two organs have moved apart and the shape of the intervening cells is now fusiform. It is no coincidence that the moving apart of the two organs coincides with the shape change of the intervening cells from stellate to fusiform.

Another example is when the neural tube expands dorsally; the surface ectoderm dorsal to the tube appears distended and stretched. The ectoderm must keep up with the dorsally expanding tube. If one is not aware that the neural tube expands dorsally away from the notochord, then the change in the overlying surface ectoderm will likely be overlooked. It is interesting that the surface ectoderm on the side of the embryo is not thin like that located dorsal to the tube but is much thicker. However, the surface ectoderm on the ventral side of the embryo stands out again as being stretched because here the heart and liver bulge deep to it.

I can understand how osteopaths are very interested in this phenomenon because force and movement bring it about. I am pleased that they are bringing to light these concepts that many developmental biologists would rather ignore. Eventually the truth of what is taking place biologically will be known.

One of the reasons I worked on the Virtual Human Embryo DREM project for twelve years was to make available to everyone digital images of the microscopic sections of human embryos at every stage and at three to four levels of magnification. Anyone who is skeptical of the concepts now can view the particular stage and sections and observe for themselves the shape changes in the cells by visiting the website mentioned above and obtaining the images. They can observe the cell shape at a particular stage, and then compare it with what they observe at another stage. I'm hopeful that developmental biologists who are interested will look at the changes. Without seeing them one might think that all the arrows in the book illustrations are just a bunch of nonsense.

M: In terms of the metabolic fields, as the embryo is expanding, different tissues and even the fields when they become paired together, there is a resistance that occurs in the growth. Can you comment?

R: Yes, there are particular areas of resistance associated with metabolic fields. A good example is the biokinetics of a blood vessel. When a blood vessel forms, no matter how big it is in the definitive state, that vessel begins as a capillary tube, which is very small and fragile. As the vessel expands, the surrounding mesenchymal cells adhere to the outer part of the tube thereby contributing to the formation of the media of the vessel. As you know, blood vessels are designed to carry nutrients to and waste products from organs and cells. Blechschmidt noticed that blood vessels do not elongate at the same rate as the structures they supply. Nerves act the same way and act as restrainers also. This is sometimes referred to as differential rates of growth.

Blood vessels that supply the early brain elongate slower than the enlarging brain and head region in general. Because of this phenomenon the cephalic part of the neural tube has to bend downward onto the heart. The first ventral bend occurs in the brain-spinal cord junction, causing the formation of the cervical flexure. Another ventral bend occurs in what's going to become the mesencephalon. Thus, there are two ventral bends in the neural tube that form precisely where blood vessels enter and leave the brain. If you study the brain as presented in standard embryology textbooks you might read that the cells on the inside are pushing the brain in the ventral direction. But if you back out of that focused view and look at where the blood vessels enter and leave the brain and also understand how the brain enlarges, you soon realize that the vessels act as restrainers on the brain and bring about the bends.

This movement occurs because the vessels are not elongating as rapidly as the brain is enlarging. The brain must maintain its blood vessels as it expands but the vessels, which are growing more slowly, are restraining its growth. As the brain grows longitudinally, it has no recourse except to bend. If one treats blood vessels as restrainers, one can then understand where bends occur in the neural tube. The blood vessels expand by forming the shape of a fan in the bends that act as restrainers of growth. This doesn't mean that they stop growing, only that they slow down their longitudinal growth in certain areas where they are bringing blood to and from a region.

Both veins and arteries act as restrainers. The arrows in the images from our book and all his other publications in English and German show this quite clearly. Stretched tissue also acts as a restrainer. As they grow, nerves also can act as restrainers of the structures they are innervating. Blechschmidt explains how the limbs bend before the muscles are formed. If you look at where arteries traverse within the limb on the ventral side it becomes obvious that the arteries are restraining the elongation of the limbs occurring on the dorsal side. The limbs bend precisely where they have to in order to maintain a blood supply. They can't outpace their blood supply, which is a basic need for continued development. Blechschmidt's drawings show where the blood vessel enters the limb and how the parts it supplies are elongating. If the artery cannot elongate at the same rate as the limb then the limb has to bend. This is an important principle of growth.

M: So you have differential rates of growth. I almost said the slower the rate of growth has more control over the growth overall, but that wouldn't be an accurate statement. It has to be in balance as a kind of polarity of differentiation. Do any of the metabolic fields act as or offer resistance?

R: Yes. There is a field that acts as a restrainer. Wherever there is stretched mesenchymal tissue or stretched ectodermal or endodermal tissue, they all act as restrainers. They are not as restraining as some structures, like blood vessels, but they restrain tissues that are deep to them. Such a field is called a retention field. The notochord forms in such a field. Stretched tissue is a spatial modification to the tissue. An example of the developmental movement that occurs in these fields is shown as stick figures in our book *Biokinetics and Biodynamics of Human Differentiations*. Two matchstick men are pulling against each other at each end of a rope. The rope does not give but retains its position. Such fields are referred to as a restraining apparatus.

The movement is longitudinal pull in one main direction that is associated with simultaneous drag caused by transverse pressure along the length of the notochord, for example, and this transverse drag becomes a detraction field at the tip of the notochord, which differentiates the basicranium. In this way the retention field differs from a dilation field where muscle forms. In both fields the tissue is pulled but the dilation field has no transverse pressure on it, thereby allowing the premuscle cells to expand and become muscle cells. In a retention field the cells cannot expand because there is a force around them that prevents them from dilating. Such fields give rise to ligaments whether they are ligaments between bones and cartilages or ligaments and tendons that hold muscles in place. They are all restrainers.

There is another late metabolic field named a suction field where there is reduced pressure on one side of a particular layer of outer or inner tissue. What develops in such fields is a diverticulum. If the diverticulum forms from the surface ectoderm it becomes a hair follicle or a sweat gland. The diverticulum is caused by the reduction of fluid pressure deep to the ectoderm. The ectodermal cells do not grow into such places unless there is a reduction of pressure that makes them grow in that direction. Initially, I wasn't keen on the term *suction field*, but I don't have a better one. The movement is a sucking motion, which is caused by a reduction in the pressure of the air or fluid. This is how fluid moves through a straw or a baby breastfeeds.

M: Right. So it's like a polarity, in the sense that one side of the structure has flexibility and the other side doesn't, and that creates the movement that he called suction.

R: The diverticulum forms from the basal layer of epithelium. The cells there change their shape and form a projection that grows into the tissue. The mesenchymal cells that are in that area take on a stretched shape, as though the diverticulum is moving into the mesenchymal tissue away from the surface epithelium. A sweat gland starts out as a solid diverticulum. Before the epithelium can grow into the mesenchymal tissue deep to it, there must be a reduction in the pressure that allows the diverticulum to form. Pressure reduction occurs throughout and deep to the skin.

M: In Blechschmidt's work, when does the earliest metabolic field begin to operate? At what age, so to speak? Are we talking about right after conception?

R: The first metabolic field occurs at fertilization with the union of the ovum and sperm. During fertilization the fertilizing sperm attaches to the cell membrane of the ovum and a process similar to a corrosion field occurs in which the outer acromosomal layer of the sperm head dissolves as its nuclear material enters the cytoplasm of the ovum. This is Stage 1a. This event causes the genetic material in the ovum to subdivide. Half of this genetic material is expelled as the second polar body. The first polar body is genetic material expelled at ovulation. The genetic material in the head of the sperm and the leftover genetic material in the ovum each form a spherical mass called a pronucleus.

The pronuclei then move toward one another. Something is causing them to move. Since there is no known electromagnetic attraction, the movement must be caused by the movement of fluid. As the pronuclei approach one another, each loses its pronuclear membrane and the chromosomes in each pronucleus line up in the equatorial plane and duplicate. The cell membrane of the ovum then begins to enfold in the equator zone on each side. The two enfoldings join in the middle of the cell causing it to subdivide into two cells. The genetic material divides very quickly.

What causes the cell membrane to enfold? Again, it's a force in the fluid that's operating to bring the membranes to join one another and then separate into two cells. The original one-cell ovum is now subdivided. Blechschmidt didn't like the term *divide.* He preferred the term *subdivide,* because the total amount of material did not increase. No true growth occurs at this stage. True growth does not occur until implantation during the second week when the embryo has access to nourishment in the endometrium. Until that time the fertilized ovum subdivides into more and more cells that become smaller and smaller with each generation. What occurs during this period is that the nuclear material is being duplicated at the expense of the cytoplasm. Eventually a ball of cells forms and then a cavity starts forming inside the ball. Toward the middle of the first week post-fertilization cells are multiplying that are progressively smaller, but each cell has roughly the same genetic information in its nucleus.

Fluid is produced that causes a cavity to form and the cells to be in different locations. This process is also a kind of metabolic field because it is caused by a compressive or kinetic force. This stage is called a blastocyst. Initially a shell called the zona or capsula pellucida surrounds the blastocyst and it is thick enough to prevent the inner cells that are subdividing from expanding. With each subsequent subdivision the cells get smaller and compressed. Toward the end of the first week, the first cell division into two types of cells occurs. Then the capsule is shed as the blastocyst enters the uterine cavity. The shedding of the capsule is sometimes referred to as hatching.

The blastocyst emerges very rapidly from the capsule and then rapidly enlarges as a result of fluid pressure increasing on the inside with little resistance now from the outside. This could be described as a type of expansion field although Blechschmidt did not give it a specific name. The cells at the periphery of the blastocyst that will become the future placenta are stretched. A clump of different cells resides on the inside on one side of the fluid cavity. These cells give rise to the embryo proper. The side of the blastocyst where the embryo proper is located is the side that attaches to the endometrium first. As this attachment process occurs a process similar to a corrosion field takes place because the uterine cells are dying, making way for the embryo to invade the endometrium. From the very beginning, metabolic fields are in operation that change the position of the cells, their shape, and their structure.

M: And then I think that the next field is the densation field.

R: As you know, embryos are 99 percent fluid. If the intercellular fluid moves out of a group of cells the cells then get closer together and become denser. This phenomenon is called a densation field. Whenever a group of cells become very dense and are very close together with very little intercellular material, then the cells are in a densation field. The matchstick drawing that illustrates this shows two men holding a strainer and fluid comes out underneath from the strainer. The structures that are in the strainer get closer together.

M: What about suction fields, which I mistakenly thought were associated with early fields in my previous volumes?

R: The suction field forms later, when growths from the overlying epithelium extend into the mesenchymal tissue beneath it.

M: I was just wondering, since the last time we talked, we discussed the late fields. Perhaps by way of ending, you could comment about the distusion and contusion fields, since they are paired fields.

R: I will be happy to discuss them. A contusion field is a metabolic field in which cells are being pressed together from an outside force. In other words, in one stage the cells are sphere-shaped and then at the next stage, they are disc-shaped in the same area. What causes the change in shape is the result of forces acting on the cells, pushing against them. This field is illustrated with two matchstick men pushing a spring from both sides. The arrows that have a transverse base line point toward one another. The forces are pushing toward one another or contusing.

A contusion field is where precartilage forms. In other words, a contusion field appears where cartilage will subsequently form. Before cartilage forms the once spherical cells become disc-shaped. When precartilage transforms into cartilage, it expands or distuses. The disc-shaped precartilage cells become large spherical cells that form cartilage. If one measures the mass of cells that are compressed to form precartilage, when the mass distuses, it enlarges tremendously. In other words, the cells are flat discs early on when they undergo contusion and become precartilage. The cells then become spherical and the mass elongates in a distusion field to give rise to cartilage.

M: It's so elegant, the whole notion of metabolic fields. It's such a different way of almost feeling the way the embryo grows.

R: When I was in Germany with Blechschmidt, I was on sabbatical leave from my university. I would attend his lectures to the medical students in the morning. He would use two or three projectors so that he could compare what's happening from one stage to the next. After his lecture he usually came to my office and for an hour or two with pencil and paper we would discuss his presentation. He knew a little bit of English and I knew a little bit of German. Together, by using mostly embryological terms, which are similar in both languages, we were able to communicate. The drawings of the matchstick men were a result of our meetings.

So the precartilage mass then elongates in a distusion field, which usually sets up a dilation field. Premuscle masses usually surround a mass of cartilage. As the cartilage distuses, the cells in the premuscle masses elongate simultaneously with the distusion. And as they elongate, they change into muscle. The distusion field sets up or brings about the dilation field. Biologists often wondered what caused or what circumstances cause the muscles and skeletal elements to be just the precise length for the muscle to act across the joints. There must be communication between the two metabolic fields to bring this about. Otherwise, either a skeletal element or the muscle will be too long or too short for smooth movement. Both elements are very precise in their lengths, so that they operate across the joints in a very precise manner.

These two fields occur early, as soon as the limb bud starts forming. The precartilage condensation is contused, which then distuses as the limb bud elongates. Distusion is the agent of motion in the developing limbs, not the muscles. The condensed mesenchymal tissues surrounding the cartilage are premuscle masses that change into muscle as a result of the distusion movement of the cartilage. If the distusion movement did not occur then the dilation field would not occur. This is a beautiful example of how one field sets up another.

M: Thank you for your generosity, Ray. I really appreciate it.

R: Anyone who understands and is willing to disseminate biokinetic development will always have my cooperation because I very much believe in this. I have observed the tissue and cell changes. I know the shape, position, and structure changes are real. This is not a fabrication. I have been very fortunate to be able to look at the embryo sections at different levels of magnification and what I see is what Blechschmidt saw. To observe the changes during differentiation is very fascinating and convincing work. I'm so thankful that osteopaths are very interested in the concepts and are promoting it. I don't know if they can utilize all of the concepts in their practice, but the biokinetic concepts remain true, nevertheless.

Postscript by Raymond Gasser, PhD: Watching the one-cell, fertilized ovum give rise in eight short weeks to nearly 95 percent of the named structures in the adult body is probably the most fascinating single event in my life. Witnessing this miracle take place has convinced me that only a higher power could bring this about. Rather than viewing development regionally or systemically in isolation from the rest of the embryo, as heretofore has been traditional, it is now possible to view developing structures as a part of the whole embryo (i.e., wholistically).

Interview and postscript included with permission from Raymond Gasser, PhD.

CHAPTER 2

Principles of Biodynamic Embryology

with Carol Agneessens, MS

At first glance, understanding Figure 2.1 might be challenging. How does the reader orient to the information being shown? Hand in hand, we will walk through this labyrinth slowly, allowing the reader time to absorb and digest the information. The intention of this chapter is to provide a comprehensive understanding of biodynamic embryology principles from the perspective of palpatory skills in biodynamic craniosacral therapy. It is an understanding and experience of biological wholeness. The embryo is a living whole and that wholeness as a living moving reality is never forgotten in the process of growth and development throughout life.

As a practitioner cultivates a full body sense of a living, breathing, fluid wholeness within oneself in relation to neverending embryonic development, a new way of practicing biodynamic craniosacral therapy emerges. This chapter also serves as a glossary of important terms used in the classroom to teach biodynamic embryology and translate that into palpation skills. We are very grateful to Raymond Gasser, PhD, for his permission to use images from his *Atlas of Human Embryos* (Gasser, 1975) so the reader has a visual reference for this chapter.

While settling in the realm of Primary Respiration and stillness, many practitioners have already sensed embryonic movements in themselves and in their clients. Figure 2.1 offers the practitioner an opportunity to review fundamental principles and developmental markers of embryonic development. The best way to learn embryology is to visualize the process being discussed in one's own body. For example, if we are talking about the heart, then pause from reading and sense the activity and movement around your heart right now and find its embryonic origins with the help of Primary Respiration and stillness. Chapters 3 and 4 go deeper into how to identify and palpate these embryonic features that exist through the lifespan. Repetition and practice are key for the depth of this understanding to sink into the practitioner's sensibilities and be incor-

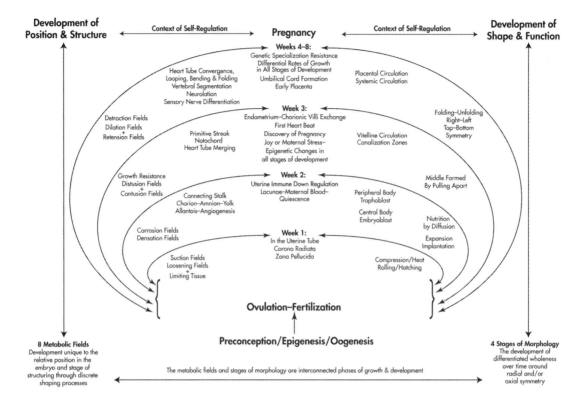

Figure 2.1. The biodynamic and biokinetics of embryonic self-regulation.

porated into a biodynamic practice. Biodynamic embryology is a deep somatic practice.

Although the scope of this chapter necessarily limits all the permutations of an embryonic reality, it can be studied as three overlapping stories of creation. One story begins on the left side of Figure 2.1 as the metabolic fields. The second story begins on the right side as the story of morphology. The third story is in the middle. It is the creation story as pregnancy. Within these three stories are a set of principles that we unfold as part of each creation story. These principles are oriented around the idea promoted by Dr. Jaap van der Wal that what begins as a metabolic reality in the embryo becomes physiology after birth and a psychospiritual reality throughout the lifespan. With this in mind, let's begin our tour of the embryo.

The Eight Metabolic Fields

Understanding of the metabolic fields has evolved since the publication of Volume One of this series. With the support of Ray Gasser and the lectures of Brian Freeman, we have evolved a deeper understanding of these forces of development. Descriptions of these fields can also be found in Volume Two, Chapter 28; Volume Three, Chapter 29; and Volume Four, the Glossary of Biodynamic Terminology.

Let's begin at the bottom left of Figure 2.1, with our first creation story. It is a story about the structure of the embryo. The eight metabolic fields relate to "development unique to the relative position in the embryo and stage of structuring through discrete shaping processes." Now notice the arrow pointing to "development of position and structure" in the upper left corner. This pathway from bottom to top covers both early and late metabolic fields over the course of embryonic development.

The metabolic fields are areas of development (position) in the embryo, with each having different gradients of density or viscosity. They are full of living water. They retain what is called spatial order because every field "knows" where every other field is located. This is a basic principle of biological wholeness. Since each of these gradients is going to be different, it means that in the case of just one field, there will be different pressures exerted from the fields surrounding it. This shaping process will be discussed in more detail when we get to the other side of Figure 2.1 and talk about morphology. One of the jobs of a metabolic field is to manage its water content, and generally losing water or displacing water causes a metabolic field to develop a form.

For example, imagine the varying metabolic fields shaping the embryo at its cephalic and caudal end (head and rump). Each field will have a different structure and density. Not only do these fields have varying densities but also distinctive motions (also known as biokinetics, discussed in detail in Chapters 1, 3, and 4). In Volume One of this series, the metabolic fields were presented as a possible explanation for Dr. William G. Sutherland's discovery of the analog of these motions throughout the body in the musculoskeletal system. He named these movements: torsion, side-bending, flexion-extension, and shearing laterally and vertically. He especially noted these motions in the sphenobasilar junction of the cranium early in his career. This means that the metabolic fields can be palpated, as the reader will discover throughout this book. The palpation we are referring to is done with Primary Respiration.

Let us now enter into the related terminology of the metabolic fields inside the four curved lines. Starting at the left column, the list of metabolic fields starts with the term "limiting tissue." Limiting tissue has an outer layer that is thicker and an inner layer that is thinner and metabolically more active. This is the first order of palpatory skills in a metabolic practice, discussed in detail in Chapters 3 and 4. The practitioner differentiates between outer and inner tissue while inhabiting a somatic attitude of buoyancy and with attention settled on the backs of his or her hands rather than the palmar surface. This contact refers to the cultivation of a multidimensional or holographic touch rather than a focused or narrower contact.

The inner layer is surrounded by loosening fields, which are known by their wateriness, as mentioned above. This is the second order of palpation and gives access to the movement and viscosity of the metabolic fields. This is where the practitioner places his or her hands for working metabolically with the client through Primary Respiration and stillness.

From bottom to top in Figure 2.1 the metabolic fields are named:

- Suction fields

- Densation fields

- Corrosion fields

- Contusion + distusion fields

- Growth resistance (a quality associated with densation, corrosion, contusion, retention, and detraction fields and thus an intrinsic part of the fields)

- Retension + dilation fields

- Detraction fields

Although these fields tend to overlap, they are roughly divided into what are called the early fields and the late fields. The early fields consist of the loosening fields, suction fields as seen in the first week, and the densation and corrosion fields seen in the second week. Remember again that a case could be made for densation fields to be present from the moment of fertilization, as discussed in Chapter 1. We highly recommend reading Chapter 1 to understand this point.

There is an inherent challenge in creating a two-dimensional linear graphic (Figure 2.1) of a three-dimensional nonlinear process. Remember that in human embryonic development, it is not possible to say that the definitive features of the human embryo arise in a specific time sequence. Although the twenty-three Carnegie stages (O'Rahilly and Muller, 1987) attempt such a description, a massive study of human embryos in Japan (Blechschmidt, 2004) has clearly shown that developmental timelines are nonspecific and one could say that the features of growth and development are expressing themselves simultaneously in many dimensions without adhering to a rigid time sequence. Human embryonic development is more like watching a garden in springtime burst forth with color and fruit.

Palpation of the metabolic fields offers a greater possibility in restoring the health of the client. The fields operate under three principles: development of *position,* development of *form,* and development of *structure.* The fields occupy a unique position in the embryo different from where they end up and they develop a unique form prior to differentiating into a definitive structure like a heart or a brain or a bone. They have different gradients of fluid (mostly water) that begin in a specific area or position in the embryo. Then the fields begin to condense into a form much like scaffolding made of jelly and gradually come into a definitive structure some time later (the sacrum, for example, does not finish ossifying until twenty-eight years after birth).

It is possible to affect the adult structure by sensing any of the three elements of a field (position, form, and structure) in which it was originally constructed. The universal fluid movements and patterns of order and organization inherent in all the fields continue to be present in the adult as both biokinetic and biodynamic forces. This will be discussed in detail in the next chapter.

Growth Resistance

The late metabolic fields beginning in the third week are denoted with the term *growth resistance,* which is a significant factor in the development of the human embryo. It also operates as a principle biokinetically and biodynamically throughout the lifespan. The most basic way of understanding growth resistance is that of observing differential rates of growth in the embryo. The drawings of Blechschmidt in all of his books use a particular type of arrow to indicate growth resistance.

It is now known that during pregnancy, both the mother and her child dance together in a biochemical type of resistance to one another. For example, when the growing embryo and fetus require additional nutrition, a hormone is produced by the embryo that raises the mother's blood pressure, thus pushing more nutrition into the embryo and fetus. In addition, the mother has biochemical factors that resist the growth of embryo and fetus within her. The entire context of embryonic development can be seen as a sequence of growth resistances either biokinetically or biochemically.

As the varying anatomical systems begin to develop, this resistance is also observed. The most obvious is the different rate of growth between the nervous system and vascular system. The nervous system is fast growing and the vascular system is slow growing. The characteristic folding of the neural tube of the embryo is due to the speed of its growth and the drag on it from the underlying vascular system causing the embryonic brain and spinal cord to fold over the heart and cerebral arteries as a way of meeting its nutritional needs. Differential rates of growth are seen frequently in all the tissues of the embryo. The theme of resistance is explored throughout this chapter because the basic principle is that there is no growth without resistance. This principle operates at a lot of different levels from the embryonic to the spiritual.

The fields seen in the third week and weeks four through eight begin to generate specific structures such as heart, bones, muscles, cartilage, etc. Now notice that in weeks one and two and weeks four through eight, that there is a plus sign (+) between some of the fields. This is an indication that it takes two fields acting together to form a specific structure. This is seen at the tip of the notochord, which forms the basisphenoid and basiocciput. It takes both a distusion and a contusion field to make a cranial base. The bottom of the notochord is also fixed in its position in the developing pelvis. This means that the notochord is functionally or dynamically still as if being held in a tug-of-war at either end of it. It is yet another type of growth resistance.

Coming into Form

The metabolic fields we have just identified in the left side of Figure 2.1 are related to the structures identified in the adjacent column as they begin to take form and transition into becoming specific structures. For example, in the relationship between the cardiovascular and nervous systems the embryo builds many intermediate forms prior to the final structure found in the fetus and adult bodies. Blood vessels are an excellent example of an intermediate form. Blood vessels arise one day to support a certain structure and the next day these vessels disintegrate as another form is expressed. Since many of these structures are temporary, the whole embryonic period is a process of structuring.

Structuring is a three-step process of coming into a position and then a transitional form and dissolution of that form as a gradual definitive structure is made. This three-step process of position, form, and structure is maintained throughout the lifespan at a physical, emotional, and spiritual level. An embryonic principle becomes a life principle in that building a life or a body is a process of constant transitions. Some transitions are larger than others. This is not simply about change. The embryo expresses an intentionality of being upright and requires a biology that is flexible and adaptive. The metabolic fields contain this intention.

Now look at the terms adjacent to the metabolic fields in week two: connecting stalk, chorion-amnion-yolk, allantois, and angiogenesis. This represents the metabolic fields coming into a form. Some of the work of the second week is to build three spheres of fluid. These are known as the chorion, amnion, and yolk (Figure 2.2). A case can be made for a fourth fluid cavity called the allantois (partially seen in Figure 2.3). The allantois becomes part of the bladder. The blood also begins to form in the second week before the heart differentiates. The blood has connective tissue cells in it that must build a connecting stalk for the future umbilical veins and arteries (Figures 2.2 and 2.3).

It is also imperative that the connecting stalk forms between the embryo and the trophoblast (future placenta) or the embryo will perish in the second week. Dr. van der Wal calls this the necessity of *rooting in the periphery*. The growth gesture of rooting is repeated during sexual intercourse and breastfeeding on one end and simply holding hands or giving someone a hug on the other. Such

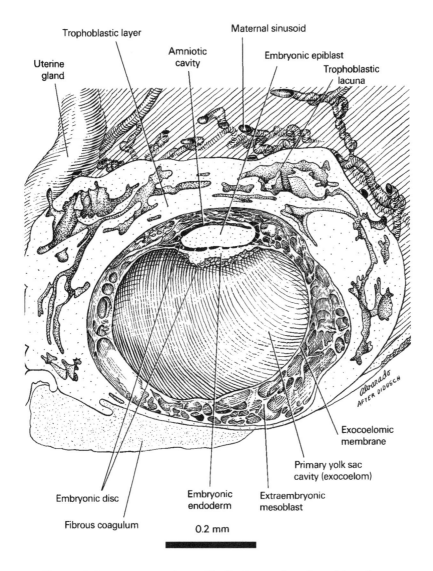

Figure 2.2. Reconstruction of half of a twelve-day-old embryo showing its internal features.

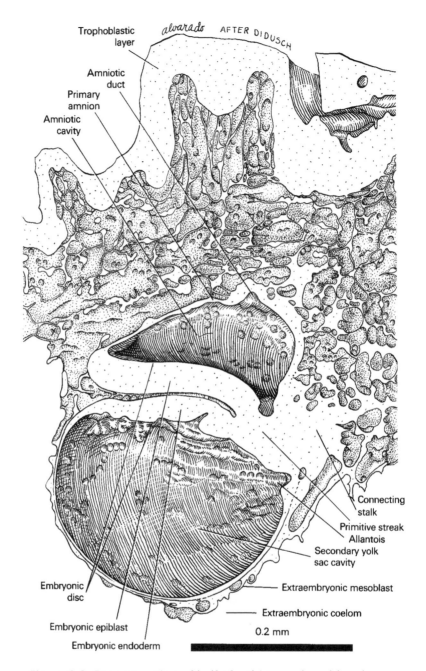

Figure 2.3. Reconstruction of half of a thirteen-day-old embryo showing the relations of its extraembryonic membranes.

connection or rooting in the periphery is a basic embryonic principle that is seen through the lifespan. Connection with other people is a basic rule of life and it starts obviously in the embryo as the embryo connects to itself as much as with the uterus.

Traversing up the column we see some of the relationships to various structures and structural processes, especially around the heart tube and its basic construction. Looking at week three the structuring shown is "primitive streak, notochord, heart tube merging." The heart arises in a canalization zone between the head and the transverse septum (future respiratory diaphragm). This is between the layers of endoderm and ectoderm. Precursor blood cells begin to move into the canal causing blood islands to appear that gradually coalesce into a heart.

The primitive streak (Figures 2.3, 2.4, and 2.5), where the early blood cells arise, is a trough that grows from the caudal or rump end of the ectodermal surface at the beginning of the third week. As the trough forms, the cells at the edge of the trough become heart cells and move into the ebb and flow of fluids at the top of a horseshoe-shaped canalization zone becoming the future heart. The

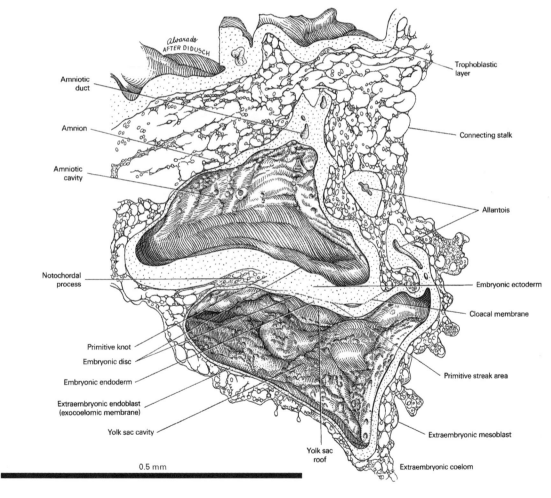

Figure 2.4. View of the right half of the trilaminar blastocyst showing its relation to the connecting stalk, fluid cavities, and notochordal process.

primitive streak grows up to the future third cervical vertebra and that termina-
tion point becomes the fulcrum for the center of the heart, which begins in the
neck region in early development, gradually growing down into the chest cavity.
At that time the primitive streak starts to recede, leaving behind a canal that will
form the notochord (Figure 2.4). The notochord is functionally quiescent and
stretched at both ends as the spine grows around it. Biological stillness is at the
core of the vertebral column.

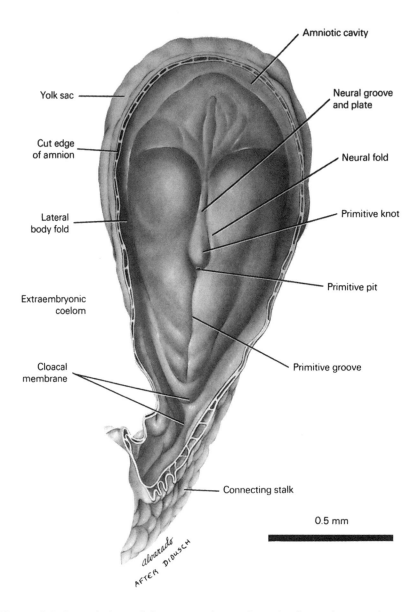

Figure 2.5. Dorsal view of the presomite embryo in the early neural groove
period showing specializations in the ectoderm.

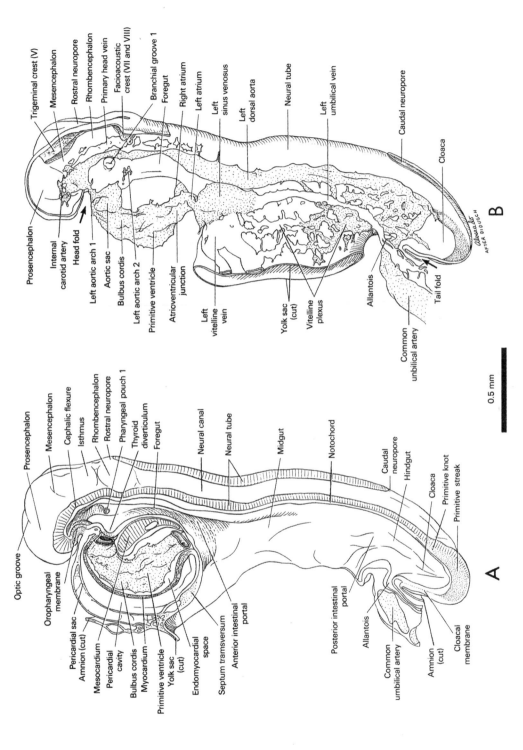

Figure 2.6. A: Midsagittal view of the ten-somite embryo showing the relations of the neural tube, notochord, gut, and pericardium. B: Left lateral view of the ten-somite embryo showing the cardiovascular system.

Moving up the chart place your attention at weeks four through eight, on "heart tube convergence, looping, bending, folding, vertebral segmentation, neurolation, sensory nerve differentiation." Sensory nerves begin to differentiate at twenty-eight days post-fertilization. From the perspective of the brain it could be said that this is when the embryo starts sensing and responding to its environment. However, the embryo is sensing its environment once primordial germ cells differentiate or sooner via a primitive intelligence in the living fluids of the embryo (discussed in Chapter 8). Embryonic cells are sentient, which means they move toward pleasure (food and nutrition) and away from pain or noxious stimuli coming through the maternal environment. There is a sensory intelligence in the fluids or a cellular sentience even at this early developmental stage. Analytical therapy and regression therapies have demonstrated this principle of pre-nervous-system intelligence since the 1930s.

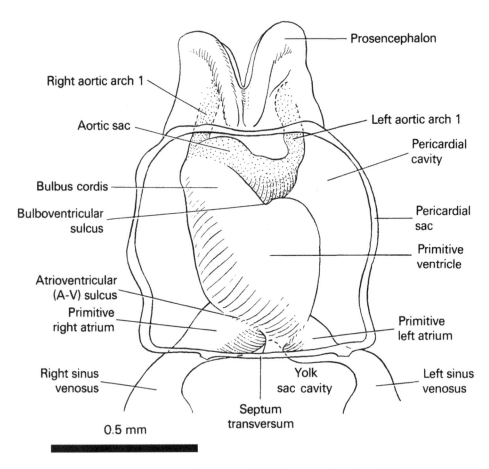

Figure 2.7. Ventral aspect of the heart and pericardial sack of the ten-somite embryo.

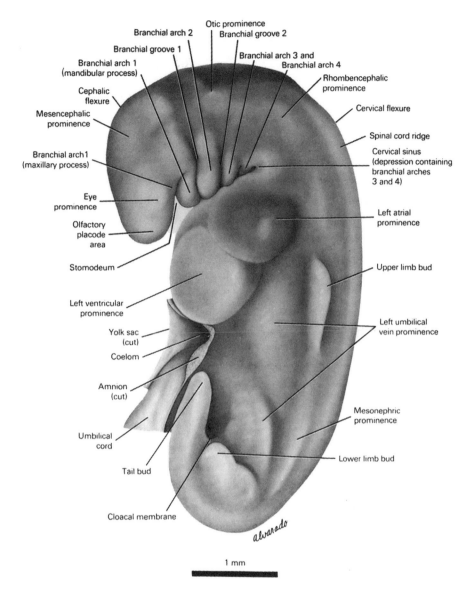

Figure 2.8 External features of the 5-mm embryo.

Neurolation describes the closing of the neural tube at the top and bottom in week four (partially seen in Figures 2.6 and 2.7 by looking closely at the top of the images where the tube is still open like two lips). Neurolation refers to the closing of the neural tube at the top, called primary neurolation, and the closing of the neural tube at the bottom several days later, known as secondary neurolation. Look at Figure 2.8 to see the closure at both ends of the neural tube. The rapid growth of the future brain reveals neurons differentiating every minute. The vascular system, however, prefers slow growth as mentioned and

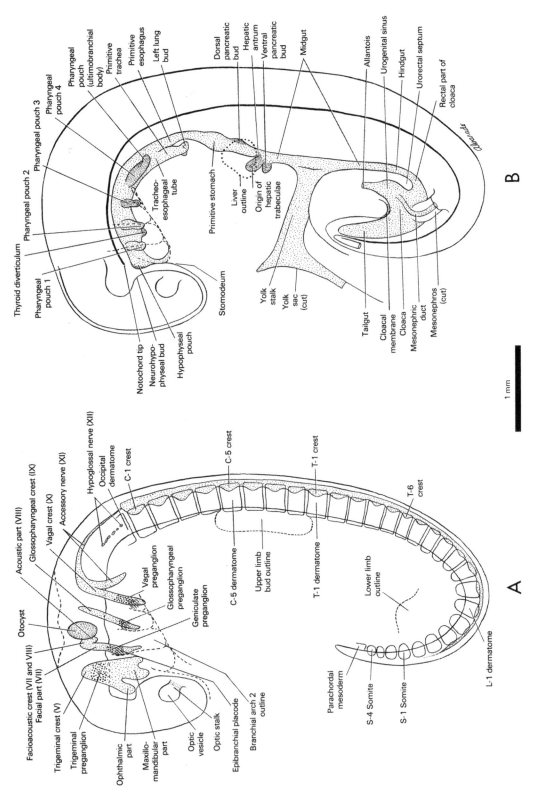

Figure 2.9. A: Peripheral nervous system of the 5-mm embryo. Preganglion cells (large stipple) are evident in the cranial neural crest and form near placodes (striped areas). B: Alimentary and respiratory systems of the 5-mm embryo.

that is the biggest differential growth rate of development between the fast brain and slow heart.

Vertebral segmentation refers to the development of the embryonic somites (Figure 2.9). Somites are the precursor structures to parts of the vertebrae and surrounding musculature, as mentioned. Vertebral segmentation is an important milestone in embryonic development. The whole must be subdivided into segments so the brain can build pathways to communicate to each area of the body and each area of the body can communicate to the brain. It is a two-way street. However, an initial communication system between areas of the embryo is located in the metabolic fields. Remember that each metabolic field knows where each other field is located and each cell in the human body knows where each other cell is located. The *knowing of the whole* is never lost. It may be forgotten but never lost.

Heart convergence refers to the movements of the embryonic heart, which ensure proper location of the intake and output tubes at the top of the heart. The embryo develops in a way that the two atria are initially at the bottom of the tube. Kinetically the heart goes through stages of looping, bending, and folding backwards and upwards in order to have the atrium converge at the top (Figure 2.7 and 2.10). In a sense the heart must be turned *down-side-up* for proper

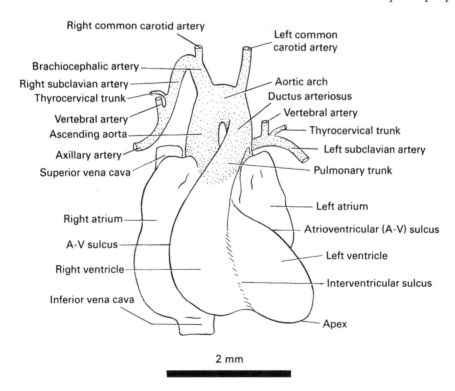

Figure 2.10. Heart of the 18-mm embryo.

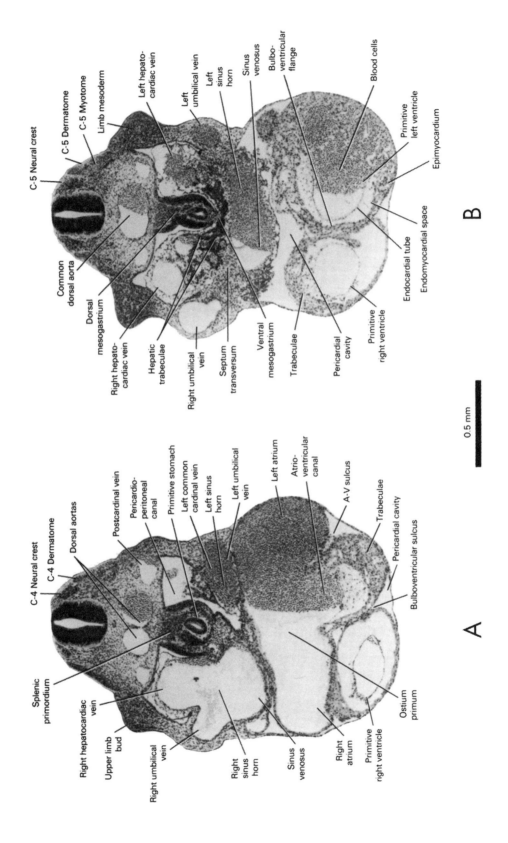

Figure 2.11. Section through the neural crest, heart, and neural tube at the level of C4.

function. Contrary to all other embryonic organs, the heart's initial anatomy does not correspond to its final anatomy because of the need for convergence. No other structure in the embryo is reversed like this as it forms. Look closely at Figure 2.11 and notice that the heart occupies the majority of space in a slice through the middle of the neck compared to the spinal cord and early nervous system. For a review of heart development, refer to Volume Three. This concludes our first story of creation of how the embryo came into form.

Morphology

Now we begin our second story of creation. It is a story about shape and movement. Let's look at the bottom right section of the chart, where the term "4 stages of morphology" is seen, and underneath "the development of differentiated wholeness over time around radial and/or axial symmetry." The arrow above is pointing to a phrase in the upper right corner called "development of shape and function," which further defines morphology.

Biodynamic embryology is a formal study of morphology rather than biochemistry. Dr. Blechschmidt was very clear about this distinction. Morphology in a general sense encompasses all levels of understanding embryonic development through movement and specific shaping and fluid flow functioning in the embryo. Many embryology books begin with chapters describing the morphology of week one, week two, week three, and finally weeks four through eight. These four distinctions comprise the four stages of morphology, which are covered in Volumes One, Two, Three, and Four. Dr. van der Wal has also written about it in Volume One.

Symmetry

Morphology is a description of the biokinetic and biodynamic movements in the embryo; it is the movement of coming into localized form and a total whole structure and shape. *Shape* refers to the surface of the three-dimensional mass of the embryo that is expanding during growth. These movements have a principle of orientation around two types of symmetry. The first is called radial symmetry, or point orientation. For example, in the second week of development, three fluid cavities form—the yolk sac, amnion sac, and chorion. Each of these fluid bubbles are growing from a central point or fulcrum. This point usually does not have an association with a particular embryonic structure, but is simply a balance point for all of the growth activity occurring at that time. This constantly shifting fulcrum of growth was discovered by Dr. Sutherland. He called it a suspended, automatically shifting fulcrum. We will continue to use the terms *point* and *fulcrum* as interchangeable.

All growth and development in the embryo has a symmetrical orientation. We like the expression: *man cognizes, God geometrizes.* The embryo is a wholistic organism. It moves as an interconnected whole shape through discrete phases of external and internal growth and development. Every single cell and metabolic field within the embryo knows where every other cell and field is located (this has been mentioned several times so it must be important). Using the example from the preceding paragraph, there is a point or a fulcrum of orientation for growth and development in the amniotic sac (nervous system), the yolk sac (intestinal system), and the chorion (cardiovascular system). See Figures 2.2, 2.3, and 2.6 for views of these developing structures. From a clinical point of view, the practitioner accesses these fulcrums within himself or herself as a way of self-regulating under the guidance of Primary Respiration and stillness in those redundant systems of wholeness. For a discussion of the three redundant systems of wholeness, refer to Chapter 2 in Volume Three. The locations of these fulcrums become the third ventricle, the heart, and the umbilicus in the fetus, infant, and adult. Gradually at the fourth week of development, axial symmetry starts to occur, where the embryo continues to grow using the primitive streak and notochord as a reference midline (axis) for all surface growth and the physical geometry of human shape.

The phrase used earlier in this chapter, referring to the embryo being *spatially ordered,* is an important one to remember. This pre-existing order, a fundamental substrate of our being that is never lost although it may fade to the background, has components of radial and axial symmetry. By settling into stillness and connecting with Primary Respiration, the spatially ordered movements of the metabolic fields and the wholeness of development can be accessed with knowing, thinking, sensing hands. This is because Primary Respiration and stillness have a functional relationship with the fulcrum and the midline of symmetry. When a practitioner senses either of these two biodynamic phenomena of Primary Respiration and stillness, he or she may immediately notice them from the place of the fulcrum or midline coming out and back from the horizon.

As can be seen on the right of Figure 2.1, each line curves around and is related to a particular stage of morphology. Remember that there are four stages of morphology, so Figure 2.1 shows these four stages and gives select information arranged by columns. Starting in week one, you can see different descriptions of morphological processes depending on which column is being studied. They are descriptions of the three-dimensional shaping movements and activity taking place within the wholeness of the embryo.

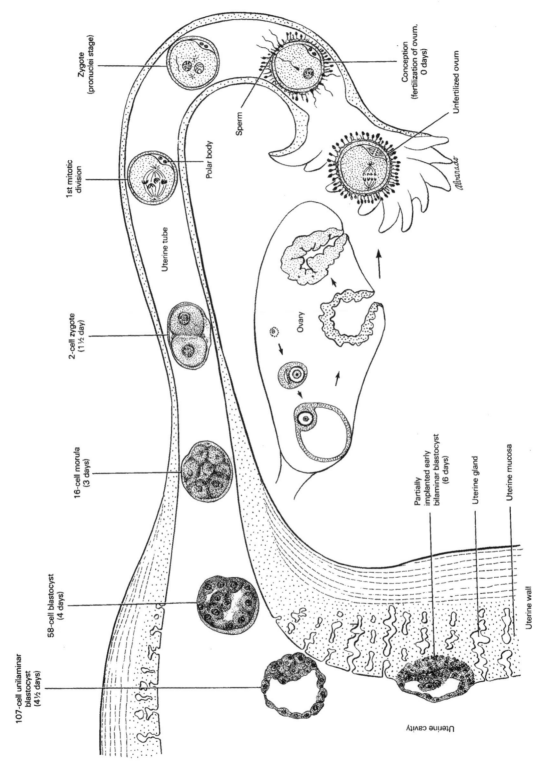

Figure 2.12. Stages of development during the first week and early second week.

These morphological descriptions are associated with the functions occurring in each of the stages. This function then disappears after several hours, days, or weeks. With each differentiation of the embryo (each cell division within its metabolic field in week one), the cells get smaller and smaller, as seen in Figure 2.12. At the bottom of the inner right column in week one is seen "compression/ heat, rolling/hatching." Part of the morphology of the first week is a significant amount of compression and consequently heat arising from the compression. The first week is very busy metabolically as is all the embryonic time. The rolling of the embryo down the fallopian tube causes the zona pellucida to develop fissures or cracks. As the embryo exits the fallopian tube, it has an opportunity to break out of the shell by a process called hatching. That brings us back up Figure 2.1 to the second week and onward.

Nutrition

Week two indicates a morphology of "nutrition by diffusion and expansion/ implantation." This is a central feature of biodynamic embryology. From many fields of medical study we know that nutrition coming in must be balanced by the waste products going out at every level of development. A. T. Still, the founder of osteopathy, said, "We suffer from the want of need and the burden of dead deposits." That is a major theme of this Volume Five. When every cell gets its needs met and properly discharges its waste products then physical health is in balance. When this balance is compromised at any level of cell aggregations, tissues, or physiological systems, the health of the body of the embryo, fetus, child, and adult is compromised.

The most basic understanding of a metabolic approach to biodynamic craniosacral therapy is to understand the importance of this balance of flow from nutrition coming in and waste products going out. This is accomplished by normal blood flow and fluid flow in general (such as water, lymph fluid, and cerebrospinal fluid). This principle operates in each of the stories presented in this chapter. Recently, a previously unknown waste removal system in the brain was discovered. It is a system of microscopic tubes running along the blood vessels filled with water and cerebrospinal fluid that removes toxic proteins from the brain. This is another reason why the canalization zones arise prior to blood vessel formation because of the spontaneous need in different areas of the embryo to receive nutrition and remove waste products in a water-filled canal. The brain also has the largest and most dominant need for nutrition in the embryo. Whatever comes into the heart is distributed to the brain first, then the heart. Whatever is left over is distributed to the structure in most need in the embryo

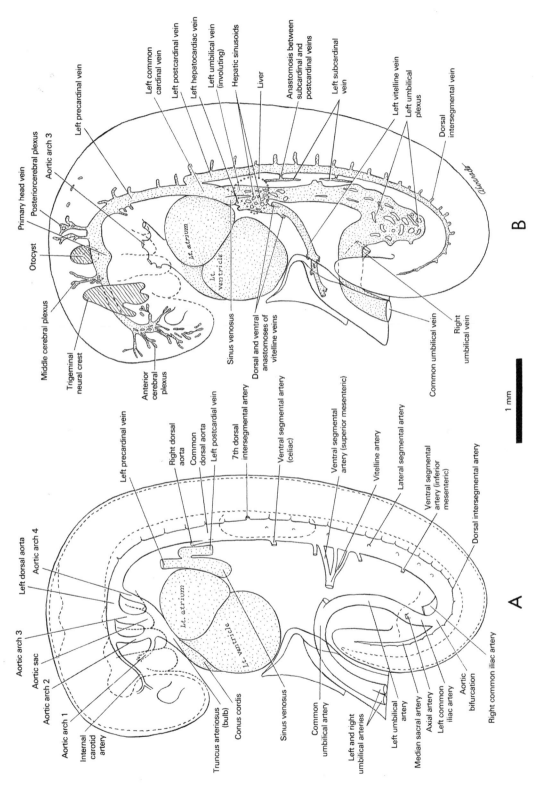

Figure 2.13. Cardiovascular system of the 5-mm embryo.

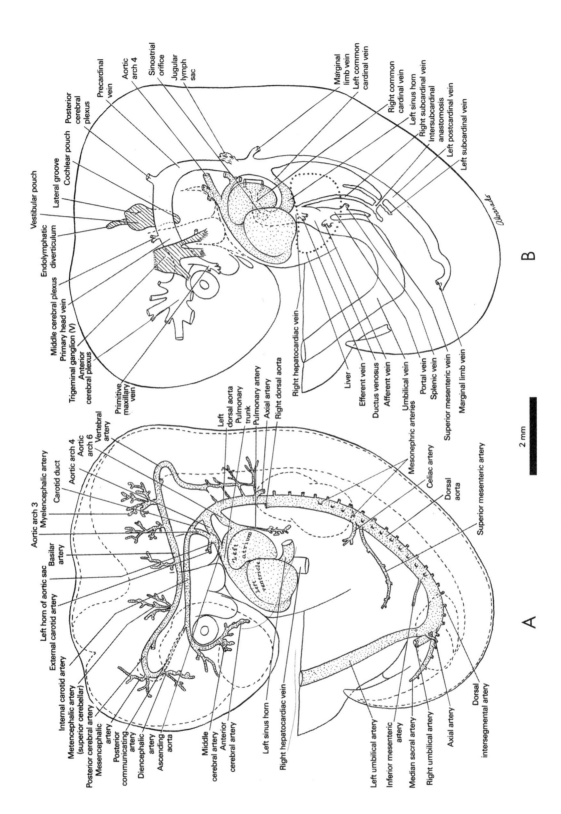

Figure 2.14. Cardiovascular system of the 10-mm embryo.

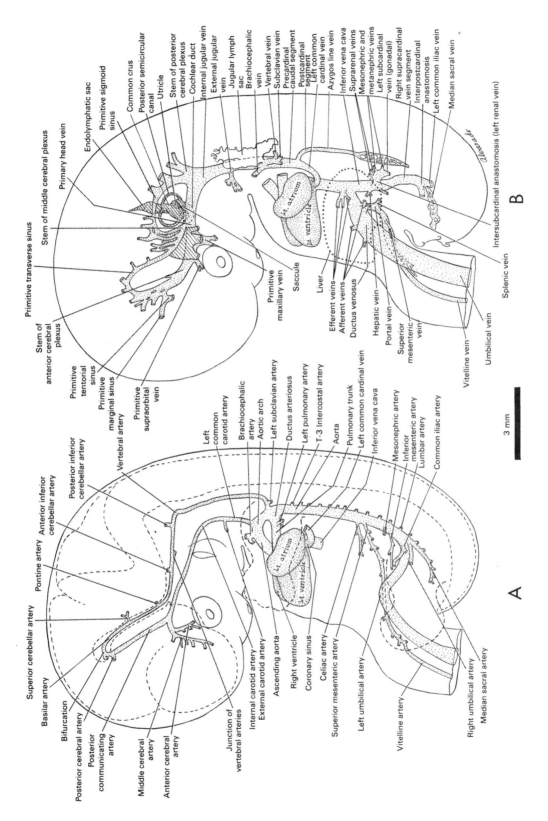

Figure 2.15. Cardiovascular system of the 18-mm embryo.

at that time. Obviously this requires a positive source of nutrition coming in through the mother's diet. If the mother's diet is inconsistent then the embryo will be malnourished and possibly not develop normally (Nathanielsz, 1999).

At week three is "middle formed by pulling apart." During the third week of development, the ectoderm and endoderm begin to pull apart as a normal part of growth. This process leaves many cells behind to change their developmental trajectories. It is ironic that one's position at any given time in life sometimes leads to some dramatic change. Along with the incursion of cells differentiating

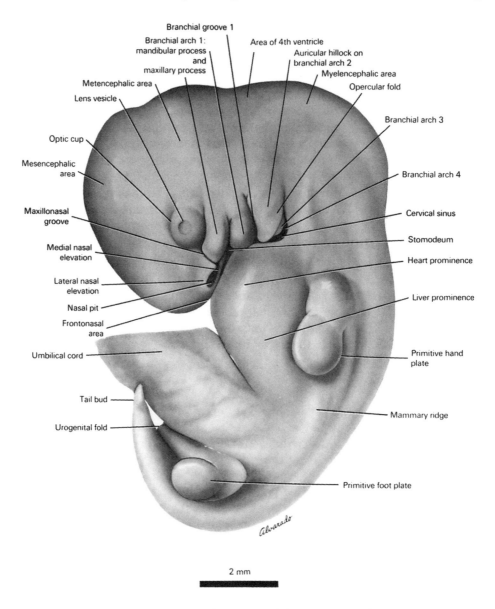

Figure 2.16. External features of the 10-mm embryo.

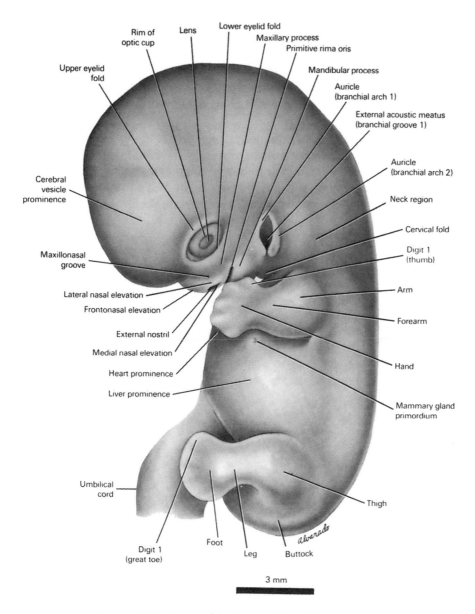

Figure 2.17. External features of the 18-mm embryo.

from the primitive streak, more cells join those left behind and together they change into mesenchyme, the undifferentiated precursor of mesoderm (from the Greek *meso* meaning middle). Some embryologists call this third week "the development of a middle" or the arising of a midline associated with the primitive streak. Because such a middle has diverse contributions coming from all other parts of the embryo, it is perhaps more appropriate to say that the embryo is one homogenous wholistic organism without a biodynamic midline. Certainly the discussion about symmetry above is about biokinetic fulcrums and midlines.

The embryo is more of a series of overlapping whole spheres of fluid. The whole continues to arise and differentiate with very transient fulcrums or midlines. This could be why Ronan O'Rahilly and Fabiola Müller (2001) have suggested the removal of the term *midline* or even *midsagittal plane* from embryonic usage.

The main system being built by the pulling apart is that of the heart and aortic arches. If there is a middle or a midline in the human embryo, then it is the heart. This is seen in Figures, 2.10, 2.11, 2.13, 2.14, and 2.15. Take time to study these images and the developmental progression of the heart and its circu-

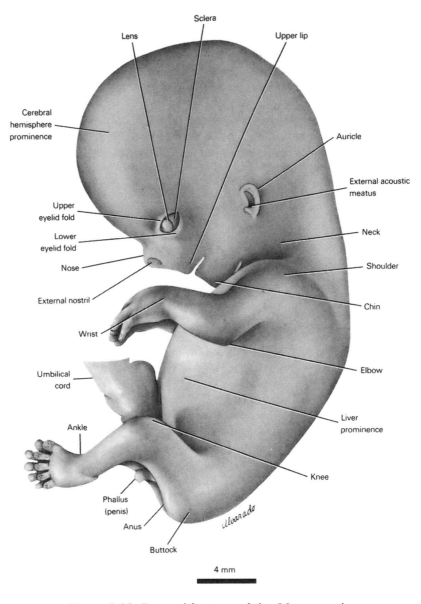

Figure 2.18. External features of the 30-mm embryo.

latory systems. The heart can handle being pulled apart, which is one of its first gestures of development. Then the heart coalesces in the middle as a bridging or coming together of two streams from its opposite sides. The two becoming one is then its next gesture of development, discussed in Chapter 3.

At weeks four through eight, we see "folding-unfolding, right-left, top-bottom, and symmetry." Gradually, at the end of week three and the beginning of weeks four through eight, there is a folding and unfolding biodynamic process taking place through the entire embryo. Take a look at the progression of Figures 2.8, 2.16, 2.17, and 2.18 for a beautiful sequence of the folding process. Since the embryo is alive it also exhibits an unfolding motion done in a rhythm with the folding that cannot be seen here but can be seen in a beautiful animated reconstruction of a human embryo from Johns Hopkins University. The reader can go to http://virtualhumanembryo.lsuhsc.edu/videos/JHUmorph.htm and download this animation free of charge.

In addition, the basic symmetries of right and left and top and bottom are forming at this time. It is a mistake to think that the symmetry of two legs and two arms, for example, are perfectly matched or balanced. Growth and development occurs like a pendulum. Nutrition is not delivered evenly to developing structures. First one arm gets something then the other arm as growth see-saws back and forth. It is true for all paired structures in the body and even nonpaired structures. For example, the heart has a field of growth on its anterior surface that is different than the posterior surface. The activity of the metabolic fields is also dictated by access to nutrition and ability to remove waste products. Nutrition, digestion, absorption, and elimination in the adult body are as important and operate under the same principles found in the growing embryo.

Now begin to orient to the adjacent column of terms to the left of those we just discussed. In week two we see "peripheral body, trophoblast [paternal genes], and central body, embryoblast [maternal genes]." These terms are an indication of a brilliant strategy that the embryo has to create not just one body but two bodies, in order to accomplish the enormous work of growing and developing. Dr. van der Wal uses these terms to describe the bifurcation of structure and function in embryonic development that begins in the second week of development. Of course, *the central body becomes the adult body. The peripheral body becomes the placenta,* which dies at birth. We will discuss this in more detail below during the story of pregnancy.

Going up that column, in week three is seen "vitelline circulation, canalization zones"; continuing up this column, in weeks four through eight is seen "placental circulation, systemic circulation." Vitelline circulation, placental circulation, and systemic circulation are terms referring to the complexity of the embryo in the process of developing three types of circulatory systems necessary to manage the relationship of the peripheral body to the central body (placenta to the embryo). Figures 2.6, 2.13, 2.14, and 2.15 show the progression of systemic circulation in the embryo. A review and complete discussion of these circulatory systems can be found in Volume Three. It is crucial to remember that the embryo has three overlapping ways of *knowing* wholeness: the fluid body that appears in the first two weeks as chorion, yolk sac, and amniotic sac. The vascular systems that appear in subsequent stages and then disappear (vitelline and placental) know wholeness as does systemic circulation that persists throughout life. Finally, the nervous system knows wholeness, especially in weeks four through eight.

Finally, in this second story of creation, canalization zones refer to fluid currents in the embryo at all stages of development. The heart develops in a canalization zone, as mentioned earlier. This is why the term was placed in week three on the morphology side of Figure 2.1. Before there are definitive veins and arteries, there are canals and currents of fluid, like rivers in the protoplasm. Recent research has shown that it is the actual flow of fluids in the vessels of the body that create the vessels themselves. This brings us back to the central theme in the first and second stories of creation: there is order and organization in the fluids of the embryo and thus in the adult body sensed with the slow tempo of Primary Respiration and stillness.

Pregnancy

This brings us now to the central column having to do with pregnancy (see Figure 2.12) and the terms "context of self-regulation" lateral to the word pregnancy. It is our third creation story of the relationship between the embryo and the mother. What is biodynamic self-regulation? It is the ability of this small human organism to swiftly and positively adapt to the changing circumstances of its growth. This requires both an inner body-centered resilience and an outer or interconnected resilience with the placenta, uterus, and maternal environment. This embryonic resilience is followed by physiological and psychological resilience after birth in the form of autonomic nervous system (ANS) adaptability, capacity to modify arousal in the ANS, breathing, heart rate, and attention. Self-regulation develops into an ever widening spiral of potential health and well-being. This is one side effect of the infant-mother attachment and bonding that begins well before birth. Self-regulation is the work of a lifetime to become swiftly adaptable to the complexities of one's own biology and social connectedness. Such adaptability is a moment-to-moment process in the embryo and the adult. To self-regulate is to develop more and more body awareness of heart rate, breathing, arousal, and attention states in order to modify them as quickly as possible when not in a normal range of well-being.

Thus, self-regulation is defined as having two components. The first and most obvious component of self-regulation is concerned with relationship. In the case of an embryo, the relational context is the pregnant mom and the effects of her pre-conception stress or joy on the developing embryo. The second aspect of self-regulation is called autonomy. The metabolic autonomy of the embryo must be balanced with the external relationship to the mother's pregnancy for healthy self-regulation. These two aspects of self-regulation are observed in human development from pre-conception through the lifespan. To reiterate: what starts as a metabolic reality becomes a psychological and spiritual reality during the lifespan.

The new field of epigenesis has provided a wealth of information regarding stress imprinting on the egg and sperm as they mature in the ovaries and testes of adolescent boys and girls. Some research has indicated that if our great-grandparents as adolescents endured a period of sustained stress such as starvation, the genes of the female egg and male sperm could be altered in a way that supported the appearance of a disease process or the appearance of physical disorders in embryos that were conceived from such sperm and eggs. The effects of these stress imprints could manifest at any time during the lifespan of their offspring and their offspring. This research holds true for the descendants of individuals who survived the Irish Potato Famine in the mid-1800s or lived in Belgium during the long winters of starvation during World War II. We are related to our ancestors in many ways, especially through the imprints they carried. At the same time pregnancy is designed to be a time of joy and love for a woman and her partner. This possibility revolves around the creation of a family and the fulfillment of a biological dream or destiny.

Two Bodies

The second aspect of self-regulation is autonomy. This is clearly seen in the embryo, which has two metabolisms. The first metabolism relates to nutrition coming through the blood from the mother's uterus and the placenta. This metabolic process informs the self-regulation of relationship. The embryo is rapidly adapting to a changing environment. But there is also an autonomous self-regulation, a unique metabolism occurring within the embryo, as seen through the structures created in the eight metabolic fields already discussed. At the right of the chart are the four stages of morphology and secondary movement activity or gestures made by the developing embryo. We call these stages of morphology *functional* because they are based on qualities of both wholistic and localized movement patterns shaping the container of the human body as it evolves through successive stages of growth and development. The embryo has the capacity to express its autonomy through its morphology. Its morphology is the way it gestures to the world, as discussed in the next chapter.

These two types of self-regulation found in the embryo are described by a metaphor that Dr. van der Wal uses. He talks about the central body and peripheral body of the embryo in Volume One. Figure 2.1 shows this just above the arrow of pre-conception/epigenesis at the bottom center of the chart. At the end of the first week, the embryo divides itself into two bodies. The central body is the embryo itself, which exhibits a great deal of autonomy in its metabolism. The peripheral body, or what will become the placenta, is initially invested in relationship and union with the maternal blood vessels of the mother's uterus. Even though these two bodies function differently, they are part of an integrated whole.

Another reason that the two-body self-regulation principle is important is because the embryo develops different functions without an associated structure in development. One example is the presence of liver enzymes in the future placenta before the initial presence of a liver structure in the embryo. There are many such examples but the point again comes back to self-regulation. The embryo projects its functional needs out to the peripheral or relationship body until it can build the structure necessary for the integration of that function within itself. The placenta receives many such projections. But again, it is crucial to point out that what starts metabolically in the embryo becomes physiological and psychological later in life. The relationship of a mother and her baby is a prime example of the physiology of projected functions, especially around the development of the brain. Thus later in life difficult emotions are projected onto someone else like a partner until a psychic structure can be built to own and integrate complex emotions.

Wholeness

It is important to make the distinction that a single-cell, fertilized human egg exhibits undifferentiated wholeness. The fertilized ovum is a single-cell human body. With each new phase of growth, however, and each developing structure going through numerous phases to get to its endpoint, which in some cases might not occur for thirty years, is the unfolding of a differentiated wholeness. This is a very important sensibility regarding one's body, whether it is an adult or an embryo. The embryo is working proportionally a thousand times harder metabolically than an adult body. This is because all new structures are being built every day and, in some cases, these structures are only temporary housing that then disintegrates and something else needs to be built.

A central theme in developmental biology during the last century was the observable conservation of wholeness that the embryo maintained through successive stages of development. The conservation of wholeness through increasingly complex phases of growth and development is called differentiated wholeness. As adults, we are called upon to manage the complexity (self-regulation) of numerous levels of input physically, emotionally, and spiritually. It is through the orientation to the slow tidal movement in the embryo and adult, and the metabolic stillness necessary for two vascular systems to connect and nurture one another, that a biodynamic practice is built. Once this level of self-regulation in relationship is established in therapeutic practice, then the client can self-regulate autonomously without the practitioner interfering with that autonomy but simply witnessing it.

Working our way up the central column of terms, we first encounter "the metabolic fields and stages of morphology are interconnected phases of growth and development." As much as this chart is busy breaking down the embryo into many different parts and functions, it is still one interconnected whole. This wholeness as a living experiential reality contains a biodynamic principle that needs to be restated: there is organized movement of the fluids throughout all stages of growth and development. It is the slow tempo of Primary Respiration that biodynamic practitioners feel is one source of that wholistic organization.

The Primary Period

Let's continue looking at the bottom middle of the chart where we see "preconception/epigenesis/oogenesis." At this point, it would be very helpful for the reader to reference Chapter 14 in Volume Three, written by Wendy McCarty, the dean of the pre- and perinatal psychology doctoral department at the former Santa Barbara Graduate Institute. The chapter is entitled "Supporting Human Potential and Optimal Relationships from the Beginning of Life: Twelve Guiding Principles of the Primary Period."

Biodynamic embryology is contained in the context of what Wendy calls the *primary period*. The primary period is the new emerging developmental model. Wendy states: "The primary period for human development occurs from preconception through the first year of postnatal life. This is the time in which vital foundations are established at every level of being: physical emotional, mental, spiritual, and relational" (Shea 2010, 204–205).

Epigenesis refers to stress imprinting on the egg and sperm, as mentioned earlier. It also refers to epigenetic changes in the fetus and placenta due to maternal stress. This can cause genes to be turned on (expressed) or turned off (suppressed). Unfortunately, it is the unhealthy genes that get turned on and the good ones that can get turned off. The most important thing to remember about imprinting at the genetic level is that even though these genes may be turned on or off at the pre-conception or even during pregnancy due to stress, they still need to be activated by maternal stress during pregnancy and life experience after birth. Maternal stress has the capacity to alter the expression of these genes causing long-term consequences such as obesity, ischemic heart disease, type 2 diabetes, and more than a hundred other disorders and diseases including learning disorders. In fact, maternal stress will also raise the risk of interventions during labor and delivery.

There is also a blueprint for health that is occurring in the embryo. This original blueprint relates to Dr. Blechschmidt's observation that there is ordered and organizational movement in the fluids. Developmentally, the slower the movement, the better it is for development. Ask any mother about the importance of stillness and raising her baby. There are very fast movements occurring during development and the embryo must operate in a balance that is provided by the slow tempo of Primary Respiration and a biology of stillness. Stress always speeds things up in the body and mind and can diminish the availability of Primary Respiration as a catalyst that converts the heat of the speedy processes to available life force or potency. The antidote is mindfulness of slowness and stillness, which are metabolic realities in the embryo. We have stressed earlier in this chapter how the second week of development depends on stillness in the future placenta for proper connection to maternal blood nutrition. Likewise, the heart is the organ of stillness par excellence during development. Stillness is a metabolic and biological reality in the embryo (and adult) and normal development cannot proceed without it.

Conception

Moving up you will find "ovulation-fertilization." Fertilization is a synonym for conception (see Figure 2.12). Recent research by Jonathan Tilly at Harvard University has refuted a basic tenet in the biology of the female egg and ovaries. His work demonstrates that human female ovaries have stem cells that can transform themselves into viable eggs at any time after birth. This flies in the face of conventional thinking that a woman is born with all the eggs she will ever have in her ovaries and only releases up to 400 during her lifetime.

We call this new research the *paradigm of fresh eggs*. What if you or I were conceived from an egg that only came into being several moments or days before our individual conception occurred? What if there was no pre-conception or maternal stress on the egg that each of us came from? This offers a complete possibility for transformation and self-regulation. It also begs the question that we might be spending way too much time trying to discover meaning from a history that might not even be ours. Therefore, we would like to go on record that any of us might have come from a fresh egg without familial imprinting. Everyone has the possibility to be free from their past right now. Chapters 3, 4, and 14 go into detail on how to integrate this information on the paradigm of fresh eggs into clinical practice.

The zona pellucida is the hard covering or shell around the embryo during the first week. Because the embryo has a hard shell, all the cells that are multiplying on the inside of the conceptus are squeezed and compressed as the overall space is not expanding. It is important to consider the zona pellucida as a form of resistance to the embryo at this time. As we mentioned earlier, resistance is vital to the growth and development of the embryo and happens in so many ways even the resistance of a hard container is necessary to ignite the embryo in the first week of development. How often have we bumped up against a seemingly unmovable barrier in life only to have it magically disappear later?

Week One

Now we get to week one in the middle of the chart. Here the term "in the uterine tube" is seen. The first week of embryonic development takes place for the most part in the uterine tube, as seen in Figure 2.2. It is known that if the conceptus implants in the uterine wall, an ectopic pregnancy occurs, which is very dangerous and can cause the death of the mother. This journey down the fallopian tube takes place by the embryo essentially rolling down the tube.

The term "corona radiata" describes a cluster of feeder cells surrounding the embryo. At a microscopic level, it can be seen that these cells have miniscule tubes like pipes going into the cytoplasm of the conceptus. They are providing nutritional support for the fertilized egg and removing waste products. Another important feature of the corona radiata is that the shape of its mass as it surrounds the conceptus is very eccentric. In other words, there are more of these cells clustered together on one side of the conceptus than on the other. It is felt by some embryologists that this eccentric shape initiates the rolling process down the ovaries and if this eccentric shaping does not occur after fertilization, then the conceptus will die. The rolling motion is extremely crucial and creates cracks in the zona pellucida. These cracks allow the embryo to hatch and implant on the uterine wall in the second week of development, seen in Figures 2.2 and 2.12. Research indicates that up to 80 percent of all human embryos do not come to term. Many conceptuses die during the first, second, and third week, and without rolling down the fallopian tube in week one, death is inevitable.

Week Two

Moving up the middle of the chart, underneath week two, we see "uterine immune down-regulation." This is the story of implantation seen in Figure 2.12. Implantation describes the beginning of the second week, when the embryo hatches itself and attaches to the uterine wall. As it attaches to the uterine wall, it secretes an enzyme that begins to destroy the cells of the mother's uterus. As these cells rupture, nutrition is drawn in from the cytoplasm for the embryo. It might be said that the embryo eats its way into the uterus, rather than implants itself.

The Biology of Stillness

Growth resistance has a fulcrum of biological stillness. Of particular interest are the lacunae that arise starting in the second week of development (seen in Figures 2.3 and 2.4). Lacunae are characterized by the stillness in a pocket of fluid. This stillness in the second week surrounds the entire embryo and is responsible for inviting the maternal blood vessels to connect with the future placenta. The stillness or lack of movement is a fulcrum around which the resistance of growth and development occurs at different rates or speeds, in this case between the uterus and future placenta. Each of the somites (precursors to parts of the spine and spinal musculature) arising in the third and fourth weeks post-fertilization has a lacunae in the middle. Thus our entire musculoskeletal and cardiovascular systems, at one level of understanding, are biologically oriented to a deep sense of stillness.

The research of Donald Ingber (2006) indicates that whenever an embryonic vessel bends or folds, it causes the cellular structure in that bend or fold to change its shape into that of a wedge. By this change of shape, one edge of the wedge will be small and the opposite edge much larger. By definition, the small edge of the cell becomes quiescent. It is this Dynamic Stillness that becomes an inducer and orienting factor for growth and development in that area or position of the embryo. Growth resistance and the fulcrum of stillness are significant aspects of embryonic formation and influence the relationship between all the developing physiological systems and related structures. The biological importance of still-ness in embryonic development cannot be understated.

One important component of the second week, however, is in regards to the "lacunae-maternal blood-quiescence." The term *quiescence* describes an incred-ibly important biological reality in the development of a human embryo and body through the lifespan. Although much can be said about the second week of development, the most interesting component that can be applied readily in therapeutic practice is the stillness function of the lacunae (Latin for lagoon, a still body of water where fresh and salt water meet). The lacunae are pockets of still fluid in the protoplasmic mass surrounding the embryo that will shortly become the placenta.

This mass of protoplasm is called the trophoblast (Figures 2.3 and 2.4). This mass develops pockets of fluid that are "still" and hence the Latin designation of being like a lagoon. The stillness of the fluid in the lagoon invites the maternal blood vessels in the uterus to begin connecting directly into the lacunae. Now an additional function of the lacunae begins to occur, that is, the meeting of two bodies of fluid with varying salinity. I (Michael) live close to the Indian River Lagoon in South Florida where inland fresh water meets ocean salt water and this is what occurs in the world of nature as well as the world of the embryo. Dr. Brian Freeman (2010) uses the term quiescence to describe its importance for the orientation of growth and development. This quiescence or Dynamic Stillness is a fundamental component of human embryonic development. This quality is noted both in the surrounding fluids but also within the embryo during the second week and later stages of development. Another notable structure possess-ing this quality of Dynamic Stillness is the notochord, which is the precursor of parts of the spine.

With this information in hand, it becomes imperative that practitioners reflect a quality of quiescence or serenity within themselves and their connection (connecting stalk) to the client. This is the foundation of self-regulation. The practitioner cultivates and orients to these pockets of stillness three dimension-ally within and surrounding his or her body and that of the client. These areas of stillness in the zones of perception can extend through the office and all the way out to the horizon. This perception allows a panoramic stillness that permeates the session, especially in zone C, the office space. It is like being in the ocean. The lacunae surround the entire embryo three dimensionally and thus the embryo is surrounded by stillness in the second week of development, inviting connec-tion. This becomes zone C in clinical practice. The sky, the clouds, and the trees outside the office become the lacunae of the uterine-placenta space.

Week Three

At week three we see "discovery of pregnancy, joy or maternal stress—epigenetic changes in all stages of development." Please refer to Volume Three for an in-depth discussion of pregnancy. Pregnancy involves an emotional spectrum from the joy of motherhood, all the way to the metabolic struggle associated with maternal stress. The field that studies maternal stress is called bio-behavioral perinatology and is discussed in detail in Chapter 19 by Ann Weinstein. A lot is known about maternal stress causing an inflammatory condition in the placenta that alters and changes the milieu of the embryo epigenetically. It is wise to advocate for pregnancy massage, prenatal craniosacral therapy (see Chapter 24), and relaxation strategies for pregnant women and their families for the future health and well-being of our planet.

Then we see "endometrium-chorionic villi exchange." Endometrium-chorionic villi exchange is one of the ways in which nutrition and the basic building blocks of growth permeate the chorionic walls. It is a process of diffusion. The small molecules of nutrition travel through the porous membranes of the chorion into the yolk sac, feeding and nourishing the growing embryo.

Weeks Four through Eight

The next term is "differential rates of growth in all stages of development" in weeks four through eight. This relates to an earlier statement regarding the fact that there is no set or precise timing sequence for the development of structure in the human embryo. In addition, all the different metabolic fields have varying rates of growth. It's a bit like the cacophony of an orchestra tuning up at first, but gradually all the different parts of the orchestra become synchronized. The synchronization process is a function of ordered movement in the fluids. This dynamic organizational movement is associated with slowness and stillness and provides the optimum conditions for normal growth within a wide range of possibilities. These tempos allow for the orchestra to play in sync with each other. Wholeness, which underlies health, is the tune that is being played.

Next is "umbilical cord formation and early placenta." Finally, at the end of the embryonic period, we get a definitive placenta and an umbilical cord with functioning arteries and veins (Figure 2.16). These arteries and veins plug directly into the heart of the embryo. The heart is of special interest as all incoming nutrition goes directly to the heart. Figures 2.10, 2.11, 2.13, 2.14, and 2.15 show the gradual development of the heart and vascular system between weeks two, three, and four through eight. Note the size of the heart in relationship to different structures around it.

At the top of the column in weeks four through eight is seen "genetic specialization resistance." It has been said that a human being is a perpetual embryo. Figure 2.18 shows an embryo at the end of the embryonic period. Another way of understanding this concept stems from the unceasing metabolic function sustaining the health and wholeness of both the embryo and the adult. In addition, a human does not finish its embryonic period by developing special features for survival after birth as all other animals do. Human embryos resist all types of survival specialization and thus must rely on caregivers for years after their birth. Specialization, such as in athletics and or the pursuit of career or excellence in an academic field, occurs years after a child's survival needs have been met by their caregivers.

We just finished watching the televised 2012 summer Olympics in London. Even though the American women did quite well in the gymnastics competition, it was difficult to watch the stories of their childhood being consumed with gymnastics. They had to overcome their childhood and adolescence to specialize in gymnastics. The notion philosophically is that this resistance to such specialization is a hallmark of human freedom or perhaps more openness to a huge human potential. Is it possible that the more specialized one becomes the less freedom one has? This, of course, is debatable but worthy of mention. Resistance is a key to healthy growth in the embryo at a metabolic level, as discussed in Volume One of this series. We notice in ourselves and in clinical practice that resistance is not a constant but rather is designed to be in balance with a certain freedom or openness of the body to express the potency of life moving through its fluids.

Genetic resistance to specialization takes it a step further. Genes offer a type of resistance to human growth because they can change the way a cell or a whole body functions usually in an unhealthy way through mistakes during DNA replication, shifting of DNA sequences, mutations, deletions, substitutions, translocations and crossing over, and the integration of foreign DNA. Even identical twins have different health outcomes over their lifespan. Ultimately, a human embryo and therefore an adult is always free to overcome any limitation or resistance, even at the genetic level. It is hard work. One reason for this is that the primary influence on the cell nucleus is the cytoplasm of the cell. We observe in our sessions and experience in our own bodies that the deepest influence on the cytoplasm is Primary Respiration, the Long Tide. The biggest influence on this slow tide in the cytoplasm is the ocean of stillness it is connected to in the placenta of the world around us. When we maintain a sensibility around biodynamic wholeness in and of our fluid body, we can overcome any resistance. This ends the third story of creation.

Conclusion

We are frequently asked in class whether these eight metabolic fields and four stages of morphology are important in terms of clinical evaluation. We once thought that, if we studied embryology, we could put hands on a client and sense exactly where the problem began to occur in the embryo, or how it began to occur. This turns out to be a romantic fantasy. The knowledge and understanding of metabolic fields and morphology in general is to inform the adult practitioner about his or her own body, not only as it exists in the present moment as a continual shape-shifting organism, but to provide a deep sense of wonder regarding one's origin from a single cell. It is a road map of the beginning of the primary period. It keeps us in touch with our original wholeness in the present moment. It allows us to hear the authentic story of our being that existed before the stress and trauma story. It gives us the felt sense of love. This is the new healing paradigm.

When we put our hands on a client, our job is first and foremost to sense the client's wholeness with Primary Respiration and stillness. As a metaphor, we could say that our first intention is to touch the embryo. So our question to our students is: if the client lying on the table is indeed an embryo (and certainly retains a significant amount of embryonic metabolism), how do I put my hands on an embryo without interfering with the enormous work of creation, repair, and maintenance happening under the guidance of Primary Respiration and stillness? This is health. This is the importance of studying biodynamic embryology. The health is pre-existing in the body. It changes the way we touch our clients and how we perceive the world in general. As Dr. Sutherland said toward the end of his life, if one is going to do this work, one must have an enormous amount of respect and reverence for the self-regulating forces already present in the human body. We need to cultivate a broad and novel understanding of the human body. This is the embryo as it exists inside of us as a relationship between the living, palpable, wholistic forces of stillness and Primary Respiration.

The metabolic forces spoken of in biodynamic embryology are the same as in biodynamic practice at the level of biokinetics (refer to Chapter 1). They are related to a modifying influence coming from outside the cell or outside the adult body toward the inside. In biodynamic practice this influence has a reciprocal motion of returning from the inside to the outside. To Dr. Sutherland and the lineage holders of cranial osteopathy, one layer of this self-regulating force was named the Breath of Life, from the Book of Genesis. We prefer to say that our experience is about Primary Respiration, which includes the Breath of Life (as a spark at the beginning of primary inhalation). Primary Respiration is related to the biodynamics of biodynamic practice. This will make more sense to the reader in Chapters 3 and 4, as the distinctions between biokinetic and biodynamic palpation are covered.

Primary Respiration is a biodynamic, wholistic force or wave or breath (choose your metaphor because it is personal and experiential) moving back and forth from the natural world or the visible horizon. This can come from the sky above or the earth below, moving into, organizing, maintaining, and repairing the human body, and then moving out, much like a tide some days and a breathing other days. The stillness is indivisible from Primary Respiration and is a unique perceptual state that is like an ocean surrounding and inside of us. All of this, of course, depends on numerous factors in the therapeutic relationship, but none is more important than a relaxed, peaceful state of mind in the practitioner.

Figures 2.2 through 2.18 are reprinted with permission from Raymond Gasser, PhD.

CHAPTER 3

Categories of Embryonic Movement

with Carol Agneessens, MS

The art and science of palpation have a long history. The enormous expansion of manual therapies in the past 100 years has produced a wealth of written material on how to properly make contact with a client's body. The field is dominated by orthopedic considerations of how joints and soft tissue move and respond to manual therapy, from osteopathy and chiropractic to massage therapy and craniosacral therapy, not to mention numerous other derivatives and offshoots of the original schools. It is truly a very creative time at this moment in the ever expanding field of the therapeutic touch arts.

At the core of the skill of therapeutic touch is the simple question: how does a therapist come into relationship with the motion present under his or her hands? A second question is: how does a therapist discern the relative value of the motion present in the client? This entire series of volumes explores these questions in the light of embryology and the link between embryonic movement processes and adult movement. This chapter will continue in that direction of exploring motion present in the body with a summary given in Figure 3.1 at the end.

Categories of Movement

This chapter discusses two categories of embryonic movement. The first category of movements describes fluid flow that is ordered and organized, as first described by Erich Blechschmidt and Raymond Gasser (1978, revised ed. 2012). In general, fluid flow is the delivery system for nutrition in the body and the removal of waste products. With so much metabolism in the embryo there must be a significant amount of nutrition delivery and waste removal going on. It must have order, or chaos and disintegration manifest as disease and disorder.

The second category is related to the movements of growth and development. We will separate this second category of movement in order to differentiate growth from development. Of course these two broad categories of movement are made for the sake of palpation but in reality everything is happening at once in the embryo with some important sequences that will be noted. Clinically speaking, it depends on the practitioner's relationship with Primary Respiration that determines any category of movement perceived. The embryonic and adult bodies are constantly growing and actively structuring, maintaining and repairing parts of the body. Blechschmidt said that proportionally the embryo works 1,000 times harder metabolically than the adult and even then there are ten million cell divisions occurring every second in the adult body. In either body, this indeed is a very active growing and developing process.

As stated, all such palpation of the embryonic forces depends on the practitioner's perception of Primary Respiration. It is probably not possible to describe all the movements associated with the embryo or adult. Nor is there any discussion of biomechanical movement in this chapter that is available in many other texts. This chapter must be considered as an introduction to how the embryo moves or at least how biodynamic practitioners perceive such movement with their hands and body. This chapter is an interpretation of the science of observation by transposing the embryo observed into the embryo palpated as a conscious perceptual process. These movements also happen in dynamic phases of wholeness, which means in relationship with each other over a span of time in embryonic development. If the practitioner forgets this principle, the palpation may cause compression that is not normal.

Basically the embryo builds a body by condensing itself and removing water from its various structures via the metabolic fields described in the previous chapters. We are writing this chapter based on our personal experience from a phenomenological point of view. This means how each of us experiences our embryo that lives within us. It is a living three-dimensional experience of the continuum of wholeness and its absence. It is completely subjective. The practice of biodynamic craniosacral therapy is primarily about the practitioner's perception of his or her own body and the space around it, including nature, from the point of view of Primary Respiration and stillness. Primary Respiration and stillness are the constant in this equation. Secondarily, biodynamic practice is about the discernment of motion present in the client. A basic principle of biodynamic practice is that the metabolism of the embryo is still linked to the metabolism of the adult body and it can be sensed consciously in one's self and palpated in the client.

We teach palpation based on one's personal experience of slowing and stilling and that gives students more ways to describe their own somatic experience and then to teach clients how to relate to their own experience in their own language. We have been studying embryology for the past decade and there is an abundance of new information or more precisely a clearer understanding of the original information in Dr. Blechschmidt's embryonic morphology. His terminology is now accepted internationally in the scientific community (see http:// www.unifr.ch/ifaa/Public/EntryPage/ViewSource.html for the newly approved Terminologia Embryologica) and his books are now being edited and reprinted, especially the book he co-authored with Dr. Raymond Gasser (2012).

Buoyancy

We would like to describe the basis for the perception of all the movements described in this chapter. It is called buoyancy. It is the simple lived experience of the human body being a fluid body that is 92 percent living water. This creates a discrete sensibility of a life under the skin and immediately around the surface of skin that is aquatic in nature. For the nine months of gestation inside the mother's womb, the child is surrounded by fluid. Fetuses breathe fluid in and out of their lungs and intestines, so there is a fluid memory in and around every body that can be accessed any time. It is also a memory of wholeness. Thus buoyancy also means the felt sense of wholeness. It is a three-dimensional awareness, as if the body is one drop of fluid pulsing slowly with micromovent from bottom to top. The general flow of fluids in the embryo was from bottom to top and this upward movement provides a sensibility of both being lifted up and pulled down by gravity at the same time.

Buoyancy is defined by the weight and density of an object such as a human body and the weight and density of an equal volume of water when the body is in it. If the weight and density of the body are heavier than the water, the body will sink. If the body is not heavier than the water or denser, the water effectively lifts or provides an upthrust causing the body to float. Certain fish have what are called buoyancy organs—flotation devices that they use to maintain buoyancy. One such organ can be the spaces in the body that fill up with air, thus providing more buoyancy, which everyone who has been in water knows when they fill their lungs with air. We liken this to the capacity to sense Primary Respiration in the adult body when synchronizing primary and secondary respiration during a session. Such synchronization is a buoyancy device in clinical practice.

Flotation devices in fish that are heavier than water are usually the dorsal and ventral fins that can provide lift. The hands and arms of the practitioner need to be buoyant as if lighter than the water element of the client's body. In biodynamic practice weight corresponds to the actual pounds that one carries when standing on a scale. It is the density issue that can be worked with more readily in biodynamic practice. We prefer to use visualizations such as the skin becoming more porous and all the layers of fascia and tissue under the skin being more like the layers of a tubular sea sponge. This is the basic practice of dedensificaton and becoming porous in the unification of zones A and B. Practitioners need to decrease the density of their body without giving up the weight of their body. This is accomplished by also including awareness of the unification of zone A and B together as one continuum of the fluid body. Chapter 14 covers this in detail.

Metaphors are frequently used in class, such as the skeleton being seaweed or the skin being a tubular sea sponge. To access this information, one must be able to form an image or sense of the body being whole as if one drop of fluid. The body can be viewed as a single continuum of transparent fluid. We have found through trial and error that to get to this quality of buoyancy in the body, it must be done slowly. Each system of the body, from the surface to the core, must be dedensified from its solidity that resulted from years of misunderstanding and wrong beliefs about body function and structure. Solidness of the musculoskeletal system, for example, returns to its normal buoyancy when the body is at rest physically, mentally, and emotionally. The experience of buoyancy is facilitated by the perception of Primary Respiration and practicing movement disciplines from yoga to dance therapy that support buoyancy. Please refer to Chapter 12 for a meditation practice on buoyancy.

The shape of a living human body is constantly changing and the conscious discernment of buoyancy is a defining feature of biodynamic practice as we teach it. Self-buoyancy is one of the first orientations made when beginning to come into relationship with the client. It is simply the experience of fluid wholeness. By sensing one's own buoyancy with decreased density and a porousness that gradually opens to all the zones, the practitioner is much more easily able to receive the held stresses and trauma in the fluid body of the client. They may cause a ripple or a wave in the practitioner's buoyancy, but it readily dissipates because of the relationship to Primary Respiration and stillness. The practitioner's buoyancy dissipates fluid imprinting in the client as a form of self-regulation. Because the therapeutic relationship is an interconnected state, the capacity of the practitioner to be buoyant is very important.

Development

Embryonic development of the various structures and functions of the human body occurs in three stages regarding the morphology of structure and function, as described in the first two chapters. The first stage is called development of *position.* For example, the human heart begins as a flow of nutrition across the transverse septum (future diaphragm), which in the early stages of the embryo is located below the face. At this position a flow of nutrients from both sides of the embryo is moving into canals that conveniently converge across the transverse septum. So the initial position of the heart is somewhere between the face and the neck in an incredibly small embryo no bigger than a lentil.

The second stage is called the development of *form*. Again taking the example of the heart, the three-dimensional growing embryo causes the transverse septum to stretch downward. At the same time, cardiac cells are entering the canals crossing the bridge of the transverse septum. These cells actually form blood islands. Imagine islands of blood that are ebbing and flowing in the canal across the ever widening bridge of the transverse septum. They gradually loosely connect with one another to give a very fragile plexiform, a loose web-like structure. It is much like a system of fragile blood capillaries. Gradually, stage 3 emerges in the development of *structure.* As this web of loosely interconnected blood islands receives stretching pressure from the overall growth of the embryo and especially the rapidly growing brain above it, a definitive heart tube is formed. The heart tube is attached at the top by the face and bottom by the future respiratory diaphragm. This allows for the central portion of the tube to grow freely in a dilation field and begin to loop and bend in the progress toward forming a four-chambered heart.

Everywhere one looks in the embryo at structure and function, one can see these three stages of development. Thus the study of human anatomy should include the study of embryology to understand these three stages and their importance. Each of these stages requires an inflow of nutrition and an outflow of waste products. This is our first category of movement, the delivery and removal system for the construction site. This is the subject of the various canals and currents discussed next.

Canalization Zones

It is interesting that the term *canalization zones* comes from Blechschmidt's work in the 1950s. In contemporary German language, a canalization zone refers to a sewer line. In the embryo, that is only half the story. This is because a canalization zone will also be carrying nutritional products. A canalization zone is a channel between two layers of tissue. Gradually, the main source of nutrition is going to come through the arteries and the main sewer lines will be the veins. In the beginning there is just an inflow and an outflow through canals oriented to the chorionic wall, which is receiving nutrition from the uterus via diffusion.

Lateral Fluctuations

Blechschmidt sometimes refers to the basic organized movements of fluids in the embryo. These movements occur in an organized canalization zone, as mentioned above, but they also occur as rivers such as a movement perpendicular to the plane of tissue at any given area in the human embryo. Early cranial osteopathy discovered this fluid motion and called it lateral fluctuations. Again, lateral fluctuations need to be considered to be a vehicle for moving information that includes nutrition and waste products. Initially, it is just an ebb and flow of water in the embryo. In-depth discussion of lateral fluctuations can be found in the previous volumes in this series.

Longitudinal Fluctuation

Blechschmidt refers to another type of organized movement that is parallel to the long axis of limiting tissue. Once again, cranial osteopaths have referred to this movement as the longitudinal fluctuation. The longitudinal fluctuation, however, is just one of the main longitudinal movements since it is associated more directly with an axis between the coccyx and third ventricle. Every plane of tissue in the body, whether it is skin, fascia, or muscle, will have a longitudinal fluctuation of fluid along its surface. Even the fluid properties of the fascia are now considered more important than its elastic qualities. It has the same purpose as the main one from the coccyx to the third ventricle which is the delivery and distribution of energy and information and the removal of waste.

Transparency

Blechschmidt goes on to describe fluids moving through the tissue. This implies the water molecule—the smallest molecule in the body, capable of moving through any tissue. This is a very important clinical consideration. (The reader is advised at this point to look at the transparency meditation in Chapter 13.) Transparency is an important experience associated with Primary Respiration. When the practitioner can sense Primary Respiration moving through his or her buoyancy from the horizon in back through to the horizon in front without interference from a barrier, a greater sense of wholeness is generated—students frequently report "finding their embryo." Transparency, however, requires a dedensificaton of the musculoskeletal system and the cardiovascular system for starters. This is because those two systems hold so much stress that has caused the fluid body to solidify.

Streaming and Surging

There are undoubtedly many other movements associated with fluid flow that one can perceive in one's own body and that of the client. We feel that if practitioners can consciously focus on the movement and activity of their own heart, a wide range of therapeutic fluid movements become apparent. Even the term *automatic shifting* from cranial osteopathy can be an indicator of integration of the cardiovascular system and the autonomic nervous system. When we sense automatic shifting, there is a felt sense of streaming and surging, usually from bottom to top in the body. These movements are initiated in the fluid body and sustain it. By themselves they are possibly related to terms describing movement in the metaphysical body such as Kundalini and Shakti. These movements are initiated in the pelvis also and are rather simple rather than anything profound. The basis of perception of streaming and surging or Kundalini and Shakti is buoyancy and transparency. They are expressions of aliveness and integration.

Growth Expansion

Now let us turn to the other category of movements associated with growth in general. We have already covered developmental movements above. Growth means the three-dimensional expansion of the whole mass of the embryo and more localized fields of metabolic activity causing expansion and contraction of the surface ectoderm of the embryo. The first type of embryonic movement is called *growth expansion,* which is the three-dimensional mass of the embryo or adult expanding at its surface in relation to a point or fulcrum (radial symmetry) or a midline (axial symmetry).

One of the first functions of biodynamic practice is to sense the three-dimensional body of the client expanding and contracting in the tempo of Primary Respiration. Such a growth expansion is the actual foundation for the subsequent growth movements discussed below. Growth expansion has a reciprocal growth contraction and during the embryonic, fetal, and postnatal times, it is a constant until adulthood. Even in adulthood, the body continues to expand three dimensionally or contract in rhythmic phases, especially with breathing and heart rate. It is usually our adult clients who come in with significant stress, trauma, and/or related disorders in which growth contraction is the prevalent dynamic. Primary Respiration allows the contraction to balance itself with the necessary growth expansion.

Growth Oscillations

The second type of growth is called *growth oscillations.* They are biokinetic movements. One example is the growth of the arm buds. Because the vascular supply of the arm is located on its ventral or under side, that side is slow growing because the vascular system under the surface of the skin is known for its slowness. But on the ventral surface of the arm, fast growth is occurring in the ectodermal covering because the ectoderm is known for its fast growth. Thus the arm movements of adduction and abduction oscillate back and forth as the arm grows. This is also true for the legs.

This type of growth oscillation is caused by differential rates of growth on the two sides of the arm, for example. This means that in biodynamic practice, one hand may be sensing a different rate of movement than the other hand, wherever the hands may be located. The hands of the practitioner switch from sensing wholistic movement to more local and individualized movement under each hand. This is biokinetics, discussed in Chapters 1 and 2. The work becomes an allowing for the different rates and maintaining a balance between both hands with Primary Respiration. Growth oscillations are common during the embryonic period and become more eccentric in the adult body, and thus may be overlooked in terms of their importance.

Local Growth Gesture

The third type of growth is called a *local growth gesture.* This is also a biokinetic movement. The arm eventually grows in a distinctive pattern of flexion for grasping objects and pulling them close, as with food. So the ability to grasp fruit growing from a tree and bringing it to the mouth is actually a function of embryonic growth. The future ability of the hands to grasp objects is pre-exercised as a function of how it grows embryonically. Thus the growing movement can be considered a gesture because it contains an intention for the growth as well as the growing movement itself. In this way, the embryo is very expressive and communicative. All organs and parts of the embryo have this capacity built into its cells and cell aggregates starting as metabolic fields. Growth oscillations usually precede localized growth gestures as well as occur simultaneously. Thus, it depends on the practitioner's perception of events unfolding under his or her hands that help notice the movement and its potential therapeutic value. This is done with the aid of Primary Respiration and stillness. There is really nothing to do with the movement but simply notice it. The health manifests in the noticing.

Later in embryonic development is when these definitive localized growth gestures begin to become visible. Gradually, it can be seen that an arm and hand are built for grasping (or thumb sucking). The legs are built for locomotion. Growth oscillations and growth gestures are a normal sequence in development. In terms of palpation, the growth gesture, especially of the limbs, incorporates a rotational movement. In the case of the limbs, the overall rotational movement is 90 degrees, so when the practitioner is palpating the client's limbs and senses a rotational movement, he or she will know that this is a localized growth gesture and allow Primary Respiration to allow the movement to fulfill itself with added potency.

Another important local growth gesture is found in the development of the heart. The heart starts under the chin of the embryo and above the future respiratory diaphragm, which at this point is around where the clavicles are in the adult. In this position the lumen of the heart begins its three phases of growth and development. First is the plexiform stage in which blood islands begin to ebb and flow into this area from either flank or side of the embryo along with a lot of water. We like to call this the stage of transparency as Primary Respiration can breath through this mesh-like configuration. The second stage is the tubular stage, in which the blood islands have coagulated, so to speak. Since the future respiratory diaphragm is pulling downward, the heart elongates into a tube in which the future atria are at the bottom and the future ventricles are at the top. We like to call this the elastic heart stage, in which the heart learns how to stretch itself. It will need this capacity all through life. Finally, in the third stage the heart begins to loop and turn downside up so the atria and ventricles can get into their normal position. We like to call this the upside-down-heart stage. It is another quality needed and experienced throughout life. Whenever these developmental movements are encountered it is so important to practice the transparency meditation in Chapter 13.

Global Growth Gesture

Dr. van der Wal, in his Chapters 6, 8, and 9 of Volume One in this series, speaks of a fifth morphological gesture that needs to be accomplished in each of the four stages of morphology. We call it a *global growth gesture.* This is another type of growth gesture in terms of the whole rather than the parts. Thus they are biodynamic movements and occur over longer phases of time in growth and development.

- Week one is associated with the development of an internal world of compression and rolling.

- Week two is associated with the external world of expansion and connection.

- Week three is associated with the middle world, or world of the heart that occurs between the ectoderm and endoderm layers of the embryo.

- Finally, folding and unfolding is the global growth gesture of weeks four through eight. This is the morphology of the whole in terms of its three-dimensional movement and developmental functions.

Secondary Growth Gestures

There are not only four types of growth movements but also numerous subcategories. Each stage of morphology has primary and secondary global growth gestures, which were discussed in Chapters 2 and 6 in Volume Three. To review them:

Week one is associated with:

- Compression

- Rolling

- Cracking (cracks appear in the shell of the zona pellucida)

Week two is associated with:

- Hatching (escape)

- Negotiation/death with the endometrium

- Embracing/attaching with the endometrium

- Expanding

- Rooting of center to periphery via a connecting stalk

Week three is associated with:

- Rotation of the heart

- Right/left symmetry of the heart and body

- Top/bottom symmetry of the heart and body

- Heart flow and bridging, looping, folding, rotating, bending, and convergence

- Covering of the brain and heart

- Fragmentation

Weeks four through eight are associated with:

- Curving/uncurving
- Lifting/unfolding
- Flexion/extension

All of these gestures have a fulcrum of Dynamic Stillness. All of these gestures are felt when engaged in one's buoyancy. Buoyancy and Primary Respiration are the keys to sensing any growth movements or gestures. It is through

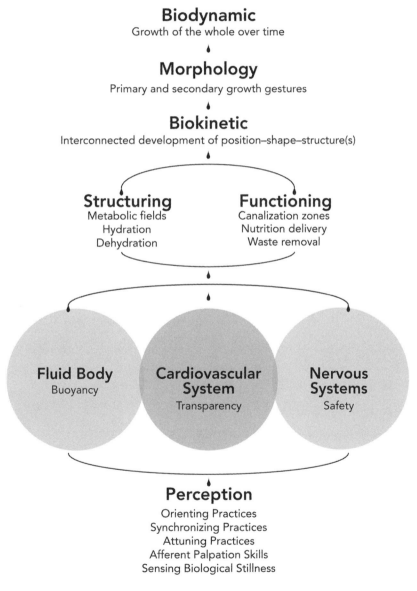

Figure 3.1. Summary of biodynamic embryology.

one's buoyancy that the practitioner can perceive all of the movements described above and many more that spontaneously occur in the practitioner's body and the client's body. Palpation is not a linear process. We ask the reader and practitioner to not follow this chapter as if it were a protocol. Rather, simply come into relationship with Primary Respiration and let it direct your perception. Just be in the noticing.

CHAPTER 4

Palpating the Embryo

with Carol Agneessens, MS

This chapter is written with the goal of transitioning the morphological language of observing the growth and development of the embryo into a language of palpating the embryonic forces present in the infant, child, and adult body. Palpation now listens for both the biodynamic and biokinetic movements of development as differentiated in the previous chapters. In this chapter we will make further distinctions with these two terms (biokinetics and biodynamics), as a way of bridging the science of observation with the art of palpation. We highly recommend reading the preceding three chapters before this one to be grounded in these distinctions.

The scientific study of embryonic morphology describes four essential components: first, the growth and maintenance of the whole, which is the totality of all structure and function throughout embryonic time (biodynamics); second, the local position and space available for development (biokinetics); third, the three-dimensional shaping processes of individual metabolic fields beginning to create a mold for a structure to fill in (biokinetics); and fourth, the eventual definitive structure being built from those fields (biokinetics) that becomes recognizable (such as the early liver, heart, arm, etc.). These are the categories of biodynamic growth and biokinetic development from the observations made by Drs. Blechschmidt, Gasser, Freeman, and others.

Basic Competencies

Can the biodynamic and biokinetic forces of the embryo that continue to sustain the health of the child and adult be palpated? We believe the answer is yes, based on the development of four competencies, described below.

With the *first competency,* the practitioner periodically settles into a whole-body sense of Primary Respiration moving through him or her, the zones, and the client. The practitioner develops a panoramic awareness of this therapeutic activity as it becomes the sustaining factor in treatment.

The *second competency* is the cultivation of a full-body sense of the transparency of Primary Respiration in a balanced rhythmic exchange with Dynamic Stillness contained in all the zones of perception (A+B+C+D). See Volume Four for a complete explanation of the biodynamic zones of perception. The zones are a holding environment for transformation to occur within and the practitioner is the manager of the container.

The *third competency* is the discriminating attunement with one's own and the client's nervous and vascular systems as the basis of contact and relationship. This is called interoceptive awareness and includes mindfulness of breathing, heart rate, and the felt sense of the body from a nonjudgmental point of view. This type of attunement and resonance is the basis of empathy and compassion as attention is moved slowly toward and away from the client. We believe that biodynamic practice is a protocol for compassion.

The *fourth* competency is the capacity of the practitioner to have buoyant hands and a buoyant body. The buoyancy of the client's fluid body is imprinted with stress and it dissipates into the practitioner's fluid body upon physical contact.

Up to now we have been teaching biodynamic palpation based on these four competencies. This chapter helps the practitioner enter a new phase of practice in which the palpation of the local biokinetic forces is balanced with the perception of a three-dimensional whole breathing biodynamically.

Principles of Order and Organization

The wholeness or total shape of the embryo is maintained through successive stages of complex development (biodynamics) by the interconnected order and fluid organization of the metabolic fields (biokinetics). The metabolic fields are fluid fields with different levels or gradients of viscosity and movements that precede definitive structures in the embryo. Order unfolds first in a discrete position (space) and then form (mold), which precedes a definitive structure. One might consider the metabolic fields to be very flexible, jello-like scaffolding around which structure fills in or condenses. The scaffolding around the heart is actually called cardiac jelly. Thus the scaffolding contains the blueprint of the definitive form of what is being generated in any given location in the embryo. It is a gradual process of condensation and shaping by the adjacent metabolic fields and fluid flows between them.

Every field knows where every other field is located in the whole, just as every cell in the body knows where every other cell is located. Each field has an adjoining or neighboring field that shares in the shaping process locally and globally. The metabolic fields are a web or matrix of interconnected wholeness. Consequently, biodynamics is both a study of wholeness and biokinetic inter-relationships. To see how this works in life, just spend time in a shopping mall or airport and observe the clusters of people in different degrees of separateness or compaction.

The organizational dynamics or local physical properties (biokinetics) of living wholeness experienced by the whole over time (biodynamics) can be restored by "thinking, knowing, feeling fingers," as Dr. Sutherland said. The following skills are related to positional or localized development of a form occurring simultaneously within a reciprocally expanding and contracting three-dimensional growing organism—the human embryo. The practitioner's hands are localized but at the same time he or she maintains a perception of the whole by periodically orienting to stillness and synchronizing with Primary Respiration while in contact with the client. This is called the *macro cycle of attunement,* taught in the previous two volumes. The steps to learning biokinetic palpation and perception eventually flow into a single continuum guided by stillness and Primary Respiration.

For understanding order and organization in the fluid body we have these three levels of understanding and palpation—position, form, and structure. We have repeated this notion to stress its importance. Position, form, and structure are the sequences of all human development in the embryo and adult body. The physical metabolism of this early positioning and form precedes the structural anatomy and physiology of the body. Therefore, making contact with these formative forces in the tempo of Primary Respiration can restore order and organization to the body at a very deep level. This is a key principle in an integrated biokinetic and biodynamic morphology: we observe order and organization in the fluids of the embryo at these three levels and palpation is synchronized with the tempo of Primary Respiration by a practitioner who is consciously aware of global and local stillness when it arises.

The Skin

We would now like to point out some of the important features of Figure 4.1 regarding the different layers of skin, fascia, and blood vessels. This is where a biodynamic practitioner places his or her hands for either biokinetic or biodynamic palpation. The figure shows that there are two layers of skin, two layers of fascia, and two layers of muscle. Between these layers are canals with veins and arteries moving longitudinally. What cannot be seen but palpated is a significant amount of fluid from water, blood, and lymph surrounding the fascia and skin. The fascia itself is a gel-like substance and it has more fluid properties to it than elastic properties. Furthermore, it has been discovered that a substructure of the fascia conducts a wave moving at a rate of 80–100 seconds. This of course is in the experiential range of Primary Respiration that is essential for palpating embryonic forces.

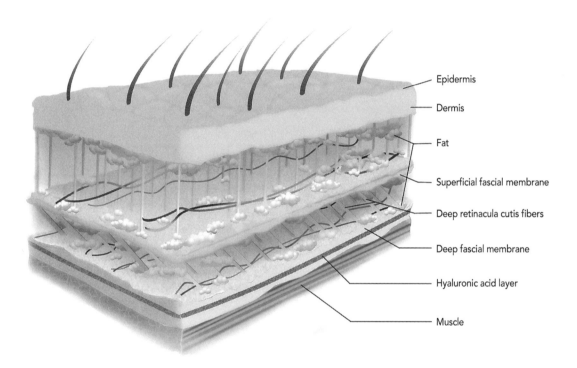

Figure 4.1. Layers under the skin where loosening fields are located.

Returning to Figure 4.1, recent research has indicated that there are three different types of touch receptors in the hair follicles that send information to the sensorimotor cortex of the brain to discriminate the sensation and the insular cortex of the brain to discriminate the context of the touch as safe and nurturing or not. This part of the brain was discussed in previous volumes, especially the research on the insular cortex. It connects the amygdala or fear center of the brain to the left prefrontal cortex and thus is critical in self-regulating fear-based emotional states. The amygdala is also monitoring the space around the body out to a distance of 15–20 inches. This of course is zone B and the practitioner must be acutely aware of both his or her zone B and that of the client to be effective both biodynamically and biokinetically. Chapter 14 covers this in detail. This is because of the tendency to concentrate with one's hands so that they become compressive or become confused about the difference between sensing biokinetic movements versus biomechanical movements, which are exclusively structurally related but lack a sensibility around early developmental position and form. All a biomechanical practitioner needs to do is switch from efferent hands to afferent hands and listen to Primary Respiration in whatever hand position is being used. It is really a rather easy transition into biokinetic and biodynamic palpation.

The Micro Cycle of Attunement

A four-step *micro* cycle of attunement is taught for contacting the metabolic fields of the embryo. This does not replace the *macro* cycle of attunement mentioned above. This is a preparatory practice done deliberately before and during contact with the client until it becomes spontaneous. Initially the practitioner performs a macro cycle of attunement. The micro cycle of attunement is a refinement of the macro cycles as follows:

First, the practitioner periodically maintains awareness of his or her zone A and B being homogenized as one drop of fluid.

Second, the practitioner maintains a three-dimensional sense of buoyancy, lift, and micromovement in the buoyancy of the unification of zone A and B.

Third, the practitioner feels his or her heart pulsation at the center of zone A and B and the pulsation spreading three dimensionally out to the edge of zone B. This can include visualizing arteries extending out to the edge of zone B. The heart is the fulcrum of biokinetic and biodynamic practice as we teach it.

Fourth, the practitioner synchronizes his or her breathing with Primary Respiration, as taught in Chapters 11 and 15.

These four steps comprise a micro cycle of attunement. This micro cycle of attunement is practiced periodically after the macro cycle of attunement. Once contact is made with the client and the practitioner has allowed his or her fluid body to dissipate the client's stress, the practitioner considers the location of his or her zone B and that of the client. Now that we have covered the basic principles and intentions of biodynamic and biokinetic palpation, we will start to develop a sensibility with our hands. These layers and levels of palpation are presented in a linear fashion here but we can assure you that it is a very nonlinear process in the office.

Corrosion Fields

This level of palpation is about what are called corrosion fields. The more time that a practitioner is in contact with one location on the client's body, the closer the practitioner's perception moves to what is called a corrosion field. More heat will build at the surface between the palms of the practitioner's hands and the skin of the client as two bodies are connecting in one small area. At a metabolic level, there will also be a decrease in nutrition and waste removal and the possibility for a breakdown of the tissue. Remember what your skin looks like after having a Band-Aid on it all day long. The redness of the skin is a corrosion field and it sometimes takes a couple of days for that redness to go away. When the practitioner's hands are buoyant, they not only float but each hand has variable intermittent micro pressure and release (IMPR), covered below, responding normally to the metabolic activity right under the hands. Conscious hands avoid being adhesive like a Band-Aid.

At a deeper level, it may feel as if the above distinctions disappear and the layers of tissue cannot be sensed. Corrosion fields occur when nutrition and waste removal are compromised by compression of the inner and outer layers of tissues, causing a blending together. Consequently, the tissues begin to dissolve and die. This opens the area to a different flow, as if a dam has broken. Since the whole is the smallest subdivision of life, all life is attempting to merge together constantly. One mechanism that maintains wholeness is a corrosion field. It allows us to sense the interconnectedness of all beings. Something that dies always opens the door to something new to follow. The therapeutic relationship itself is like a corrosion field since the neurology of empathy is exactly that. Each of us can sense the other person inside of our body. Thus the layers and filters of our brain, heart, and body are designed to be corrosive in life and death.

When the practitioner makes contact with the client, however, the fluid zones of practitioner and client overlap. This is a type of a corrosion field in which the boundaries of each of the edges of zone B have dissolved. It is important that the practitioner periodically focus on the stillpoint located where the two zone Bs overlap. In order to down-regulate the amygdala of the client, it is helpful if the practitioner is able to recognize the client's zone B and sense the contact boundary between him- or herself and the client. Not only does this settle the nervous system of the client but lends itself to a sense of safety, allowing Primary Respiration more expression of its therapeutic priorities.

Intermittent Micro Pressure and Release (IMPR)

Biokinetic palpation means that the practitioner is able to sense something different in each hand when in contact with the client. Typically, biodynamic palpation uses hands that are synchronized together to sense the whole breathing with Primary Respiration. That capacity remains in the background for now as a new skill is learned with the practitioner's hands. The first biokinetic differentiation is discovering which layer under the hands is thick and which is thin. The image of the skin and fascia shows multiple layers. In embryology, these skin and fascial layers are called limiting tissue. Wherever the hands are located on the body of the client, it is helpful to distinguish thick or thin. It is like trying to sense the density of a wet sponge or the edges of a tubular sea sponge in the ocean. Hands are buoyant and floating on the client's skin, exploring the subdermal layers with a natural intermittent micro pressure and release (IMPR). It is like the hands are on the surface of the ocean that is gently rising and falling with waves. The hands naturally seek this distinction.

Tim Shafer, a biodynamics instructor, put together an analogy of the metabolic fields for the use of palpation. One of their characteristics is the gradient of viscosity from very loose to very thick. As a metaphor for these varying densities, recall your experience with the following:

- Apple juice—represents the viscosity of the early metabolic fields
- Apple sauce—as growth and development continue, new fields arise and become thicker by losing water
- Apple butter—here, a degree of greater thickness has occurred
- Apples (or apple mash)—the apple itself and its firmness, coming into what is called pre-cartilage
- Dehydrated apple chips—often spongy and not completely dry, representing the cartilage
- Dried apples in granola—in this analogy, the bones, since many minerals get added to the metabolic field to make it a bone and thus the last and most dense of the metabolic fields

Deliberate use of IMPR is used at first to wake up this natural capacity for buoyant contact until it becomes a spontaneous way of contacting the client. It is then revisited frequently as a way of staying afloat on the ocean. The intention is still at the surface of the body, but now the surface is porous and has many sponge-like layers. In the adult body it must be remembered that the thick tissue may be denser and damaged from such things as surgery, diet, constipation, lymph edema, or simply lack of hydration.

IMPR is a discovery about viscosity and fluid density under the client's skin. It is critical in sensing the correct level of buoyancy in the contact with the client's skin. The practitioner's hands must be capable of regularly making micro adjustments when in contact with the wateriness under the client's skin. Surrounding these subdermal tissues is a body of living water, blood, and lymph that must have an adequate canalization system for nutrition delivery and waste removal. This is called a loosening field in embryology. Remember that one hand typically perceives differently than the other in biokinetic work. The depth of each hand in the client's tissue also varies naturally with IMPR. Periodically, both hands synchronize when working biokinetically. The synchronization of both hands is an indication of the whole moving biodynamically. The practitioner is aware of this distinction between his or her hands during a session and deliberately readjusts his or her hands during a session to maintain contact with the loosening fields below the skin. It is like surfing as the waves are constantly changing depth, length, and direction.

This intention includes sensing the vascular system, especially the blood capillaries under the skin, which move independent of the heart and the arteries. In this way the practitioner develops a discrete palpatory sensibility of the different layers of tissue and fluid immediately under the hands. This level of palpation is about viscosity and tempo of the motion present around the tissues. Surrounding these limiting tissues is a body of living water that must have an adequate canalization system for nutrition delivery and sewage elimination, as discussed in the previous chapters.

Nothing in the shape of the body is straight or linear. The convolutions and curvatures associated with the skin and its coverings shapes the cells into a wedge-like form at the deep bends of the fascia holding them. This is also true for any vessel in the body that bends. When cells take on this type of shape, narrow at one end and wider at the other like a slice of pie, there begins the possibility for appositional growth. This means that the inner tissues and associated fluid fields where the cell shape is narrower will generally be growing slower and relatively quiescent while the outer layers with the wider broader end will be growing faster or more intensely. This type of polarity creates a direction of ease between and around each layer for the flow of nutrition and waste removal. The rhythm of Primary Respiration sets the underlying tone and tempo upon which these developmental functions arise. Primary Respiration is like a catalytic converter since so much growth is so fast and Primary Respiration is so slow.

Resistance

Another level of palpation is sensing growth resistance in the tempo of Primary Respiration. Connective tissue functions as a restraining and resisting force via its contractile elements starting in week two. When the motion present is slow under one hand and fast under the other, that is an indication of growth resistance. This tissue polarity creates canals and direction of flow in response to differing areas of resistance. Resistance is not considered a barrier or obstruction preventing growth and development, but rather part of normal local kinetics in which both dynamics of growth and development are palpated as a whole. One hand may be sensing the resistance of a retention field and the other the expansion of the dilation field. The next moment both hands may be synchronized with the global movement of Primary Respiration. The metabolic field within will have a biodynamic pattern of wholistic movement and a slow tempo when the practitioner is synchronized with Primary Respiration and stillness. The metabolic field will then be able to self-correct without interference from the practitioner. In the adult, when a metabolic field self-corrects it allows the localized stem cells to fully repair, maintain, and/or generate new structure.

Balance of Incoming Nutrition and Waste Removal

The direction of ease in the growth resistance creates what are called canalization zones and consequently a direction of flow in response to the differential rates of growth. The limiting tissues are the borders of the canalization zones. According to Blechschmidt and Gasser (2012), there are three basic directions of flow: perpendicular to the tissue, through the tissue (diffusion of nutrients, water, and the effects of Primary Respiration), and longitudinally along the plane of the tissue. The general overall direction of fluid flow in the embryo is from bottom to top or from the rump end of the embryo up to the cephalic or head end. These canalization zones in the embryo are the substructure or template for the developing blood vessels whose definitive arrangement can be seen in Figure 4.1 of the different layers of skin and fascia, especially the longitudinal canals or vessels.

This level of palpation is about the superficial fascia. Once the practitioner begins to get a sense of the watery loosening field, then he or she can tune into the entire three-dimensional shape of the body as it extends longitudinally from the hands. The practitioner can begin to sense the longitudinal canals and the entire fascial matrix as if it were a bed of plankton. The plankton is moving in rhythmic waves of around a minute up and down the body or from the midsagittal plane of the body out to the lateral borders of the body. Imagine sitting at the beach and palpating the waves moving perpendicularly into and away from the hands. Then get into the water and sense the current moving longitudinally up and down the length of the beach.

Included in this sensibility are the blood vessels conducting the flow of nutrition and waste removal in the adult. The blood vessels are embedded in the fascia and surrounded by fibers of the autonomic nervous system. In this way the blood is considered to be the active element of the fascia. Palpating the metabolic fields contacts a very deep level of metabolism via the blood and fascia. It is the back door, so to speak, into the autonomic nervous system and thus can reduce high sympathetic tone. The sympathetic nervous system via the cardiovascular system is responsible at its deepest level for delivering oxygen everywhere in the body. Too much sympathetic tone restricts the blood vessels from delivering the oxygen via the blood. A basic principle of practice constantly being repeated is that the nutrition coming into the body must be balanced with waste removal, even at the local level of the hand placement. The macro and micro cycles of attunement are one way that waste products have an opportunity to be recycled so to speak and the channels opened for more nutrition to come in. This principle of balance is found at every level of the body, especially the cardiovascular system.

The blood vessels are the primary conductor of nutrition and waste removal in the embryo fetus, infant, and adult body. The blood vessels are gradually embedded in the fascia and surrounded by fibers of the autonomic nervous system. Thus biokinetic work involves contacting the blood vessels, especially the arteries, to more deeply influence the metabolism of the body. This is discussed in the next chapter. Sometimes the resistance is experienced as a suction field in which an organ or tissue is sensed as being pulled in one direction without a reciprocal return. The early heart-liver relationship is a good example, where the heart has a strong pull or suction on the liver and pulls it into growing bigger as the liver resists the pull.

The limiting tissues in the adult will be the fasciae, especially the superficial fascia and subdermis under the skin throughout the body. The practitioner may be able to sense Primary Respiration moving through the fascia, especially longitudinally. This will help rehydrate damaged fascia from surgery or other trauma. Chronic inflammatory conditions in the gut will alter the ability of the fascia to recover and must be considered part of any client evaluation, as discussed at the end of this volume. Clients must reduce the toxic load of waste products from inflammatory processes and other conditions such as mercury amalgams in the mouth. Enemas, colon hydrotherapy, and infrared saunas are several valuable means to reduce the toxic load in the body. Please refer to Chapters 31–38 for information on detoxification.

Review

Now we would like to review or summarize the steps just covered in this chapter. Please consider this a brief ready reference guide to entering into biokinetic palpation.

Step 1. Practice orienting and synchronizing with Primary Respiration, allowing this rhythm to shift your perception to the horizon and back, at the beginning as well as throughout the session.

Step 2. Let your sensibilities open to the inner and outer layers of tissue in the client.

Step 3. Sense the wateriness around the inner tissue.

Step 4. Begin to use intermittent micro pressure and release (IMPR).

Step 5. Notice your breathing and sense the expansion and contraction of the shape of the client through the zones as if he or she were breathing beyond the body.

Step 6. Notice the longitudinal flows that might arise, both like canals and/or an entire bed or blanket of seaweed that is moving rhythmically.

Step 7. Allow your attention to cycle back to the immediate skin-to-skin contact placement, noticing any heat or other phenomena present.

The Intelligence of Touch

Each hand perceives and contacts tissue differently. If you are right hand dominant, allow your left hand to sense, feel, and feedback the quality of information received from the tissues. The depth of each hand in the client's tissue also varies naturally. Only periodically do both hands synchronize. Listen to what each hand is sensing through the tissues and fluids.

There are two levels of understanding the palpation of the embryo mentioned in this chapter. One is from the biodynamic point of view and the other is from the biokinetic point of view regarding the growth and development of the human body. The biodynamic model of craniosacral therapy includes both sensibilities into an integrated metabolic model. Working with the physical movement of the metabolic fields is working with the deepest level of development called biokinetics. By placing attention on these dynamic moving and interrelationship processes, the practitioner helps the client synchronize with the order and organization present in the fluid metabolism of the body. These are key components in palpating the metabolic fields of the embryo in the adult and the restoration of wholeness. They are profoundly healing.

CHAPTER 5

Working with the Blood and Heart

This chapter is the result of working with the information in the first four chapters. A missing skill in the field of manual therapy and craniosacral therapy in general is the ability to sense the blood, the tubes it moves through, and the heart. The cardiovascular system is the interface between the fluid body and central nervous system. It is in the blood and heart that the autonomic nervous system can be influenced in such a way that physiological resilience results. This means that the structure of the brain changes for the positive, simply by paying attention to the movement of the heart and blood. In biodynamic practice, this level of post-advanced work requires a delicate and subtle palpation skill. The blood is the active element of the fascia. Thus Primary Respiration moves through the fascia just as waves of the ocean come to the shore of the beach. Primary Respiration also moves through the arterial system three dimensionally away from the heart and returns to the heart via the venous system every fifty seconds.

The heart and the blood become the new midline of the body in this sensibility. The fluid body is able to resolve its imprints through the interrelational dynamics of a client and therapist working heart to heart. Primary Respiration moves between two hearts and generates the felt sense of love and happiness. This is not so much a sexual intimacy as it is a basic human condition. It is actually the pre-existing condition of our empathy and compassion-based heart, brain and body. These protocols are very beneficial in the recovery of one's embodiment. As a note to practitioners, my recommendation is that you thoroughly acquaint yourself with Chapters 3 and 4 regarding the palpation and movement of the embryo when sensing Primary Respiration. I would then only recommend doing two of the practices outlined below at any given time with a client, and usually in the middle of a session.

The vascular work is considered biokinetic work. This is an important distinction. In these practices function is being related with, rather than specific structures, although the practitioner must know the anatomy to have precision with hand placements. The arteries have blood moving through them and the walls of the arteries are managing pressure dynamics just as the ventricles of the heart are managing pressure, At its deepest level, the autonomic nervous system is helping the blood deliver oxygen to every cell in the body. Since much of the work with the contemporary client is stabilizing the autonomic nervous system first, then working biokinetically with the heart and vascular system can change the set point of homeostasis in the autonomic nervous system and thus reduce fear and help generate resiliency when under stress. Working biokinetically requires competency in zone practice, as described in Chapter 14.

The *vascular tree* is the place I always start and then work with one or two specific arteries. The heart in its location is associated with the respiratory diaphragm and thus can also facilitate a diaphragm release.

The Vascular Tree

First, practice several cycles of macro attunement with the window.

Sit at the side of the table and, after settling with a cycle of attunement, negotiate permission to make contact with the vascular tree of the client.

Then practice a micro cycle of attunement when making contact.

Contact is made with the radial artery with one hand cupping under or over the wrist of the client and the other hand is placed over or under the lower leg, just above the ankle in order to contact the venous return from the foot. Thus both hands are in contact with the peripheral end of the entire vascular system.

Focus attention on your own zone B and the pulse of the client's vascular system under your hands.

Vary the depth of contact in both hands with intermittent micro pressure and release. This includes sensing the loosening fields under the skin.

Allow the pulse of the radial artery to come and go. The blood is the active element of the fascia.

The interconnecting factor is the way in which Primary Respiration moves through the fascia that holds the vascular tree. You may sense Primary Respiration moving like a bed of plankton on the ocean surface. It is a slow wave moving through the fascia.

Lightly bring attention to your own heart and both zone Bs, and then wait for the vascular system of the client to clarify its direction of flow, increased flow, three-dimensional flow, and so on.

Either you or the client, or both of you, may experience an accelerated heart rate. In some cases this is simple awareness, even though the heart is not moving faster. Or the heart may actually be moving faster and the client should be taught how to do a relaxing breath into the abdomen to lower the heart rate. This is the autonomic nervous system going through a process that leads to stabilization.

The Subclavian Artery

The next window involves making contact with the subclavian artery in the client. Ask the client to turn the head to the right while you are gently restraining his or her forehead on the right in order to make the anterior scalene muscle activate.

Sit at the head of the table and gently place a fingertip of either the index or middle finger bilaterally in the gap between the anterior and medial scalene muscles as they attach onto the first rib. This is the space of the subclavian artery. Alternatively, use your thumbs to palpate this artery by contacting the edge of the client's clavicles and rolling the thumbs gently under the clavicles in the gap between the scalenes.

Repeat the process of finding the anterior scalene on the left and settle into a bilateral contact of the subclavian artery.

Wait for harmony and communication between the two arteries while sensing your own heart rate periodically.

Initially you may not sense the artery but must wait until the artery comes to your fingers. It is wrapped in the inferior cervical sympathetic ganglion and thus protected from intrusive palpation. Arteries are often sensed as a flow rather than a pulsation and they will vary in terms of sensation from side to side.

The Common Carotid Artery

The third window involves making contact with the common carotid artery bilaterally. Again, you are sitting at the head of the table. Place one or two finger pads on the anterior border of sternocleidomastoid muscle a centimeter or two above its attachment on the clavicle.

Sensing the pulse of the common carotid artery is valuable in lowering the tone of the autonomic nervous system. This is because the contact is located around the inferior and middle cervical sympathetic ganglion that innervate the carotid artery and close to the carotid sinus.

Wait for harmony between the two pulses bilaterally and also for Primary Respiration to move through the fascia and loosening fields under the skin.

Occasionally you may sense the flow of Primary Respiration through the entire vascular tree of the client, and likewise the client may sense this as well.

I ask clients to make a slight smile on their face when they sense this level of wholeness.

The Occipital Artery

The next window is to make contact with the occipital artery in the suboccipital triangle of muscles. This is a modification of the atlanto-occipital joint releases taught in almost every school of craniosacral therapy. This area at the base of the occiput is the doorway into and out of the cranium.

The occipital artery comes from the carotid artery and has a pulse or a sense of flow. The practitioner waits to sense it and also for the same softening and opening that occurs in the fascia with Primary Respiration. This leads to more space for the fluid body to expand and balances the superior sympathetic ganglion with the vagus nerve exiting the jugular foramen.

The occiput of the client may begin to gently and slowly flex and extend, which indicates a deep release and settling.

Practice the vascular tree on the opposite side of the client's body.

Finish with the pietà, sacrum, or feet. (All of these hand positions are shown in detail in Volume 4.)

The Iliac and Femoral Arteries

Sit at the side of the client and palpate the iliac/femoral arteries on one side. The pulse/flow of the iliac artery is located midway to two-thirds of the way down the inguinal ligament toward the pubic bone from the anterior superior iliac spine on the superior border of the ligament. The finger pads of one hand are above the inguinal ligament palpating the iliac artery and the finger pads of the other hand are inferior to the inguinal ligament palpating the femoral artery. The femoral artery is the continuation of the iliac artery below the inguinal ligament. This palpation balances the legs to the pelvis and the pelvis to the trunk.

Repeat on the other side of the body.

The finger pads of both hands are lined up in such a way above and below the inguinal ligament that they form a V-shape. This is because the iliac artery is at an angle coming from the central abdominal aorta and the femoral artery angles back toward the medial side of the lower leg.

Abdominal Aorta

The next window involves making contact with the pulse of the abdominal aorta. You can ask the client to flex the knees if there is too much tension in the abdomen. Place your finger pads lateral of the umbilicus at the border of the rectus abdominus muscle. Use intermittent micro pressure and release to sense the aorta. Wait for the aortic pulse to come into your fingers. Check the other side and see which side has more potency. The client's legs can be extended once you sense the aorta.

Practice moving your fingers inferiorly to where the abdominal aorta bifurcates into the iliac arteries somewhere on the level of L3 to L5.

The other hand is supported and reaching toward the other side of the client's umbilicus in order to sense the aorta bilaterally. If this is uncomfortable, the practitioner can do one side at a time. All arteries must be palpated bilaterally.

Once contact is made with the abdominal aorta, then Primary Respiration can be accessed through the mesenteries. This also is very helpful for the celiac, as well as the superior and inferior mesenteric arteries.

Practice the vascular tree on the opposite side without repeating the several cycles of attunement as you did at the beginning.

Finish with the pietà, sacrum, or feet.

Remember in all the hand positions to practice finding the loosening field under the fingers. This means practice intermittent micropressure and release as if each hand or finger is like a cork floating on water.

Primary and Secondary Heart Fields

Review the anatomical location of the adult heart and pericardium. Note that the heart is resting on top of the diaphragm, slightly to the left of the midline of the sternum. The heart is lying on an axis roughly between the right shoulder and spleen.

Sit on the left side of the client and place one hand under the rib cage, approximating the position of the posterior portion of the heart. The other hand is on top of the rib cage, approximating the location of the anterior structure of the heart.

Embryologically the heart develops from what is called a primary field, which consists of the majority of structures on the anterior chambers of the heart and associated inflow and outflow vessels. The posterior portion of the heart forms from what is called a secondary heart field. This means that the cells making up the posterior heart came from a different location in the embryo. In addition, there is a structure in the embryo that attaches the posterior heart to the posterior body wall or coelom of the embryo.

The intention is to come into relationship with the embryonic movements of the heart, which consist of looping, bending, and folding in the context of Primary Respiration. This is very valuable for balancing the autonomic nervous system.

As an alternative, you can place both hands under the secondary heart field and then both hands on top of the left side of the rib cage over the primary heart fields. Listen with Primary Respiration.

The Aortic Arch

Sit at the side of the table by the shoulder of the client, who is supine.

Place the heel of one hand over the sternal angle between the manubrium and the sternum. The fingers are pointing toward the opposite shoulder. This hand senses the aortic arch on a curve from anterior to posterior.

The finger pads of the other hand are palm up under the client's neck at C3–C4. Gentle contact is made with the spinous processes of the vertebra with only a finger pad or two. This is known as the area of the heart fulcrum window. Alternatively, the bottom hand can be placed under the upper thoracic vertebra. Find which lower hand position works best and for which client. This is very beneficial for the subclavian and carotid arteries.

Sense the fascia that suspends the aorta.

Both hands synchronize together with Primary Respiration in the artery or in the fascia.

These hand positions are incredibly valuable for stabilizing the sympathetic branch of the autonomic nervous system.

The Carotid Sinus

The client is sidelying. You can approach the client from the front or back of the client's neck.

Imagine that all ten finger pads and tips are on a piano.

Contact is made with the entire length of the carotid artery especially the area of the carotid sinus at the junction of the common carotid and internal carotid artery.

Since the carotid artery is under the sternocleidomastoid muscle, the practitioner may find it easier approaching from either the front or back.

The intention is to sense Primary Respiration either in the artery or fascia suspending the artery. This stimulates the carotid sinus, which lowers hypertension according to research.

The Thyroid Artery

The client is supine and you are sitting at the head of the table.

Make contact with the index fingers almost touching together starting at the hyoid slightly lateral of the midline of the client's neck. Gradually palpate the anterior neck until contact is made with the thyroid gland, which is more dense.

Then make bilateral contact over the thyroid gland area of the client. This is just above the manubrium of the client. The thyroid extends under the sternocleidomastoid muscle bilaterally. Keep your fingers medial to the sternocleidomastoid muscle.

Use the pads of both index fingers and sense the thyroid artery (it is coming from the carotid artery). Primary Respiration will reveal the metabolic field of the thyroid. Wait for the interchange of Primary Respiration and stillness through the zones.

This skill is very valuable in stabilizing the hypothalamic-thyroid axis. It reflexes into the hypothalamic-pituitary-adrenal axis and the hypothalamic-gonadal axis. It must be practiced with Primary Respiration guiding the hands of the practitioner.

For a more in-depth exploration, I highly recommend *Visceral Vascular Manipulations* (Barral and Croibier, 2011). This is a thorough investigation that supplements the skills of my Volume Five. In addition, there are ample photographs and anatomical images to help the practitioner navigate what I present in this chapter and elsewhere. I believe that the palpation of the cardiovascular system is the cutting edge of biodynamic craniosacral therapy and healing in general.

CHAPTER 6

Palpating the Bones

This chapter is a series of palpation exercises designed to make contact with the living skeletal system of the client. It takes into account the metabolic fields in the embryo from which bones and cartilage arise. Bones and cartilage are the last structural elements that are formed in the embryo. Palpating the bones can be considered as a doorway into the embryo. Living bone is highly vascularized and filled with fluid. One intention of these palpation exercises is to differentiate between intraosseous motion and interosseous motion. This, of course, occurs with the practitioner's perception of Primary Respiration.

Intraosseous motion specifically refers to how the bone breathes by itself with Primary Respiration. For example, when palpating the sacrum, the sacrum and its intraosseous motion will feel much like a flower opening and closing. Interosseous motion refers to bones that are connected to one another through whatever types of joint or sutural system move in relationship to each other. As with all palpation oriented toward localized biokinetic movement, one should also toggle attention to the dynamic whole periodically. Have fun.

Practitioners' hands encounter the bones of the client's body frequently. When encountering a bone, there may be several metabolic fields associated with it, depending on its location in the body (near the viscera, the brain, muscle tissue, etc.). When the practitioner's hands encounter a bone, considering a pause to sense its metabolic field is appropriate with Primary Respiration.

Remember, when sensing metabolic fields there are adjacent fields that come into play. These adjacent fields have their own shape and location. It is likely that your hand just passed through one field to get to a bone. Then the question becomes where is the other field(s) located. This requires three-dimensional thinking and feeling fingers.

A key principle is that the fields all have polarities, which means one hand is sensing one shape and density while the other hand may be sensing a different shape and density (field). Both hands must stay in the polarity for as long as possible, guided by the tempo of Primary Respiration. Metabolic fields and their palpation are covered in Chapters 3 and 4.

Windows for palpating the developmental aspects of a bone go through a sequence of stages.

- Simple contact with the periosteum of the bone allows for palpation of Primary Respiration moving through the fascia. This is in a loosening field, which means there is a watery element present.

- The density of the bone is then sensed in terms of its fluidity.

- The vascular and fluid parts of a living bone are then palpated with Primary Respiration in order to sense intraosseous motion. This intraosseous motion has a fulcrum around which it moves like a flower opening and closing.

- If the bone has marrow in it, then this midline of the bone is sensed again with Primary Respiration. If it is a long bone, such bones typically breathe on their long axis. The marrow will also have a fulcrum related to the vascular system and the communication channels through the bone made up of veins and arteries, which travel on an oblique pathway that may feel like a spiraling movement.

- Palpation of the bones with Primary Respiration is exceedingly valuable in helping to stabilize the endocrine system of the client. The neurohormones serotonin and testosterone are metabolically linked to the healthy functioning of the skeletal system of human beings. This is all new medical research detailing the important relationship of the skeletal system to the endocrine system.

Some of the following bones are involved in this palpation exercise.

- The tibia-fibula bilaterally
- The hip bones ipsilaterally or bilaterally
- The rib cage and sternum
- The frontal bone and parietal bones
- The parietal bones bilaterally
- The sacrum and floating ribs

Each of these bones or osseous areas are then palpated with the sensibility discussed above.

Now let's take this palpation into clinical treatment by working with the extremities.

Lower Extremities

1. Stand by the side of the table next to the client's pelvis. Gently make bilateral contact with the trochanters of the client's femurs. This is the area where the leg bud was initially located. Synchronize with Primary Respiration.

2. Now sit by the side of one of the client's legs and place one hand under the lower leg and the other hand under the upper leg. Imagine you are cradling the client's leg. Tune into Primary Respiration and any available growth or developmental movements. Repeat on the opposite leg.

3. Sitting at the side, choose one leg. Make contact with the greater trochanter of the client with one hand. With the other hand, make very buoyant contact with one or more tips of the toes of the client. This area is called the apical ectodermal ridge. You will need sufficient props under the wrist and arm in relationship with the tips of the client's toes. Wait for Primary Respiration to breathe the leg. If there is time, repeat on the opposite leg.

4. Now switch hand positions so that one hand is under the gastrocnemius of the client's leg. The other hand is over the top of the quadriceps of the same leg. Each hand is perceiving a different growth or developmental movement. Come into relationship with these differences and wait for them to balance with Primary Respiration.

Upper Extremities

1. Sit at the head of the table. Make gentle bilateral contact with the heads of the client's humerus on both arms. This is the general area where the arm bud was first located. Wait for Primary Respiration.

2. Now sit by the side of one of the client's arms and place one hand under the lower arm and the other hand under the upper arm. Imagine you are cradling the client's arm. Tune into Primary Respiration and any available growth or developmental movements. Repeat on the opposite arm.

3. Sitting at the side of one arm, as with the leg exercise above, allow one hand to make contact with the head of the humerus and the other hand to make contact with one or more tips of the client's fingers (apical ectodermal ridge). Again remember to let the arm breathe with Primary Respiration.

4. Switch hand positions so that one hand is under the radius and ulna of the client's forearm. The other hand is on top of the upper arm midway between the elbow and the shoulder. Whichever way the client's arm is

resting, whether it is pronated or supinated, makes no difference; you have one hand under the forearm and the other hand on top of the upper arm. The intention is to notice different growth movements occurring under each hand. Then wait for Primary Respiration to balance the arm.

I hope you had fun!

CHAPTER 7

Palpating the Core

This chapter contains two protocols that I developed for sensing and decompressing the coelomic cavities of the body. The coelomic spaces are embryonic spaces relating to the pleura, pericardium, and peritoneum. These two protocols could be considered to be a variation on the traditional diaphragm releases, but actually they are quite different. One reason they are different is because of the perception of Primary Respiration; a second reason is the knowledge of the biokinetics of the embryo, as detailed in Chapters 3 and 4.

The first protocol deals with the pericardium and the pleura. The second protocol begins with the peritoneum and finishes with the feet. I do not recommend practicing both of these protocols at once, but rather one at a time. I developed these protocols specifically as a way to decompress the fluid body. I gradually discovered that not only the core of the body needed to be decompressed, but also detoxified, and thus the chapters on detoxification at the end of the book were added. As with any biodynamic protocol, the priority is Primary Respiration and the sensing of wholeness. Local biokinetic movements must always be joined with the whole.

In both protocols, the practitioner is doing zone practice.

Zone Practice

Orient and synchronize to Primary Respiration out to the horizon and back.

Establish contact with your own zone A and B, breathing with the potency of Primary Respiration.

Zone B is continuous with zone A. Sense the surface of your skin and then the membrane between zone B and C.

Sense zone B filling up with air, warmth, and the potency of Primary Respiration known as the Reciprocal Tension Potency and the longitudinal fluctuation.

Pericardium and Pleura

1. Focus the zone practice on your own zone B.

2. The pericardium portion of the protocol is usually done with a water bag placed over the sternum, xyphoid process, and epigastric area.

   Approach the client from the side. Place one hand on top of the water bag and the opposite hand underneath the client between T5 and T12. The hand underneath only needs a little bit of contact with the spinous processes of the thoracic vertebra.

   When a water bag is not available for practice, the hand placement should be over the lower part of the sternum.

3. Working with the pleura can be done either standing or seated. Either way, it requires good props for your wrists and arms.

   Make contact bilaterally on the lateral aspects of the lower ribs. The fingers can actually be in contact with the table as they curve around toward the back of the ribs.

   Primary Respiration breathes the lungs during development from their initial buds that appear between C3 and C7.

   Visualize or sense the location of the hand bud in both hands while staying in the tempo of Primary Respiration.

   Sense Primary Respiration around the horseshoe shape of the pleural cavity in its embryonic form.

   There are other access points for assessing the pleura and pericardium that are also valuable for this assessment. Useful tips: For working with the pericardium and pleura, maintain your attention between zones A and B. For the shoulders, move your attention between all the zones.

4. Bilateral shoulder assessment is the next step.

   Sitting at the head of the table, place both hands palm up under the client's (or practice partner's) right and left shoulder. This does not have to be all the way underneath the scapula.

   As an alternative, you can make bilateral contact with the partner's clavicles, placing the pads of your index to small fingers around mid-clavicle. Not all finger pads will fit on the clavicle, so just choose the fingers that are most comfortable while in contact.

   The thumbs can be making contact around the transverse processes of C5–C7.

   In either or both hand positions, a determination is made regarding the quality of movement of Primary Respiration through each shoulder. You must decide which shoulder to focus upon.

5. Ipsilateral shoulder contact takes place now.

   Choose one shoulder to work and change position to sit perpendicular to the shoulder to be worked on.

   Place one hand underneath supporting the scapula and place the top hand, supported, so that it contacts the head of the humerus and the clavicle.

   Wait for Primary Respiration to inflate the shoulder.

   If you are in a class or a practice session, it is not necessary to treat the opposite shoulder, although it might need it in clinical practice.

   Now repeat steps 1 and 2 from above while in contact with the one shoulder.

6. Finish with the sacrum. Make contact with the sacrum in the primitive streak hold. Sitting at the side of the table perpendicular to the client's pelvis, place one hand around the coccyx and the other hand around the sacral base.

Peritoneum

1. The client is supine; you are sitting at the side of the client facing his or her abdomen.

   Sense into your own abdomen and breathe between the pubic bone and umbilicus slowly.

   Place both hands palm down above the pubic symphysis of the client. Do not cover the umbilicus of the client with your hands.

   Sense the client's respiratory and pelvic diaphragms synchronizing. Then sense the entire peritoneal cavity of the client breathing with Primary Respiration.

2. Give your attention to the primitive streak.

   Place both hands under the client's sacrum. One finger of one hand is near the coccyx and the other hand (small and ring fingers) is near the sacral base.

   Sense your own pelvic floor and periodically squeeze your pelvic floor muscles gently as if holding back from urinating. Following the short muscle contraction, sense your own zone B for it filling up.

   Then sense interosseous or intraosseous motion of the client's sacrum and/or related phenomena around the primitive streak and pelvic cavity.

   You are synchronizing with Primary Respiration in the client's pelvis.

3. Evaluate the innominate bones.

Standing or seated, place your hands bilaterally on the anterior superior iliac spines (ASIS) of the client to sense which side to start with. This is a brief assessment.

With the client supine, move to a seated position at an angle facing the lower extremities of the client by the side of his or her abdomen.

Make contact with the ischial tuberosity of one of the client's innominate bones with one hand. Place the other hand palm down over the ASIS of the same innominate bone.

Listen for the innominate bone to breathe and reshape itself in relation to Primary Respiration. This may include a decompression of the pelvic floor, causing eccentric motion to occur in the bone.

Repeat the same process on the other innominate bone of the client.

Maintain attention on your own zone B and that of the client by focusing on the stillpoint in the space between the client's body and your sternum.

4. Repeat steps 1 and 2, for the peritoneum and primitive streak, and evaluate for increased range of motion and potency within Primary Respiration in zone B.

5. Finish by holding the feet.

Please remember to practice one of these protocols at a time until more experience is gained in their effects on the client. As with all the skills that I teach, the practitioner must sense his or her own core prior to sensing that of the client. This can be simply listening to the movement of one's heart or being mindful of the movement of the respiratory diaphragm. Decompressing the core builds resilience. Resilience is the key to self-regulation. Self-regulation develops a deeper sensibility of love and happiness.

CHAPTER 8

Slime Mold Study Guide:
An Image of the Fluid Body
and Primary Respiration

This chapter is an annotated transcript of a 16-mm movie from 1954, which is available from Pacific Distributing at www.booksandbones.com. To me this film is a study of the fluid body and Primary Respiration and, as I show it to students in class I point out how Primary Respiration changes directions. The flow that is observed between Primary Respiration changing phases is likely in the range of the Mid Tide since it appears faster than fifty seconds in one direction. At one point, the narrator points out that there are multiple rhythms occurring simultaneously in the slime mold and that is the second teaching point: it depends therefore on the practitioner's quality of attention which rhythm he or she perceives. Biodynamic practice is a study in perception first and foremost.

In this transcript I have made some annotations. First, I have italicized certain passages in the transcript that I feel are important for biodynamic practitioners to notice. Second, I have placed my own comments in brackets throughout the text and summarized highlights at the end. In addition, I added time stamps for the film run length at the end of this chapter.

Title Screen: Seifriz on Protoplasm

Photography and Commentary by William Seifriz, Professor of Botany, University of Pennsylvania, 1954, produced by J. M. B. Churchill, Jr.

First Screen

Protoplasm is the basic material of which all living things are made. It is nearly always found organized into cells. One of the most extraordinary qualities of this "stuff of life" is the similarity of its appearance and activities wherever found, whether in lowly plant, elephant, or man. [One osteopath calls protoplasm *the first moldable substance.* This describes the human embryo.]

Second Screen, and Onward

In this film is seen one of the most primitive forms of life, a slime mold. The protoplasm of this organism is not composed of cells, but forms and extended living mass with many nuclei. This is a study of life in one of its simplest forms—yet how complex it still is!—where the most fundamental questions are those of life itself, and are yet to be answered.

[The question that Seifriz finally asks later in the film is "what causes the motion?" He then goes on to make a case for electrical stimulation as cause even though the slime mold has no nervous system and thus no electrical system present. I don't think one can say that Primary Respiration is a cause for movement either. I believe that it is futile to look for cause. It is enough to synchronize with Primary Respiration in clinical practice and observe its therapeutic priorities.]

I want to tell you about a very lowly form of life, a slime mold. It's the present-day counterpart of the primordial ooze that appeared on earth many, many eons ago. The descendant of this primordial ooze, the substance that gives life to all plants and animals, we call protoplasm. Now, let us go into the woods and collect the protoplasm of a slime mold. You'll probably find it growing on an old stump, such as this one. Or if the first stump reveals nothing, we'll search for another. And now, here's better luck, golden yellow protoplasm glistening in the sun. No shape to it, for it's always changing shape. No cells, no tissue, just protoplasm, one protoplasmic mass, with many living nuclei.

Having collected the protoplasm in nature, we can now grow it in the laboratory. Here's a culture of the slime mold physarum, growing so luxuriantly that it's crawled out of its culture dish. [There are two kinds of slime molds—acellular, or without cells, and multicellular. Physarum is of the acellular type.] Note here this hanging thread protoplasm on the left, with a mass of protoplasm on the end of it. It reveals the tensile strength of the living substance. [The fluid body of a human has tensile strength in various gradients of density.] And all the while the protoplasm is flowing up and down in this living thread. Here we have a closer view of the culture. In the center is an island on which the food is placed. Slime molds are very fond of oatmeal. And surrounding the island is a moat of water. And here a still nearer view of a small part of the whole, such as we would see if we used a hand lens. Remember this is not tissue, not an aggregation of cells, but just protoplasm. And through it all there is constant streaming.

And now [here is] the protoplasm as seen through the microscope. The movement never ceases as long as there is life, except during hibernation in winter time. Here is a younger portion of the plasmodium [the first change of direction of Primary Respiration is observed]. *Could we but understand the cause of this constant movement, we should be nearer to an understanding of what life is.* The protoplasm here flows all over the surface. Later, definite channels will be established. The granules you see are nuclei, fat droplets, vacuoles, and bits of food. Here the plasmodium assumes its mature form. But even now, the arteries are transitory and soon the whole picture will change. *Note particularly the reversal in direction of flow, with a rhythmic period of fifty seconds.* [Primary Respiration is seen when the flow changes directions. In other words, the flow is moving at the Mid Tide rate, which is faster. Primary Respiration, which is slower, is only visible when it changes directions. It appears that there is a slowing down of the flow, a pause, and then a change of direction. Note that in this image and others that follow, Primary Respiration begins to slow down and even begins to change direction in one area and gradually other areas of the protoplasm slow down and change direction within a 5- to 10-second time frame. This means that Primary Respiration is not like a switch being flipped and the whole organism reverses direction. I have found this helpful in my own personal explorations with Primary Respiration in my body and around my body. So that is what is visible regarding Primary Respiration. In clinical practice Primary Respiration may not always be perceived as changing directions and thus I like to say it is changing phases, which allows for different metaphors to describe its activity.]

We shall now indulge in some work in microdissection. Here are several types of micromanipulators in which glass needles are clamped and controlled. Our problem is to prove that protoplasm is elastic. We prove it by tearing protoplasm with needles, just as a surgeon dissects the human body. And for this operation, we must have a pair of delicate needles, made either in a tiny flame, such as this, or better yet with the aid of hot platinum wire. And now let us compare this microdissection needle with a good new sewing needle.

We have all sorts of instruments for microdissection. Here is a double needle holder used as forceps. But we must get to work and tear the protoplasm to see if holds together or if it is simply a fluid, like water. And for this purpose we need a culture on a microscope slide, which becomes the roof of a small moist chamber with open ends, with the protoplasm on the inside. Here we are putting the needle into one of the open ends and you will see the protoplasm on the underside of the roof of the moist chamber. We move the protoplasm aside for a moment in order to find the needle. And here it is. Now we are ready to dissect. And to prove how tough and elastic protoplasm is … [images of the elasticity of the fluid body].

We can not only dissect, but we inject with this delicate hypodermic needle, which is here merely blowing a bubble. Let us inject a toxic salt and you will see the protoplasm suddenly stop. Beyond, out of the picture, the protoplasm flows on as before. Thus the protoplasm meets contingencies, heals itself, and thus saves itself. [The fluid body enters a phase of stillness for repair.]

We turn now to a typical medical problem, anesthesia. When the normal protoplasm is treated with carbon dioxide, it slowly goes to sleep. Here is another specimen. Now, it, too, is slowly going to sleep. Now, a few minutes later, we get the first indications of recovery. And a quarter of an hour later, almost the same culture back again: healthy, normal protoplasm. And an hour later, we can't tell any difference between this protoplasm and that before anesthesia. [Here is] another specimen. It doesn't matter what I use to anesthetize protoplasm—ether, chloroform, cold, or I can even hit it on the head with little droplets of water. *There you just saw the normal reversal [of Primary Respiration] in this culture.*

But in this case it is carbon dioxide. Now the gas is on. Watch it, so sudden a cessation of flow could occur only if the protoplasm has solidified. Here's still another patient, under high magnification. *We made a discovery that the rhythmic forces [of Primary Respiration] in protoplasm are even more basic than the flow [Mid Tide]. For when the protoplasm recovers, it doesn't just start flowing. It resumes as though it had been flowing all the while.* [Primary Respiration does not stop even in the stillness. Clinically, practitioners observe that Primary Respiration exchanges places with the perception of stillness. Even though Primary Respiration does not stop, the stillness frequently becomes a more dominant perception three dimensionally in the treatment room. The instructions at this point are to wait in the stillness without moving until Primary Respiration returns from the background of perception.]

In a moment now, the protoplasm slowly quiets down. *Note that there is a slight nervous shock just before anesthesia takes place.* [The fluid body is an intelligence and capable of being startled just before the shock since it knew it was coming. Thus the fluid body has a startle reflex mechanism. This is why it is important for practitioners to remain buoyant in their own body so that as the startle dynamic releases in the client's fluid body it can ripple through the practitioner's fluid body and release.] Let me illustrate what I just said, that when the protoplasm recovers, it will be on the same curve. *The rhythm [Primary Respiration] has continued underneath, so to speak, even though the protoplasm has been asleep* [in a state of reparative stillness]. *There is still something going on. We must be very close indeed to the question, what is life?* [Or, what is Primary Respiration?] The theory applies no matter what anesthetic agent is used. With the dentist's laughing gas, nitrous oxide, we also get a quick stop. And in time, full recovery.

Anesthesia by electric shock is known, but never used on man. It is too dangerous. Electrical setup is a little complicated for we must know voltage and amperage. The electrodes are of platinum wire, which are now being put into position. Thirty volts are first administered, but the shock is insufficient. You see the electrodes coming into place, now the upper one, and now the shock. Sixty volts produce complete anesthesia with little injury. You will note that there's no streaming anywhere now in the picture. But there is no permanent damage. You get full recovery a few moments later. Let us see what a higher voltage will do. This isn't anesthesia. It's electrocution. [The slime mold was killed by the shock.]

I have done most [of my] work on toxicity, observing the effects of poisons. Here is what sulfur dioxide does to protoplasm. If anesthetic agents gelatinize protoplasm, stimulants [caffeine] should have the opposite effect, and so it proved. They liquefy protoplasm. The protoplasm here is literally pouring out into the surrounding medium, going into solution. All continuity and structure are lost and, of course, that means death. [Death by caffeine!]

Thetabromine is a close relative of caffeine, a stimulant, and it too disintegrates protoplasm. As before, the slime mold is going into solution in the surrounding water. So you have two pictures, on the one hand, anesthesia and solidification. [The fluid body of some clients feels like tissue when under stress] On the other hand, stimulation and liquefaction. As this curve depicts, normal protoplasm lies between the liquid and solid states. The solidification in anesthesia is not coagulation, for that would mean death. You cannot unclot blood, or as the chemists say, you can't unboil an egg. Anesthetized protoplasm gelatinizes and becomes quite firm. If the gelation goes too far, death by coagulation results. At the one end of the curve, we have liquefaction and at the other end of the curve, solidification, which in both cases can result in death. [The longitudinal fluctuation in the fluid body is greatly damaged from drugs, stress, and abuse. In addition the fluid body has multiple gradients of density in a human from liquid to gel, as Seifriz states. This is because of the sheer complexity of the nervous and vascular systems. With clients, practitioners are looking for a sense of buoyancy, lift, and floating of the tissue while the whole is breathing with Primary Respiration.]

In order to test the theory, I tried heroin and this was a surprise. I'd always thought morphine and heroin to be depressants and so I expected the protoplasm to gelate, to become firm. And when we saw this, we thought our theory would fail. Until we got hold of Goodman and Gillman, and read some five pages telling us that the opium derivatives are stimulants, not depressants. So the reaction we see here upheld my theory after all.

An extraordinarily interesting problem is the fusion of two droplets of protoplasm. Now egg and sperm readily fuse, while two amebas can crawl all over each other but they never fuse. Two drops of slime mold protoplasm frequently go together. But when and why they do and when and why they don't is a problem. Sometimes they go for each other in a big way, as you see here. And sometimes, there is merely a caress. They touch each other and retreat. But after all, their caress may lead to complete union and then the protoplasm fuses with absolute compatibility. *It's important that the direction of the flow in the two cases should be synchronized. One or the other must give way and until we have a wholly harmonious flowing together.* [Upon contact the practitioner withdraws attention from his or her hands and becomes receptive. This acknowledges that the two nervous and vascular systems are in a merged state and the practitioner must begin the process of differentiation from the client by focusing on his or her own body, which then resonates with the client and builds the client's capacity for self-regulation. I believe that both fluid bodies are also in a merged state and the practitioner by sensing his or her own fluid body processing with micro movement the fluid body of the client that this also enhances the self-regulation of the client.]

Frequently, two plasmodia will gaze at each other literally for hours on end, as those two did, and then finally cross at one point. Once they decide that they like each other, then the fusion is complete. Notice between these two you have a strip of no man's land, where fusion never occurs. It took quite a lot of thinking to understand why that should be true. But I believe there's a toxic substance secreted that fills in that space and they simply won't cross each other's toxic area. [As a joke in class, I like to say that this is a good instruction for marriage in general!]

We come now to one of the greatest problems in biology. What makes protoplasm flow? To say it is life is no answer. The biologist wants to know the physics and chemistry of protoplasmic streaming. I had an idea. Perhaps the outer layer of protoplasm pulsates and pumps the inner substance, just as does the human heart. Here is my proof. What you see is the same protoplasm, but now speeded up by time lapse photography. *The rhythmic period of the pulsation is, as one would expect, the same as that of the rhythmic flow [Primary Respiration]. Here's a primitive heart, one drop of protoplasm pulsating out, in, out, in.* [This shows that Primary Respiration is breathing three dimensionally around a central vertical axis. This axis is the longitudinal fluctuation of the fluid body and not a cellular structure.]

If our theory is a really good one, it should fit all cases. I therefore studied chaos, a giant ameba with many nuclei, and hunted for rhythmic pulsations. I speeded up the photography, but still no evidence of a rhythm. Rhythmic movement, but not rhythmic pulsation. At least we couldn't find it. The theory is an excellent one. But it isn't true. Mind you, the rhythm is there. *Rhythmical motion is a fundamental property of living matter, but is not the cause of the protoplasmic streaming. Both are the result of a rhythmic force that we have not yet discovered.* [Amebas have a primitive nervous system which can cause eccentric motion. A slime mold does not have a nervous system. Perhaps Primary Respiration is the cause of the streaming?]

Then around came Professor Kamiya [a researcher from Japan]. And he said, let's measure the horsepower of this living machine. I'll do it by applying pressure or suction just as one breaks-in an engine. He built a double-chambered box and put on each side of a central wall droplets of protoplasm connected by a fine living thread. When the flow of protoplasm was in one direction, Kamiya applied pressure and held it quiet. When the flow was in the opposite direction, suction was applied to stop it. The pressure applied is a measure of the vital force [Mid Tide]. Here he's holding the protoplasm quiet. [The pressure of the practitioner's hands can shut down the movement of the Mid Tide but not Primary Respiration. Primary Respiration will simply disappear from the practitioner's perception.] And then he would record the force necessary to do this. And here he lets it go. *And here we have the normal reversal* [of Primary Respiration, which keeps going even when the Mid Tide has stopped], showing that there's been no injury caused by the experiment. Now he holds it quiet again, and each time, applies the pressure or the suction necessary to hold it quiet.

From these measurements, Kamiya drew curves that depict the rhythmic flow of protoplasm. These curves, such as this one, Dr. Kamiya analyzed as a physicist would a curve in harmonics. I felt that biology had at last become an exact science. *Note, in this curve, the little irregularities at the top to the right [Primary Respiration changing directions]. Note that they always recur [every fifty seconds]. This led to a remarkable discovery: that there is not one rhythm in protoplasm, but many rhythms. Protoplasm is a polyrhythmic system.* [All rhythms are happening at the same time. It is up to the practitioner to synchronize with one or the other, especially Primary Respiration, as I said at the beginning.]

Later, in Japan, Dr. Kamiya measured the electrical force or potential of flowing protoplasm and found the same rhythm there as he had found when he measured pressure. In short, mechanical pressure and electrical pressure parallel each other. The meaning of this is far reaching, for just what it is, we have not yet found out. Though I have an idea and I shall tell you about it in a moment.

About this time, when biologists and chemists were thinking in terms of polymer chemistry, of macro molecules and long molecular fibers, my friends in Europe said the power driving this living machine is in the machine, not at the surface. It is the flowing molecules themselves, the long, accordion[-like] polypeptide chains that move the stream, or rather they are the stream. These folded molecules open and close and move forward like a caterpillar. If you can imagine seeing at a distance an army of caterpillars coming down the Champs d'Lysee, the procession would appear to flow. This is another beautiful theory, but I don't believe it. You can't open and close these molecules so easily.

I want to show you now the nervous activity that [frog] muscle fibers display, first shown to me by colleague Dr. Cookson. Notice the rhythmic procession of waves, which represent impulses radiating from nervous centers. These I like to call excitation foci. Remember too, that in a plasmodium, there is not one rhythm, but many rhythms such as [the one] you see here. I concluded that all forms of motion in protoplasm are the result of nervous impulses emanating from excitation foci. These rhythmic waves and muscle fibers are basically the same as those you saw in the protoplasm of a primitive slime mold. Synchronized with these visible waves are electrical impulses, which can be measured and recorded. Electrical impulses therefore are responsible for protoplasmic movement, for the contraction of muscle and the transmission of messages along nerve fibers.

This is my theory. And this is as near as we have gotten to a physical interpretation of life forces. [You cannot compare electrical stimulation of frog muscle in a chemical solution, as shown in the film, to a dynamic living organism such as a slime mold, which has no nervous system even though a human body is also composed of protoplasm. Biodynamic practice is an exploration of one of the life forces called Primary Respiration and of course many teachers have many interpretations of it including me!]

I've always been interested in the twists and spirals in living things. And so I thought protoplasm must have a twist in it. And I went in search of it, even though some of my friends say, pooh, another one of Seifriz's mystical rhythms. You know, Darcy Thompson, who was a great student of form and growth, studied spirals in animate nature with great care. I, like every biologist, have long wanted to meet Darcy Thompson, but the opportunity to do that did not come until later in life, and of all places, on the dance floor, at the city hall in Aberdeen, Scotland. Darcy Thompson, a fine old man, then 80 years of age, was there dancing with a lovely young lady, whom I suggest to be about 18 years of age. But the hour was late, past my bedtime, and I took the matter in hand and went onto the dance floor and simply interrupted. Darcy Thompson glared at me and said, "You can't have her." And I'm afraid I was rude, but I said "I don't want her." Then he asked, "What do you want?" And I replied, "I just want to meet Darcy Thompson." said he asked, "All right, who are you?" "Oh," I said, "that doesn't matter, you never heard of me." He said, "Well, who are you?" I said "I'm Seifriz." "Oh, yes," he said, "you're the fellow that thinks everything goes in spirals." And I said, "Well, you're an authority on growth, doesn't it?" He said, "Of course it does, but you thought you discovered something."

And now this is how we prove that protoplasm goes in spirals. We attached a tiny mirror to the end of a thread of living protoplasm and reflected a beam of light on to a circular scale. Dr. Kamiya did the experimental work with his usual brilliant ingenuity. One day he called me into his darkened room and all that I saw there was this spot of light traveling back and forth on this circular scale. [You can see a cycle of Primary Respiration on the circular scale even though the film was edited. This is important because the spiral is itself moving in the tempo of Primary Respiration not the Mid Tide. This is another visual display of Primary Respiration and an important therapeutic perception in clinical practice. It does not mean that perceiving spirals is the goal but rather one of numerous perceptions and possibilities when synchronized with the therapeutic activities of Primary Respiration.] But I knew what it meant. Protoplasm has a twist in it.

As the protoplasm flows up and down the living thread, the mirror on the end of the thread slowly turns and reflects the spot of light. And so we show that all life has a twist in it. [The spiral is the basic movement pattern of the fluid body and of the blood in the body.] I think that you will agree that protoplasm is a very remarkable substance. Often I talk about it as if it had intelligence and my colleagues raise their eyebrows. *I don't say it is intelligent, but it does often do the intelligent thing.* And after all, we are made of protoplasm. [I say it is an intelligence. The fluid body is a five-hundred-million-year-old intelligence. This is what exists just under the surface of the skin in ourselves and our clients.]

Summary for Biodynamic Practice

- Primary Respiration is seen changing directions at least ten times. Commentator says, "Note the reversal in a rhythmic period of fifty seconds."

- Primary Respiration is seen breathing three dimensionally, like a heart.

- The majority of the motion observed in the flow of the protoplasm between changing phases in the tempo of Primary Respiration is part of the Mid Tide and could specifically be called the fluid drive.

- The fluid body is seen several times accessing a state of stillness when placed under stress while Primary Respiration continues underneath.

- The fluid body is seen in a startle response that occurs before a shock takes place. "Note the nervous shock that occurs before…." This phenomenon is seen at least one more time in the film.

- The fluid body is described as having a range of different tempos, all occurring simultaneously. "We made the discovery that the protoplasm has a polyrhythmic harmony." All activity in the fluid body is occurring simultaneously.

- The reason the ameba shown in the movie does not have similar motion to that of the protoplasm is because an ameba has a primitive nervous system, which changes the vector of observed motion in the fluid body.

- The fluid body can repair itself while in a self-induced state of stillness. Primary Respiration does not stop, but keeps going on during the Stillness.

- When two fluid bodies meet, one must be receptive to complete the coming together. The fluid bodies must be "synchronized." "One or the other must give way for a fully harmonious coming together."

- The fluid body has different gradients of viscosity.

- A core movement of Primary Respiration in the fluid body is that of a spiral.

- From the point of view of biodynamic practice, Primary Respiration is the mind of the fluid body and likely the catalyst for its motion, rather than "excitation foci."

Postscript: While finishing the manuscript for this book a new piece of research on slime molds came out of Australia (Reida, Lattya, Dussutourc, and Beekman, 2012). It was discovered that slime molds have an external memory by sensing the trail of slime on the path left behind as they move. In this way a slime mold remembers not to retrace its steps, so to speak. The slime mold moves by expanding a network of pulsating tissues. It does not retrace its steps to someplace it has already been. What it interesting to me as a teacher of biodynamic craniosacral therapy is the comment by one of the authors of the study about the biokinetics of the organism and how it communicates internally: "The pulsating parts are also influenced by the throbbing of their neighbours within the cell (slime mold), which means that they can communicate with each other, to pass information through the organism about what is happening in the environment outside. The different speeds of contraction directly influence which direction the cell will then move in." To me this speaks of the conversation earlier in this book about metabolic fields and how a fluid body knows its wholeness as a quality of interconnected movement within itself. As Dr. Sutherland said, "every part knows the whole."

Time Stamps

1:23 The substance that gives life to all plants and animals …

2:26 The tensile strength of the living substance …

3:30 First turning of Primary Respiration observed

3:43 Should we …

4:17 Note particularly the reversal of flow with a rhythmic period of fifty seconds …

6:20 And to prove how tough an elastic protoplasm is …

6:52 The protoplasm meets contingencies and thus saves itself …

7:13 The patient slowly goes to sleep … [stillpoint]

7:56 There, you just saw the normal reversal …

8:21 Reversal observed again

8:25 The forces are more basic …

8:41 Nervous shock

9:07 Something is going on …

10:40 Full recovery a few moments later

11:20 Nervous shock

11:40 Death by caffeine

12:52 Solidification and liquefaction (gradients of density in the fluid body)

14:15 Fusion

15:10 It is important that the direction of flow be synchronized

16:06 I believe there is a toxic substance

16:25 Reversal

16:43 Pulsates and pumps

17:03 Primitive heart (midline)

17:20 Ameba (it has a primitive nervous system and thus eccentric movement overriding the deeper pulsation)

17:49 Both are the result of a force we have not yet discovered

18:23 Holding the fluid body still

18:33 The pressure applied is a measure of the vital force (observe the oscillation of the fluid body while it is being held)

18:54 And here we have the normal reversal

19:12 Curves on the graph depicting the 100-second cycle

19:29 Irregularities that recur (every 100 seconds)

21:47 Many rhythms such as you see here (the fluid body is a polyrhythmic harmonious system)

22:03 I concluded …

22:47 Torsion-chapter stop

24:20 And now this is how we prove that protoplasm goes in spirals

24:42 Three cycles

25:49 I don't say it's intelligent, but it does do the intelligent thing

SECTION II

...

Biodynamic Practice

CHAPTER 9

New Perspectives on the Therapeutic Relationship

A significant amount of research is pointing to a redefinition of the therapeutic relationship. Previously, terms such as transference, countertransference, and projection were part of the description of the interpersonal relationship between a client and a therapist. These terms have also been applied to manual therapy. With the advent of research on infant-mother attachment and prenatal development, a new understanding of the therapeutic relationship can be observed. There are six aspects that I would like to outline in this chapter for the reader to understand the new therapeutic relationship. Some of this will be a review that I have covered in previous volumes. I am attempting to simplify the information, something that my students ask me to do all the time.

First, the term *interpersonal central nervous system* refers to the merged state of two nervous systems, specifically those of the mother and her newborn baby. Each nervous system is mirroring the other and the infant is trying to learn to connect its higher centers for optimal functioning in life at this early time. It has been suggested by one researcher that this dynamic is actually a two-person biology and the rules of this interpersonal central nervous system can be applied throughout the lifespan to any therapeutic relationship or any relationship in general.

The actual process occurring at the root of the interpersonal central nervous system is called *attunement.* Attunement specifically refers to the way in which a practitioner moves his or her attention toward a client, which is sympathetically motivated, and moves attention away from a client, which is parasympathetically motivated. It is very important to understand that normal attunement occurs at a very slow tempo.

Along with attunement, the next important understanding is that of *resonance.* Resonance is what occurs once the therapist recognizes that he or she is involved in a two-person biology. This information usually comes from a heightened awareness of your sensory processes in his or her body. Once this recognition takes place, the therapist creates a resonant field by distinguishing his or her own sensations simply by paying more attention to his or her body, rather than that of the client. With attunement, the attention will ultimately pendulate or swing back to the client. That is the beauty of attunement: it swings back and forth between client and practitioner.

The second term in the new therapeutic relationship is called *interpersonal cardiovascular system*. New research has indicated that when the therapist is paying attention to his or her body, a significant portion of that attention should be on the movement and activity of the heart inside the trunk. I like to call it taking your own pulse without using your hands. This is called *interoception* or *interoceptive awareness* or *cardioception*. All those terms mean the same thing. It is simply paying conscious attention to the movement and activity of one's own heart. Such interoception has been shown to change the brain structure, called the insula, that helps to down-regulate fear.

The interpersonal cardiovascular system is also based on the discovery of mirror neurons in the brain and heart. These neurons create a "mirror" image and sensation of the client or whoever one might be in relationship with at any given time. Mirror neurons are responsible for generating empathy, which is the capacity to feel what another person is feeling. To deepen into the resonance of empathy, the therapist simply pays more attention to the movement and activity of his or her heart and the pumping of blood through the body. This type of attention enhances empathy into a compassionate response. Compassion, in this case, is the right knowing of when to move the hands in a therapeutic bodywork session.

The third aspect of the new therapeutic relationship is called *intersubjectivity*. Intersubjectivity is a function of the brain that monitors present time in every given situation and especially the therapeutic relationship. The reason this is important is because focusing on present time can actually change memories of the past for the positive. In addition, intersubjectivity over time generates a feeling of being felt by the other person. This is a deeply intimate state in which the client knows the other is perceiving him or her, and vice versa. This type of intimacy builds safety and trust in the therapeutic relationship. It begins to help regulate fear, which is frequently present in the contemporary client. Thus intersubjectivity is linked to the reduction of fear. It must also be remembered that a lot of research is being done on mindfulness-based meditation practices. Mindfulness is simply the ability to pay attention in the present moment, usually by concentrating on one's breathing, for example. I think it is important to restate that staying in present time changes the past and reduces fear. This is significant in the therapeutic relationship.

The fourth aspect of the therapeutic relationship has to do with what I call interconnected nature or *green time.* This is a unique aspect of the therapeutic relationship in biodynamic craniosacral therapy. Research has indicated that only five minutes of time focusing on the natural world will generate more empathy and compassion. How does one accomplish that sitting in a treatment room with one's hands on a client? This is done by the practitioner periodically moving his or her attention out the window and, if there is no window, to imagine that attention being outside in nature, looking at the trees, the clouds, or the sky. All this contributes to the generation of empathy and compassion and helps to remove the guesswork from knowing when and where to move with the client during a session. It requires that the therapist spends more time with his or her own perception during treatment. That means spending more time sensing one's own body before sensing the client's body.

The fifth aspect of the new therapeutic relationship is what is called *process versus state-bound therapy.* The world of Western therapy revolves around what is called state-bound practice or therapy. The client comes in with a specific state or expression of symptoms. The goal is to simply remove this state from the client with the intention that this will make the person feel better. Sometimes it does, and sometimes it does not. Process-oriented therapy is an exploration of the shape and sensibility of the living experience and context within which a client is having a physical experience. It is much more multidimensional than state-bound practice and can be as simple as making a dietary change to feeling an emotion that has been blocked for some time.

The sixth aspect of the new therapeutic relationship is what I call *inherent not knowing.* It is not possible to know what the client is really holding in terms of the presentation of a symptom complex. So, first of all, the therapist has to be willing to let go of any sense of knowing about the client's inner dilemma. This means that the therapist is going to make mistakes or be forgetful or get spaced out or feel completely incompetent occasionally in a session. This is normal practice unless it is an avoidance pattern and only the therapist can know that context within himself or herself. One researcher said that sloppiness was an important part of the therapeutic relationship. That means that whenever the therapist knows he or she has made a mistake, he or she is willing to readily admit it to the client. Even if I am not sure if I've made a mistake, I always say something like, "I am so sorry you are having to go through this experience."

There are several specific applications in the practice of biodynamic craniosacral therapy that are important implications from the above information. The first is to stay related to Primary Respiration and stillness. The second is to cycle one's attunement and attention through the zones from one's own body out to the natural world and back until time dilates. The third is to take the pulse of the client's fluid body at the beginning of a session and at the end. One would expect the fluid body to be breathing slower at the end of a session. It is vitally important for the practitioner to practice scanning his or her own body from head to foot and teaching the client to do that. It is also important to solicit the client's comfort whenever there is a signal from the client such as fidgeting, deep breathing, skin color changes, and tearing up in the eyes. I simply say, "How ya doin'?" Then I shift the client to his or her side if there is fidgeting or discomfort. I also like to work heart to heart with Primary Respiration, whether my hands are on or off the client's body.

Finally, I would like to say that all of this is about each person learning how to self-regulate, making a commitment to one's own self-care, and deepening into a spiritual practice as much as possible.

CHAPTER 10

The Body Scan

This series of instructions is designed to help the client participate in the session with the practitioner. I typically will do a body scan with clients at the beginning of a session and encourage them to practice the body scan on their own. At the end of a session, I might ask clients if they notice any difference in their body from the beginning. This perception of wholeness is done mindfully; that is, with conscious and nonjudgmental attention in present time. The neurological benefits over time can reduce stress and anxiety.

The body scan then has two purposes. The first is to rehabilitate a client's sense of bodily wholeness via the central nervous system. The second intention is to use the body scan as a mindfulness practice. I would like to remind all practitioners to practice the body scan themselves along with giving the client instructions.

1. Before a session begins, inform the client that you will guide him or her for several minutes through a relaxation body scan. You can also let the client know in advance that you will be directing his or her attention to discrete areas of the body as a way of settling the nervous system.

2. Once the client has gotten on the table in supine position, ask the client to take a deep breath slowly and, with the exhale, to allow his or her body to settle on the table.

3. Now you can begin to direct the client's attention. I would like to remind all the practitioners reading this that you are supposed to do the body scan along with the client. This means that, as you give an instruction to the client, you will need to pause and do the same practice with your own body.

   I like to start by saying, "Bring your attention to … without judging whether you can sense that area or not."

   Here is a list of areas of the body to name, starting at the feet and working toward the top of the head:

   - The feet
   - The legs

- The pelvis
- The abdomen
- The back
- The shoulders and ribcage
- The arms
- The head and neck
- The face

Remember to pause after each location and take a breath before naming the next location.

4. Finish by saying, "Now sense your body from the bottom of your feet, to the top of your head, both the front and the back." Allow for a silent pause.

5. Proceed with the next phase of the session by saying, "Are you ready for me to make contact?"

I like to take about three minutes for this body scan at the beginning of each session. Another reason why the body scan is important is that clients will often sit up at the end of a session and ask the practitioner what he or she sensed in their body. It is important for the practitioner to refer clients back to their own body. This can be done by saying, "Let's do a brief body scan and check in with your own body from head to foot." Pause. "Now compare this body scan with the one you did at the beginning of the session and tell me if you notice any differences." In this way, you can slow down clients' need to be cognitive and have them analyze their own sensory experience during the whole session. This could lead to other questions such as, "I wonder if you noticed any changes in your body during the session." I find that it is important to be creative with the body scan and the solicitation of sensory information from the client. Even though the body scan has an element of being a protocol, it can be applied very creatively each time it is done.

The main evolution of the body scan is to ask the client more than once to breathe into the area of the body you are naming. So perhaps the second or third time I see a client, I might use four areas of their body in which I ask them to take a breath and, as they exhale, relax. This adds another sensory input to creating a container of wholeness that is a safe and reliable resource for the client.

CHAPTER 11

Synchronizing Primary and Secondary Respiration

I consider synchronizing Primary Respiration and secondary respiration a critical component of biodynamic practice. The inside presence of Primary Respiration must be regularly established and synchronized, not only in clinical practice, but during one's day-to-day experience. It begins with mindfulness of breathing. This is extended out to the whole volume of the body as it is bounded by the surface of the skin. Gradually, the practitioner synchronizes with Primary Respiration as it moves from its fulcrum around the pericardium in the body. This particular fulcrum is specifically related to not only the heart, but the heart's relationship with the respiratory diaphragm.

I have found in almost forty years of clinical practice that the majority of clients and students do not know how to breathe. That may sound like an absurd statement, but it is a biological reality. It means that stress and trauma are imprinted on the diaphragm. Even prenatal stress can imprint on the oxygen receptors in the brain, which results in restrictions in the movement of the diaphragm in breathing. One way to resolve these problems is to notice how Primary Respiration and secondary respiration are actually one thing operating at different tempos. The other most apparent breathing dynamic is that Primary Respiration actually controls or is in charge of secondary respiration. This is purely experiential and a subjective experience of the living reality of Primary and secondary Respiration. I have spent many years doing and developing the practice below. It has brought me and my students and clients a great deal of relief.

1. Sit up like you are going to do a cranial session.

   Sense or see your skin from the bottom of your feet to the top of your head.

   Sense the activity of your respiratory diaphragm.

2. As you finish inhaling, move some attention to the surface of your skin to see if Primary Respiration continues inhaling even though your diaphragm has begun to exhale.

Or, as you finish exhaling, move some attention to your skin to see if Primary Respiration continues exhaling, even though your diaphragm has begun to inhale.

3. Practice synchronizing Primary Respiration and secondary respiration until you notice the need to take a deep breath.

Take the deep breath and notice if the amplitude of Primary Respiration has increased.

Once you are familiar with this synchronization process, you can continue to build potency during the inhalation cycle by subtly increasing the inhalation of air.

Likewise, you can continue to build potency on the exhalation cycle of Primary Respiration by subtly increasing the exhalation of air.

Stay relaxed, stay three dimensional, and do not hold your breath.

Learn how to toggle your attention very gently from the circumference of your respiratory diaphragm to the total surface volume of your skin.

Allow the skin to be very porous and, when possible, imagine both Primary Respiration and secondary respiration synchronizing zones A and B together.

It is important to be very gentle with one's self and with the client when practicing or teaching this synchronization process. The practitioner must be able to notice if his or her heart rate increases and how to lower the heart rate. If the practitioner is going to teach this process to the client, then I recommend the first protocol on palpating the core in Chapter 7. Working with the breath can be very rewarding and must be done extremely slowly. Breathing is the oldest known function in the entire biological development of our body. It is said to be at least 500 million years old. So learn to treat the breath as an old friend.

CHAPTER 12

Buoyancy Meditation

This chapter is about counteracting the effects of gravity in the human body. Some biologists feel that gravity does not have a significant influence on the human embryo. Thus the embryo has an imprint of being buoyant or capable of floating while connected and routed through to the womb. In order to contact the fluid body, one needs to develop a sense of buoyancy. This begins by allowing the skin to become very porous and open, as suggested in Chapter 14. Buoyancy is also associated with spontaneous micromovement originating from the pelvic floor and moving the inner contents of the core, upper extremities, and head and neck like seaweed in slow motion. The meditation that follows begins to develop that sensibility.

One of the reasons that this is crucial in biodynamic practice is that the stress and trauma held in a client dissipates in the practitioner's body via the nervous system, cardiovascular system, and fluid body. When a practitioner is actively sensing his or her three-dimensional buoyancy and then makes contact with the client, the practitioner can sense the effect of held stress in the client's fluid body dissipating in the practitioner's fluid body. Such a level of buoyancy awareness also acts like a dousing rod. By this I mean that as the client's stress dissipates into my fluid body, my whole fluid body is pulled in the direction of the imprint in the client. The following meditation will help you develop an additional skill in relating more deeply to decompressing the client's fluid body.

1. Find the three-dimensional surface shape of your body and rest there.

2. Imagine that your respiratory diaphragm creates waves. One wave goes toward the top of your head and another wave goes toward your feet. They both are initiated at the same time.

3. Sense the weightedness of your body as it is affected by gravity. Sense the density of your body and begin to de-densify starting at the skin. Imagine the skin and the multiple layers of tissue underneath being very porous and fluid filled. The image is that of a tubular sea sponge.

4. Place some of your attention in the core of your body and sense micromovement as if a cork bobbing in water. The micromovement will be uplifting, generating a sense of floating, and may have different currents within it moving from bottom to top.

5. Sense the tide of Primary Respiration moving from inside to outside of the body and then moving from outside to inside of the body. The fulcrum for the movement can be around the respiratory diaphragm and heart.

6. Sense the ocean of stillness in zone C. Allow the tide to direct your attention in any of the zones.

Orienting to one's buoyancy and synchronizing with the spontaneous micromovement contained in the buoyancy is yet another tool in the biodynamic practitioner's medicine bag. Remember that the biodynamic process discussed in Volumes Three and Four begins with orienting and synchronizing. Buoyancy practice is an additional skill of orienting, synchronizing, and attuning with the client at the level of the fluid body. The practitioner needs different skills and competencies, which are all based on Primary Respiration for the most compassionate action.

CHAPTER 13

Transparent Heart Practice

This chapter is a sequence of instructions regarding a larger sense of buoyancy called transparency. At its deepest level, it involves connecting with the transparency of the heart, which I provide instructions for below. Buoyancy, as covered in the preceding chapter, is the lived experience of having a fluid body. Buoyancy is defined as the power to lift an object in water. Once the practitioner has a three-dimensional sense of the shape of his or her body and begins a practice of de-densifying the skin and musculoskeletal system, the power to lift and the internal micromovement of the fluid body become recognizable inside one's body. So the starting point of transparency practice is the de-densification of the practitioner's body in order to access the lift and micromovement or potency associated with the inherent activity of the fluid body. The lift and micromovement are associated with traditional terms such as longitudinal and lateral fluctuations, but those are cumbersome terms. What I am attempting is to form a language describing the actual experience of the fluid body as it lives inside the practitioner.

The Practitioner's Transparency

This practice starts by synchronizing with Primary Respiration and leads to it being able to move through a transparent body, especially the trunk and hands. I will go into more detail about transparent hands in the next chapter, on zone B. As always the first part relates to the practitioner's sensibility. This is accomplished by placing general attention on the back surface of the practitioner's body, from the occiput down to the sacrum and as lateral as the scapula at the shoulders, the floating ribs at the bottom of the rib cage, and the crest of the ilia at the hips. Then I concentrate on the spinal cord, brain stem, and cerebellum to sense Primary Respiration out the back of my body.

The back of the body, especially the spinal cord, is used as a type of antenna or receiver for Primary Respiration going and coming from the horizon and intersecting with the trunk of the body. It is important to spend time this way because Primary Respiration has two essential components. The first is its movement, which is generally described as being 100-second cycles or two 50-second phases. The second component of Primary Respiration is its spatial organization—the movement and activity of wholeness. Thus its perception starts with a two-dimensional orientation out the front of the body, as is typical when first learning how to recognize it. Gradually, the practitioner needs to build more three dimensionality in his or her perception. It seems that the biggest blind spot in human perception, so to speak, is sensing the natural world from the back of the body. (This was covered in detail in Volume 4.)

When Primary Respiration changes phases, I sense it moving from the horizon in front of the trunk of my body, once again through the body, to the horizon in back of my body. This takes some time to practice and it is important to develop a sense of porousness and openness in the skin and layers of the body. It is like living air moving through the body and thus is good to practice outside in nature.

Once the practitioner synchronizes with Primary Respiration with a transparent body inside the office or house, I highly recommend practicing out in nature when not in the office. I like to sit on the beach and do this practice since there is a very clear horizon in front of me. There is an extra added element of the air moving and the wind changing directions as it brushes up against my skin and swirls around my body almost like an embrace. Primary Respiration is related to the wind and on a regular basis the wind will also shift as Primary Respiration changes phases because the air movement comes from Primary Respiration as does breathing in the body. While synchronizing my perception of Primary Respiration with the wind, I gradually allow my body to become transparent and, once again, feel the wind blow through the body very gently, as if the pores of my skin were simply a big fish net. This took me several years to experience this, so do not give up hope if it does not happen immediately. It is as if one must learn the language of nature, with Primary Respiration as the translator.

Dorsal Pericardium

Once the practitioner has built in this transparent spatial dimension of Primary Respiration, then some attention is placed on the dorsal pericardium in back of the heart. The dorsal pericardium is a structure that is continuous from the cervical spine all the way down to the lumbar spine via the fascia. In this way, the practitioner builds in a greater spatial dimension of Primary Respiration and allows the heart and vascular system to be permeated by Primary Respiration out the front of the body and returning through the front. It leads to the experience of a transparent heart, which leads to an experience of happiness. Sensing Primary Respiration via the dorsal pericardium not only stabilizes the cardiovascular components of the autonomic nervous system, but also allows for a more direct empathetic connection with the client and anyone else around. I frequently practice this at airports, on airplanes, walking down the street, in bed thinking about the planet and especially my wife Cathy lying next to me. Dorsal pericardium practice is an essential component of building compassion in biodynamic practice because it is the experience of a heart-to-heart connection with Primary Respiration.

Once the practitioner can sustain a sensibility of Primary Respiration coming and going from the dorsal pericardium out the front of the body in relationship with the client's heart and vascular system, then the boundary between the back of the body and dorsal pericardium is gradually de-densified. The intention is to experience Primary Respiration moving through the dorsal pericardium and back of the body like a breeze blowing through the trees and then returning and blowing back in the opposite direction—subtly, of course, as mentioned above. This now is the completion of the first part of transparency practice with the practitioner's heart and back.

Heart Presence of Primary Respiration and Stillness

The next component of transparency practice is to sense Primary Respiration breathing from the inside of the heart through the entire vascular system on its expansion phase. The practitioner imagines a placenta covering the outside surface of zone B. In this way, the veins and arteries coming from the wall of the chorion (inside surface of zone B) are allowed to connect with the body's vascular system with the aid of Primary Respiration at the surface of the skin (of zone A). When Primary Respiration changes directions in the vascular system, it moves from the periphery of the body and extremities toward the heart. Students ask if there is a problem with the blood moving in the opposite direction or at a faster rate than Primary Respiration. This is no problem as Primary Respiration moves in the blood at its own pace regardless of the direction of blood flow at any given time. This takes time to sense the inside presence of Primary Respiration in the cardiovascular system and is important to balance the work of sensing the outside presence of Primary Respiration with the dorsal pericardium. It happens naturally as experience is gained in the practice.

A deep stillness will take over the room and when Primary Respiration returns into the awareness of the practitioner, the fulcrum of its perception will likely shift to the inside presence of Primary Respiration in the heart and vascular system. Another type of stillness occurs in which it feels like the heart has actually disappeared. The space inside the trunk between the lungs is dark and empty. This is actually a stillpoint in the heart. The center of the heart is a source of biological stillness in embryonic development because of all the twisting and turning that the heart tube must do to become a four-chambered organ. Thus it is dynamically still throughout the lifespan. One osteopath calls this type of stillness a neutral. This is because when the stillness returns to the background and Primary Respiration returns to the foreground of the practitioner's perception, the spatial organization and potency of Primary Respiration will be qualitatively different than before the stillness/neutral occurred. Accessing Primary Respiration with transparent heart practice leads to the experience of a larger-than-heart experience of Dynamic Stillness in the middle of the core of the body. If the practitioner can recognize this state and rest in it, the integration of wholeness and healing is greatly enhanced.

Conclusion

This level of transparency practice can be done in every hand position. It is especially recommended for the cardiovascular work detailed in Chapter 5. As I said earlier, I recommend starting with hand positions that do not have the weight of the client's body pressing into the practitioner's palms. Gradually, the practitioner can allow the weight of the client's body to be in the hands and to then imagine that the table is transparent, which takes practice. Please take time to read and practice the exercises in the following chapter for details on developing transparent hands. As a reminder, a macrocycle of attunement needs to be practiced regularly. This means that the practitioner periodically allows his or her attention to go out to the horizon and back, thus increasing the spatial dimensions of Primary Respiration into a greater wholeness. This avoids overfocusing on one's hands and creating reactions and side effects. The work of buoyancy and transparency emerges into one whole that extends out to the horizon.

Transparency practice is another meditation on wholeness and letting go of the musculoskeletal system. The fluid body becomes more free to respond to the potency of Primary Respiration. One possible side effect is that students sometimes experience fear or anxiety. This again is related to imprints held in the musculoskeletal system. It is important that this practice not generate fear and anxiety, but rather a sense of openness and well-being. Any time fear or anxiety comes up in biodynamic practice, the practitioner must ground himself or herself in being mindful of breathing and grounding through the feet, the pulsation of the heart, and so forth. The experience of Primary Respiration and stillness does not involve fear. Ultimately, it is the heart that becomes transparent, which sustains a deeper connection to the client and everyone around us.

Earlier, I mentioned that Primary Respiration has two components: its movement and its spatial dimensions. I believe it has a third component: a timeless quality associated with love, empathy, compassion, wholeness, joy, happiness, and bliss (for starters). When I look into the metaphors of the body being an embryo, a fluid body, and a heart, this is what I begin to feel with the above practices. I have experienced these qualities of Primary Respiration and its relationship with stillness and I know they exist as a living reality in my body and in the client. It is the preexisting condition. Buoyancy practice and transparency practice lead to a heart of joy. Biodynamic practice transforms into a protocol for embodied compassion.

CHAPTER 14

Working with Zone B

In this chapter I discuss several different aspects of zone B. I started this discussion in Chapter 5 of Volume Four, on the zones of perception. The reader might recall that zone B is the space immediately around the body extending 15–20 inches off of the skin. It must be remembered that zones A and B are an integrated whole and the osteopathic literature on the cranial concept alludes to this, especially in the discussion of the longitudinal fluctuation, as seen in Figure 14.1. This image shows what Dr. Sutherland called the direct current, now known as the longitudinal fluctuation, traveling from the coccyx to the third ventricle. This is a type of central channel in the fluid body that is not associated with the subdural space directly. The subdural space which houses the fluctuation of cerebrospinal fluid is a step down from the slower longitudinal fluctuation.

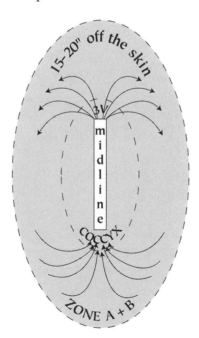

Figure 14.1. The longitudinal fluctuation cascading into zone B
and recoalescing at the coccyx.

When the longitudinal fluctuation, at the end of its 10–15-second phase, intersects with the third ventricle, it cascades like a fountain out into zone B. During this phase of 10–15 seconds, the longitudinal fluctuation recoalesces at the coccyx. Thus the cascading out into zone B and recoalescing at the coccyx takes place in zone B. Some practitioners feel that the mechanism of transport for this cascading effect of longitudinal fluctuation takes place in the electromagnetic field. I consider this a metaphor and note that different practitioners describe the sensation differently. The point is that if one phase of the longitudinal fluctuation takes part in zone A inside the fluid body and another phase takes part in zone B, then zones A and B are an integrated whole continuum. This is the sensibility I point to in Chapters 10, 11, 12, and 13. It is this sensibility that allows the practitioner to practice with a maximum degree of safety. This is because zone B is also associated with the fear center of the brain, the amygdala. Research has demonstrated that the amygdala is monitoring zone B or what researchers call the peripheripheral space. The more a practitioner rests in the awareness of the continuity of zones A and B, the better the clinical results will be.

Another aspect of the longitudinal fluctuation can be seen in Figure 14.2. The longitudinal fluctuation has a phase from the coccyx to the third ventricle extending longitudinally out into zone B and then a phase of return directly

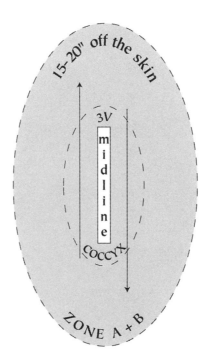

Figure 14.2. The longitudinal fluctuation moving
between the coccyx and third ventricle.

back down from the third ventricle to the coccyx. Many students ask me how this is so, since I just described in the previous paragraphs a different pathway. My answer may seem simplistic, but the biodynamic fluid body is a nonlinear system operating at many different levels. I no longer question the experience I'm having under my hands or in my body. Perhaps I should say I am no longer confused by my experience in the treatment room. I remember one of my teachers in graduate school saying that the therapist has to learn to treat strangeness with respect. Of course, Dr. Sutherland said the therapist needed to have reverence. I always let Primary Respiration and stillness figure out the paradoxes that I am presented with in clinical practice. My job is to simply notice the paradox and hold it in a larger container out to zone D and back.

Another effect of the longitudinal fluctuation is called the lateral fluctuation, as seen in Figure 14.3. The lateral fluctuation is a reciprocal wave that moves perpendicular to the longitudinal fluctuation or the so-called midline of the fluid body. It has two distinct perceptions. One is a figure eight and the other is a horizontal vector, as shown. These lateral fluctuations are used as an assessment tool in biodynamic practice. This is because if the lateral fluctuations are moving at a faster tempo than the longitudinal fluctuation, this can be an indication of traumatic stress being held in the longitudinal fluctuation. The practitioner

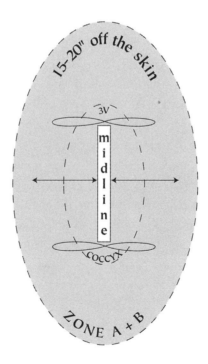

Figure 14.3. The lateral fluctuations.

must remember that the longitudinal fluctuation was called the direct current by Dr. Sutherland because he felt it was the core of the life force.

The longitudinal fluctuation, as I have talked about in my previous volumes, is absent or missing in many clients. The rehabilitation of the longitudinal and lateral fluctuations in the fluid body come about through the practitioner's awareness of his or her own zone B and the honoring and awareness of that space around the client. I find in my clinical practice that it is important to sense that interface. I tend to concentrate my attention periodically right in front of my chest where my zone B meets that of the client and it is that meeting point that is dynamically still. This is an important stillpoint to recognize in clinical practice. Furthermore, in order to ignite zone B in myself, I tend to practice chi kung or practice Kegel exercises, even when working with a client. I periodically tense the muscles of my pelvic floor as if holding back from urinating. I then relax the pelvic floor after several seconds and wait for one phase of the longitudinal fluctuation to manifest in the core of my fluid body or in zone B around me. I repeat this process several times, especially if I am making contact with the coccyx and sacrum of the client. The principle of practice is for the practitioner to ignite his or her own longitudinal fluctuation first and see if this resonates with the client.

How does the potency of the longitudinal fluctuation, once it gets ignited, move through the body? This occurs through the function of the reciprocal tension potency (RTP), as seen in Figure 14.4. The RTP has a rate of one cycle per minute. This means each phase is thirty seconds in length. It allows the life force of the longitudinal fluctuation to permeate every cell in the body. It also contributes to the felt sense of safety in the space around the body. It allows one to feel whole as a living reality. A typical biodynamic practice to sense the RTP is the scapular EV4, found in my Volume Four. The practitioner places his or her hands bilaterally under the scapulas of the client. Then the practitioner places attention on his or her own zone B and waits for the RTP to push into the hands. The timing is pretty straightforward at thirty seconds and the RTP can also stillpoint at the end of its expansion phase (and its contraction phase). The contemporary client will benefit much more from a stillpoint occurring at the end of the expansion phase because this allows the life force to thoroughly permeate the whole body and interact with every cell.

Working zone B to zone B as described above can also allow access to pre-conception imprints in the client and their possible resolution. This is because the practitioner can visualize himself or herself being an egg. The human female egg that we all came from also has a zone B, the corona radiata. In this way, visualizing the small feeder cells surrounding the egg as well as the egg itself places

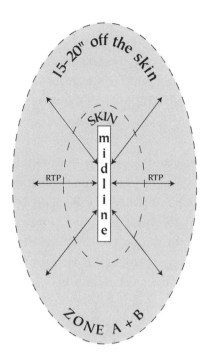

Figure 14.4. The reciprocal tension potency (RTP).

the practitioner at a time before conception. By applying this image to the client and working within the interchange of Primary Respiration and stillness, a much deeper resolution of pre-conception imprinting can take place. This, of course, is very refined work and a deeper promise that Primary Respiration makes to us. But the contemporary client has a compressed fluid body. Instead of zone A and B being a unified continuous buoyant drop of water, the vitality of the fluid body in zone B has been drained out, leaving the fluid body locked under the skin of the physical body. The practitioner needs to help the client open the window at the level of the skin and homogenize zone A with zone B.

Opening the Door of the Fluid Body

Here is a practice I use personally and with clients. It involves working with buoyancy and transparency, described in the previous chapters. At this level of understanding, transparency practice involves the practitioner shifting attention from his or her dorsal pericardium to the hands on the client. I like to call this practice Opening the Door of the Fluid Body. Initially begin the practice with the hands palm down on two locations on the client rather than beginning palm up with the weight of the client's body in the hands. I like to use a modified pietà position in which one hand is palm down around the top of the client's upper arm-shoulder area and my other hand is palm down somewhere around the knee. The practitioner is sensing the body of the client under the palms of his or her hands first. Then the practitioner shifts his or her attention to the back of the hands, sensing the fluid body in whatever way possible above the backs of the hands—the client's zone B. It is as if there are waves, currents, bioelectric phenomena, magnetic impressions, and so forth moving along the back of the practitioner's hands.

Once the practitioner can begin to sense this activity of the client's fluid body in zone B with the backs of the hands, another shift is made to the palms of the hands. Now the practitioner senses the fluid body of the client as if the hands were transparent. I recommend going from front to back of the hands several times in the tempo of Primary Respiration until the hands feel like they disappear, which means they are under water in the middle of the client's fluid body. Gradually this allows the client's fluid body to homogenize. This means that the barrier between zones A and B, where the hands are located, dissolves. The hands of the practitioner now allow Primary Respiration to flow through. It is as if the practitioner has placed his or her hands inside an envelope surrounded by water, which becomes transparent to Primary Respiration. It is important that attunement is practiced in such a way that there is not excessive concentration on the hands, but on a three-dimensional wholeness in zones A and B.

Working Zone B to Zone B

Now the practitioner again shifts attention to the transparency of the dorsal pericardium to sense Primary Respiration homogenizing the practitioner's zone A and B. I call this shifting of attention back and forth between the practitioner's dorsal pericardium and his or her hands a microcycle of attunement. This means the practitioner starts with his or her own transparency between the dorsal pericardium and back of the body. Then the practitioner shifts to the space above and below the hands while regarding the client's fluid body being homogenized as one continuum. The practitioner switches back and forth from the palm to the back of the hand in the tempo of Primary Respiration in order to open the window that has been closed in the client's fluid body between zones A and B. Then the practitioner shifts attention back to the dorsal pericardium and back of the body until a sensibility of complete transparency and homogenization with his or her own and the client's fluid body has occurred.

My sense is that the hands and dorsal pericardium become synchronized without the need to keep shifting attention. It automatically shifts and becomes evenly suspended between the hands and dorsal pericardium without needing to think about it. Then the practitioner is working zone B to zone B. Another metaphor I like is that the fluid body of zone A+B is the water. The stillness that manifests during this practice fills the office and extends out to the horizon. Then the tide of Primary Respiration is free to move and continually regenerate the client's fluid body. Water, plus the ocean plus the tide, as a living experience is biodynamic practice.

When working this way, the practitioner can access much deeper levels of stillness. The central stillness in the third ventricle will gradually extend down and through the heart. This deep inner stillness restores the whole biology of the human body. Then, when Primary Respiration returns into the perception of the practitioner, the heart is free to shift to a state of joy and happiness as fear is reduced.

Zone practice now has three levels associated with it that I cover in my books. The basic unit of work in a biodynamic practice is the cycle of attunement, covered in Volume 4. This is a practice of attuning with nature via Primary Respiration out to the horizon (zone D) and back until stillness fills zone C. This builds the container for transformation and change. In this Chapter I have taken the reader on a tour of homogenizing zone A and B which is critical for the contemporary client especially children. This I like to call a microcycle of attunement. Once the larger container of wholeness is established, then the practitioner attends to his or her own zone B and that of the client. This is covered in detail in Volume Four. Now the progression of zone practice deepens into unifying or homogenizing zones A and B together, described in this chapter.

Finally, Chapters 4, 5, 12, and 13 in this volume deal with zone A and working biokinetically. I call this phase of zone practice synchronizing with Primary Respiration and stillness in the cardiovascular system. This can only be done after attuning to nature and homogenizing zones A and B have taken place in the biodynamic therapeutic process. This is because biokinetic work when absent of awareness in all the zones can easily become mechanical and lock up the fluid body even more. These three levels of zone practice—attuning, homogenizing, and synchronizing—form the core perceptual skills of biodynamic craniosacral therapy. In my experience, each level takes time to develop competency to move through seamlessly in the therapeutic relationship. It is like opening and closing the aperture on a camera. The available light determines the diameter of the opening and, just so, the instinct of the practitioner will determine the right distance and zone to be aware of. The beauty of this practice is that it is under the guidance of Primary Respiration and stillness. Synchronize attention with them and they will lead you to the right zone at the right time.

CHAPTER 15

The Breath That Breathes Us

by Carol Agneessens, MS

Listen—Are you breathing just a little and calling it a life?
Mary Oliver

Breathing—life's most vital function. Countless writings and techniques, from ancient Sanskrit texts and yogic practices to innovative wholistic therapies and medical interventions are devoted to the cultivation, understanding, and repair of respiratory physiology. Every physical, psychological, and emotional problem is to some degree connected to a lack of oxygen and the interruption of full breathing cycles. Yet how many individuals pay attention to their personal respiratory habits? Or notice how respiratory health affects the depth and fullness of their breath and life? What happens to the breathing cycle when stressful events occur?

Too often breathing is taken for granted. Mistakenly, we assume that this function will always be working. Developing a kinesthetic awareness of breath broadens and expands our conscious participation in living. To breathe is to live, and respiratory freedom is a measure of life's potency. Maternal waves of breath transport the growing embryo from its miniscule genesis at fertilization through the birthing process. The first inhalation ignites a continuum of breaths; the last exhalation dissolves individuality into the eternal mystery at life's end.

At one time or another, you've probably experienced the sudden and shocking realization that you've been holding your breath during a stressful encounter, high-action thriller, or while waiting or anticipating news. Once you feel you haven't been breathing, do you ravenously grab for oxygen? How many notes have decorated your desktop, refrigerator, bathroom mirror, or the dashboard of your car reminding you to *breathe*? Recall the clients who describe their breathing as shallow or those who experience limited sensory awareness of the movement of their diaphragm and rib cage. With patience and guided kinesthetic directives, they may quickly begin experiencing greater excursion of their ribs and the impact that easier and fuller breathing has in their lives. Through anatomical precision and directed touch, practitioners ignite clients' felt sense of the expanding dimensions of their thorax, the depth and reach of their lungs, and the ease beneath their exhalation. We may work with athletes or singers whose beliefs about how to breathe actually complicate their quest for a fuller inhalation and passive exhalation. Or perhaps it is the child, teenager, or adult whose nervous system and breathing patterns carry the fight/flight/freeze imprint of birth trauma or the hypervigilant attitude of an early home environment lacking predictability and safety.

The respiratory control center in the brain stem demands oxygen, and thus respiration is triggered. However, bracing, slumping, accidents, injury, faulty education, or longstanding beliefs can undermine the ongoing and involuntary nature of breathing. As a longtime swimmer, I used to think that getting to the end of a 25-meter lap on one inhalation was success. I had no idea the goal was to breathe while swimming and that breathing rhythmically would increase both endurance and speed. Abalone divers know the risk of diving deep without a respirator. The body commands inhalation even when deep beneath the waters. To breathe is to live.

This chapter weaves together key areas currently igniting my interest in the movement of breath:

- Embryological underpinnings of respiration
- The interrelationship of perception, vision, and breath
- Carl Stough and his innovative work called breathing coordination
- An inquiry into the field or breath that is breathing us
- Somatic explorations on breath

The Diaphragm: The Embryological Seed of Life

All mammals emerge from a single fertilized egg cell, or ovum. Wholeness is our underlying nature and is the ground of health, adaptability, and connectivity to self, other, and the environment. The varying physiological systems and densities of our bodies arise from this beginning of "one-thing-ness." Dr. Erich Blechschmidt, an embryologist, introduced a novel way of viewing embryonic development. He felt that at every moment of differentiation, the embryo is functioning from a state of wholeness. The embryo is in relationship to its surrounding uterine environment and the fluid fields metabolizing and directing its growth. All tissues and functions arise from an origin of perfect wholeness. The embryo does not become human: it is human from the very beginning.

> Embryology does not stop at birth; we have the potential for change all along. In a sense we are embryos through our lifetime. (Schultz and Feitis, 1996, p. 3)

The embryo grows through a process of infolding and unfolding, rhythmic oscillations, centralizing fulcrums, and lengthening midlines. These expressions of form are shaped and directed by fluid gradients and metabolic forces in which the embryo is embedded. These suctioning, compressing, stretching, separating, dissolving, and germinal fluid forces shape both function and structure.

In the embryo, what emerges as the respiratory diaphragm begins development by the third week post-fertilization. Initially, the diaphragm arises as a tissue called the septum transversum. The seeds of the diaphragm are carried by mesenchyme, undifferentiated mesodermal tissue, spreading through the entire embryo. Mesenchyme is embryonic inner tissue derived mainly from mesoderm (which eventually forms connective tissue and blood). The embryonic mesenchyme reaches and merges with the potential coccyx. Take a moment and imagine the fertilized ovum as a sphere of diaphragms breathing in synchrony with each other and responding to the bellow-like pressures of a suctioning field. The action of the suction field is the major metabolic process shaping the fertilized egg. The kinetic motion of the embryonic suction field underlies the bellow-like movements of respiration.

An understanding of metabolic fields, and specifically the suction field, arises out of the extensive and detailed research of Blechschmidt, who identified epigenetic forces he understood shaped and directed embryonic development. He described this epigenetic movement as the biodynamic and biokinetic forces of embryonic development coming from the outside to inside the cell.

> Biodynamic refers to the dynamic features of development of the organism manifested in submicroscopic developmental movements. Biokinetic refers to the kinetic (spatiotemporal) forces acting on the developing organism. (Blechschmidt and Gasser, 1978, p. 270)

These metabolic forces of fluid intelligence permeate and direct the development and differentiation of the embryo. An understanding of metabolic fields arises out of a *quantum* approach to understanding the interrelationship and penetration of forces of consciousness directing development rather than a Newtonian cause-and-effect universe holding genetic determinism as the overriding rule.

Suction is one of the primary metabolic movements or fields directing embryonic formation. In the development of the diaphragm, the ascent of the brain and the descent of the viscera ignite two-directional lengthening. The rapidly enlarging brain demands nourishment (oxygen and nutrition), which are carried through the emerging blood vessels of the aorta and its branches. These arterial branches reach posteriorly and intertwine with the budding spinal nerves tethering the heart in place as the brain continues to grow. The connecting stalk anchors the embryo to the uterine wall at its caudal end.

Emerging between the polarity of a rapidly enlarging brain, lengthening spinal cord, and descending viscera is the diaphragm. As the neural tube grows, ascends, and begins to fold due to the massive growth of the brain, the future diaphragm becomes folded underneath the developing heart at the level of the cervical vertebrae. Innervations from the adjacent spinal nerves of C3, C4, and C5 are drawn into this moving potential, forming the precursor of the phrenic nerve. You've probably heard this sing-song rhyme repeated in anatomy classes: "C-3-4-5 keeps the diaphragm alive."

The descent of the viscera is closely coupled to the development of the diaphragm. The diaphragm is attached to the liver posterior [and] to the heart and arches high into the thorax. The inferior end of the diaphragm extends almost to the inferior end of the vertebral column.

The segment between the growing heart and the enlarging liver becomes compressed and taut, so that here it will be thin and tendon like [central tendon of the diaphragm]. (Freeman, 2010, p. 176)

Somatic Inquiry: The Body as a Continuing Diaphragm

Part One

1. Sit in a comfortable and upright position, with your feet on the floor.

2. Ask yourself: Is my breathing supporting me in sitting and exploring? What body-centered information emerges in response to this question?

3. Notice your breath. Sense the excursion of your thorax on inhalation and the passive release on exhalation.

4. Imagine your lungs extending beyond your back. Notice the movement of your whole body in response to breathing.

5. For the next few minutes just breathe, sensing the dimensions of your breath without control, effort, or intention to change anything.

Part Two

1. Sit with your feet on the floor or stand in a comfortable position.

2. Inquire: Is my breathing supporting the opening of the diaphragm of my feet to the life and breath of the ground? Sense the arches of your feet opening to the living planet and soils of earth. Allow a softening through your feet, as your awareness of the connection to earth touches the soles of your feet.

3. Become aware of your contact with the breathing, living ground in relationship to your breathing body. Earth's field does not stop at our feet but rises up around the body. Notice how far around and through your body space you sense earth's field.

4. Inquire: Does my breath support this relationship to earth?

With any activity you are engaged in, feel and listen to the support your breath is giving you. The simple question can be repeated: Is my breath supporting me as I work, sit, walk, study ... etc.?

Perception, Vision, and Breath

Imagine for a moment walking a mile along the ocean shoreline, hearing the thundering waves and sensing the pull of powerful currents. This meditation has nourished many twilight reveries. Walking barefoot on tide-washed sands offers a kinesthetic understanding of both the weight and ground of exhalation and the spacious lift of inhalation. The spectrum of breathing is fortified as visual senses open to include the vast horizon. The expanse of the sea, possessing unobstructed vistas, is nourishment, feeding sensibilities and imagination. The visual continuum of spaciousness births the physiological health of balance, adaptability, and gravitational security. Sensing and knowing the horizon is at the root of vestibular acuity. The secret is that you do not have to go out to meet the horizon—the horizon is always there to meet you.

Imagine the horizon is like a diaphragm—extending its horizontal reach in 360 degrees around you. Imagine yourself as the central tendon! Sense the vestibular shifts affecting your movement, rhythm, balance, and alignment as neurological intelligence attunes to the expansive environment enwrapping you. For moments at a time, depth perception can shift—the near, far, and wide of the surrounding waters and sand embrace the body in motion. A dynamic core of awareness is enlivened. Become aware of the physical shifts within your body as your central core relaxes and you begin to breathe in the openness of this vista.

The horizon touches you as you rest into this awareness. Sea air resuscitates a vital breath; as vision expands, auditory senses become heightened to the language of the waves. Balance shifts as the dynamic relationship with gravity alters with every step on the uneven shore. The sensory-based memory of our deeply rooted indigenous nature—alive, breathing, vital, and perceptually aware—rejuvenates blood, breath, and body. Sensing the horizon is key to a respiratory and spacious rejuvenation of the psyche.

The philosopher Baruch Spinoza realized that "the human mind could never be reconciled with the human body unless intelligence was recognized as an attribute of nature in its entirety…" (Abram, 1996, p. 109).

Whole-body perception of the horizon, whether we are viewing the ocean's distant edge, admiring a mountaintop vista, or perceiving the horizon even when we are enclosed by the four walls of an office, broadens a kinesthetic vocabulary. Our vestibular system is constantly seeking the horizon, whether we are aware of it or not. Yet because of the context, psychologically, emotionally, or environmentally, we limit our senses, impeding the expansiveness of our perception as well as becoming more focused in one-pointed attention. In an overly focused state, it is easy to lose touch with the presence of the horizon and the breathing expanse in which we are intimately embedded. Our industrial Western culture promotes the supremacy of the rational mind and an emphasis on the intellectual process associated with the physicality of the material world. Very little attention now orients to the invisible dimensions of intuition, spirit, instinct, and perceptions that cannot be quantified yet are inherent in the make-up of the human being.

Laurens Van der Post, author, educator, explorer, and observer of the African bushman (among other talents), wrote about anthropological concepts that have played an important role in our understanding of health and disease in society. Van der Post understood that every human being has an ancestral and instinctual spirit within him. If this million-year-old spirit is lost, modern man loses his real roots, and the source of health and wholeness.

A whole-body sense of the horizon went hand in hand with the evolution of the upright stature. The ability of early man to turn his head in a 180-degree radius, freed from limiting musculature, allowed him to scan the horizon for food, prey, or enemy. The function of the vestibular system was ignited. Imagine the "a-ha!" moments when primitive man saw the expanse of land before him, informing his actions for hunting, or running toward safety. Walking upright in gravity marked a bifurcation place in human history, from arboreal clamoring to the evolution of visual and language skills.

Cultivating perception of the horizon supports the balance of ground for our exhalation in relation to the spacious vastness of inhalation. Even if we cannot see the horizon, the deeply primal nature of our organism's vestibular system senses it as we cultivate its presence as a resource in our lives.

Somatic Inquiry: Breath and the Horizon

1. Sitting comfortably upright, notice your breath, the rhythm and ease of your diaphragmatic movement on inhalation, and the ease of exhalation.

2. Yield into the support of your chair, and the support of your feet on the floor. Follow your breath through a deeper, longer exhalation—pausing for the automatic triggering of inhalation.

3. Place your focus on something in your very near field of vision. Let your vision narrowly focus, seeing only this object. Notice any changes in your breathing, its ease or excursion.

4. Now, imagine the 360-degree expanse of the horizon around you.

5. Let the focus you are holding soften as you sense the walls to either side of you and behind you. Does your breathing change?

6. In nature: Repeat the above exploration, noticing your breathing ease or tension as you focus on the endpoint or goal (what you are walking or running toward).

7. Allow the inclusion of a whole-body sensing of the horizon, trees, and nature around you. Does your breathing change as you include the support of the horizon and its impact on your vestibular system?

Breathing changes with whatever activity we are doing. If we are hiking, biking, or climbing—breath responds. If we are hurried or confronting a difficult task, our breathing responds to accommodate. Breath is our ally; our breath is always there. The cycle of our breath is nurtured by sensing the expansiveness of the horizon and the ground beneath our feet.

> The clouds overhead are not plunging westward as the planet rolls beneath them … they themselves are part of the rolling Earth…. And we, imbibing and strolling through that same air … are enfolded within it, permeated, carnally immersed in the depths of this breathing planet. (Abram, 1996, p. 101)

Breathing Coordination: The Work of Carl Stough

Life begins and ends with the exhale. (Stough, 1981, p. 172)

A cold stethoscope on the flesh of my rib cage signals "take a deep breath." I inhale, noting the effort involved in following this directive as quickly as I can. Breathing on command is never easy.

Over this century, a multitude of breath-related therapies have come to the fore. All of these focus on breath as the primary mover of life—Carola Spead's straw technique to soften the exhale, Charlotte Selver's powerful meditations in sensory awareness, and Buteyko Breathing Therapy (among others). Innovative techniques for resuscitating the breathing cycle have exploded in the alternative health field. However, it is the work of the late Carl Stough and his emphasis on the phrenic nerve and a relaxed and effortless exhalation that piqued my interest.

Carl Stough was a singing teacher, yet because of his gift as a breathing coach in the mid 1960s, he was given access to the pulmonary ward of a military hospital, working with terminally ill men dying from emphysema. Using a new technique called cinefluography, he was able to record the rise and the fall of the diaphragm and the changes to the excursion of the diaphragm through his compassionate and gentle technique called breathing coordination.

His work at this East Coast hospital was the basis for the first major clinical study of diaphragmatic development in history. Together with his wife Reese, Carl cultivated an approach that restores diaphragmatic action and fullness of breath by skillfully encouraging a fuller and effortless exhalation and consequent toned stretching of the phrenic nerve.

Refining Respiratory Understanding

Breath underlies full-body awareness, orgasmic sensation, and living with conscious presence in this three-dimensional body of flesh and blood. A fundamental knowledge of the physiology of breathing is part of a bodyworker's education. Understanding the active and passive nature of the breathing cycle, as well as blood chemistry and circulation, are essential.

Our breathing, as well as the quality of air that we are breathing, effects changes in our respiratory rhythm's depth and activity. During normal breathing, inspiration is an active muscular process. Expiration is passive and relies on the natural elasticity of the tissues to deflate the lung. The most important muscle for inspiration is the diaphragm. The diaphragm is supplied by the phrenic nerve that is formed in the neck from the spinal nerves exiting the cervical vertebrae at C3, C4, and C5. The intercostal muscles are supplied by the segmental intercostal nerves that leave the spinal cord between T1 and TI2.

Any disease that affects the efferent or motor pathways, from the respiratory center in the brain stem to C3, C4, and C5 and the path of the phrenic nerve to the diaphragm, inflicts difficulty in breathing. Trauma to the cervical cord above C3 is normally fatal.

The diaphragm descends on inhalation and ascends with the passive movement of exhalation. The heart sitting above the diaphragm and the liver below it are intricately woven into the tissues of the diaphragm.

With each inhalation or exhalation, these organs are massaged.

One of the principles Carl and Reese Stough elaborated was that all respiratory problems were the result of high residual volume. Residual volume is the amount of carbon dioxide-laden air left in the lungs at the end of exhalation. With skill and attention, Carl would have his patients count from one to ten repeatedly, increasing the duration of their exhale with each successive out-breath *while not engaging any muscular force.* Oftentimes, the emphysema or asthmatic patient would only be able to vocally count to two. Yet gradually, with the strengthening of the diaphragm via this exercise, the count would increase. His patients at the military hospital showed improvements including vocal strength, gaining muscle mass and weight, and the ability to lift themselves out of their wheelchairs.

All this was accomplished with an emphasis on the exhalation, vocalization, and gentle stretching of the phrenic nerve by gaining a fuller diaphragmatic excursion and the restoration of tonus and strength in this muscle.

Another principle they highlighted is the diaphragm as the main muscle-organ of the body. The heart's movement is secondary. The heartbeats, via its neurological pacemaker, and are carried on the wave of the diaphragmatic movement. By strengthening this muscle, supporting a fuller exhalation and inhalation, there is a boomerang-like action that occurs through these muscular fibers. The tonus of the phrenic nerve is repaired as it stretches with diaphragmatic movement and effortless breathing emerges.

Somatic Inquiry: Breathing Coordination

Note: Adapted from the Stough approach to strengthen the diaphragm and responsiveness of the phrenic nerve.

1. Lie on your back with a pillow beneath your knees and under your head.

2. Realizing that breath is an involuntary action and that you do not need to make effort while inhaling or exhaling, let your jaw and throat be relaxed.

3. As you begin to exhale make an audible sound (ah …) or begin to count 1-2-3-4…. Allow your exhale to be easy as you count quietly until your inhale becomes a reflex. The point is to extend your exhale as long as possible with sound but without effort.

This should become a relaxing exploration.

The Breath Breathing Us

The total person is involved in the new air being welcomed, penetrating, doing its job, and then letting out what has been used. The exhalation is one of the most important things to have … to feel the going out to the very last. (Selver, 1995)

With a discussion of breath, we have to acknowledge death. Death is the uninvited guest shadowing every breath we take. According to some ascetic yogis, we are given an exact number of breaths—no more and no less. How many breaths are we given in a lifetime? Have you ever lain beside an ill partner, parent, or beloved pet, waiting with vigilant attention to the sound of their breath resuming after a longer-than-usual pause. Their life continues. Our culture shies away from acknowledging the inevitability of extinction. But as Jim Morrison said, "No one gets out alive." And it is the reality that some day we too will die, which is easily yet boldly denied. Our culture has made dying into a tidy experience. We remove ourselves from death's smells, sounds, and visuals. A death mask appears on a loved one's face—showing a visage of peace or fear as the "border crossing" nears. On a breath, they are lifted away from their earthly endeavors, sufferings, and joys, dissolving forever into spacious blue.

We enter on the wings of a life-giving breath, and we are borne from this life on our last breath. During the bedside vigil for my mother as she was dying, I found my breathing synchronizing with hers. My exhalation lingered in the pause between it and the inhale. My heartbeat and her still beating heart became one. I experienced a kind of electromagnetic field of pulsation, an ancient and archetypal umbilical connection between us. I did not know if this was the gravity of our beating hearts, strengthened through the loving field we shared, or the unfathomable intensity of the week's long vigil nearing its end, or the state of mind required for sitting quietly in the presence of death.

We shared a womb of passage, the timelessness of the in-between pauses, and the beauty of delivery into the mystery beyond. For one last treasured moment, she was here; yet as her exhalation lingered and merged with the vastness of dissolution, I realized she had passed through death's portal and was gone. The slower-than-slow primordial breath carried her through the sheer membrane between living and whatever the mystery holds. Silently, peacefully, the cycle was complete. My mother witnessed my first breath and I witnessed her last. She birthed me through struggle and pain. I became a midwife for her dying.

Being immersed in this cycle has deepened my personal inquiry and process, reorienting my own expansion, curiosities, and creative momentum. The spectrum of life, imprinted with its heartbreaking losses finds solace in the many gifts and blessings filtering through the ethers, beyond the earthly breath, showering joy and laughter in the hallows of life.

During this bedside vigil, I began appreciating more fully the gravitational weight of grief suctioning my exhale as well as moments of rising joy within my inhalation. Both ends of this emotional spectrum flowed through my senses. A deeper exhalation supports the spontaneity of a fuller breath. As I fell into the sorrow of loss, sensing-feeling the fathoms beneath their depths, I would just as suddenly be spit out into a state of expansion and light. Breath moves and guides me through a jungle of intertwined emotional, physical, spiritual and other-dimensional realities permeating my living, breathing existence.

Our life is a faint tracing on the surface of mystery.

Annie Dillard

The Breath of Life

William Sutherland is credited with using a term from Genesis, the *Breath of Life,* in describing the primary ignition that sparks the motor of life. He explained this breath as something that is not material and that cannot be seen (Sutherland, 1998, p. 147).

In applying this scriptural phrase to the study of the cranial system, Sutherland thought beyond current understandings in physics and chemistry and pioneered a novel approach to understanding the cranial-sacral system. This phrase underscores the genius of David Bohm and his theory of the implicate and explicate order, and aligns with Rupert Sheldrake's theory of morphogenetic resonance, in which fields of information are transmitted through time and space. Sheldrake's holographic understanding of resonant fields, carrying both potential and memory, corroborates with the understanding Blechschmidt brought to the fore regarding metabolic fields and rhythms that are shaping the embryo.

Intelligent and dynamic forces breathe shape, position, and form into all of life. These biodynamic fields carry the blueprint for development and are an undiminished matrix of information. They are not energy fields. This is the quantum fabric of wholeness, the implicate movement that Bohm described as the implicate order and possibly the space-time dimension that Einstein imagined. The therapeutic forces of nature, shaping the embryo, continue to shape and sustain the health, adaptability, and wholeness of the adult.

We are not only intimately immersed in the intelligent wholeness of nature, but the elements, minerals, and molecular bindings make us who we are. Skin is more like a membrane rather than an armored barrier. Our bodies, embedded in the natural world, share the intimate dance of breath with all living things. We are being breathed by the function of life infusing whole-body sensing and perception. Possessing and evolving a sensory knowledge of this implicit and natural connectivity to all that surrounds us sustains and evolves the space of "being" in the human be-ing.

> The breathing sensing body draws its sustenance and very substance from the soils plants and elements that surround it … so that it is very difficult to discern, at any moment precisely where this living body begins and where it ends. (Abram, 1996, p. 47)

This chapter is written in loving memory of my mother, Dorothy Agneessens, who passed away on May 28, 2012.

Section III

...

Pediatric Craniosacral Therapy

CHAPTER 16

My Work with Cerebral Palsy

This chapter is my history of pediatric practice and in particular my experience with cerebral palsy in young children. Cerebral palsy is a type of traumatic brain injury that can occur during the prenatal and perinatal time of life from any number of factors. I began working with traumatic brain injury (TBI) children in 1980. At that time, I was invited to evaluate twenty infants and children with a diagnosis of cerebral palsy. I remember flying to Cincinnati at the invitation of a pediatric physical therapist. I had done a series of Rolfing sessions on her and she thought that Rolfing, or what is now commonly referred to as myofascial release, would be a wonderful adjunct to her manipulation and movement therapy. She was right.

Cerebral palsy is a form of TBI caused by a variety of prenatal traumas, birth traumas, or postnatal traumas that result in significant developmental delays in children. This can be anything from an inability to walk or eat to cognitive and sensory deficits. The prenatal trauma can be on a spectrum from intrauterine growth restriction to physical abuse by a partner who kicks or punches the pregnant mother's abdomen. Birth trauma can be from overuse of forceps, vacuum extraction, and/or subsequent loss of oxygen to the brain (anoxia). It may include the shock and trauma from Cesarean section or premature cutting of the umbilical cord. Postnatal trauma to the brain can come about through a wide spectrum of experiences, including physical abuse and insecure attachments.

In my early years of working with TBI, I was using Rolfing techniques on a category of these children called *high toned*. These children had extensive spasticity in the musculoskeletal system, preventing them from standing and walking or properly walking. There were also other problems involved with feeding and sensory deficits. My first experience of seeing results were that the children could stand up and stabilize with their feet on the ground and had a better and more stable movement pattern. In addition, feeding issues were helped just from this physical manipulation, especially around the gut. All of these improvements would then change the brain and allow it to become more plastic and adaptive. These changes could be sustained over time with other adjunct therapy such as movement therapy done by the pediatric team of physical therapists, occupational therapists, and speech therapists. These wonderful therapists, such as Phyllis Aries who contributed Chapters 25, 26, and 27, eventually cross-train in each other's disciplines and recognize the importance of manual therapy.

With this level of success, I gradually developed protocols and courses for the Easter Seals Society of North America and several pediatric clinics associated with the medical schools at Wake Forest University, the University of Florida, and Ohio State University. I also traveled extensively around the United States and Canada, consulting and teaching at numerous other pediatric clinics. Once I was sponsored by the Department of Child and Family Services in New Mexico. This was a time when I had just begun studying craniosacral therapy and integrating it with the myofascial release work. Over three years of teaching courses in New Mexico, I also developed protocols for children with TBI who had fetal alcohol and fetal cocaine syndromes that also caused brain seizures and significant developmental delays. I went back on another cross-country tour, teaching this protocol to other pediatric clinics. This is still relevant as the number of fetal alcohol and fetal drug addicted babies is significant because of the increasing incidence of addicted mothers.

The results of the combination of these therapies were quite remarkable to me. The first was a significant reduction or elimination of seizure activity in many children. There was also a noticeable increase in cognition and learning. Frequently I would have to rely on the parents to give me such feedback. At the same time, I began consulting in different state institutions housing children with very severe developmental delays. I was asked to evaluate these populations for the value of manual therapy. This included infants with shaken-baby syndrome in which the parent violently shakes the baby to stop it from crying, thus severely damaging the infant's fragile brain, and other infants and children who had been heinously abused.

One such child that I will never forget had boiling oil poured over her face and into her mouth to stop her from crying. The resulting neurological insult was devastating. Even she, when I saw her at the age of nine, gained a greater degree of cognition and communication with her caregivers and me. I learned through these experiences that all children have an intact communication system and all I had to do was synchronize with it first and then start work. No matter what age, everyone has the capacity to indicate a yes and a no. This guided my hands and mind in helping these children. I must also say that these children taught me so much and especially their parents about the power of compassion and love.

Under this spectrum of traumatic brain injury, the results that I have seen further include improved feeding, which is critical, and a reduction in hyperarousal. To that end, I was invited to develop a program called integrative touch therapy at the Miami Children's Hospital, Dan Marino Center, in Westin, Florida. I worked there in conjunction with the pediatric neurologists and pediatric therapists for a year. During that time, the protocols I developed were used for a wide variety of infants and children, but especially with infants with cranial molding (misshapen heads) and other anomalies of the cranium itself, such as craniosynostosis, which is a birth defect involving premature fusion of the cranial sutures. I also worked with other forms of pediatric encephalopathy or plagiocephaly. These are misshapen heads resulting from the compressions on the baby's head during a vaginal delivery at birth. The pediatric physical therapists that I worked with were already utilizing craniosacral therapy to a large degree, including at summer camps for children with cerebral palsy in which the children would receive multiple-hands craniosacral therapy.

I began to see the value of craniosacral therapy more and more when the principal challenge was with the head itself. Entrapment neuropathies of the cranial nerves were greatly relieved, thus normalizing the suck-swallow-breathe reflex in children, including digestion and elimination and headache reduction in adults. I started to form a postdoctoral research committee to study the value of craniosacral therapy with these children, but at the end of one year, the hospital decided to go in a different direction with the program and I left. At that time I decided to focus exclusively on the use of biodynamic craniosacral therapy for the children I was seeing. This has evolved into a five-level training in pediatric craniosacral therapy and a six-level training in trauma resolution for adult clients.

Currently, I am seeing several children in Italy and Germany with TBIs. One child in Germany, who at the age of six months, was in a very bad car accident in which his tongue was severed from a severe concussion and ultimately reattached. The resulting insult to the brain caused this child to become quadriplegic. Leo is very communicative and talks. He is on a respirator, though, and gradually has become very responsive to biodynamic craniosacral therapy. I even taught his mother how to perceive Primary Respiration and sense it in Leo therapeutically. After the first session I worked on him, his parents told me that I was the first male therapist he allowed to contact him since his hospitalization. I attribute this to working with Primary Respiration, which creates a very safe place for children with brain injuries.

As I work biodynamically more often in these past few years, I see children such as Leo becoming much more able to self-regulate both emotionally and physiologically regarding feeding and communication, including speech improvement. I also learned several years ago while working with a severely handicapped child in Italy about the value of metabolic testing. I learned that any child with a TBI should also have metabolic testing for specific allergies such as gluten, sugar, and dairy products. Children with TBI who have proper metabolic testing and are fed a diet that matches their metabolism get better across all parameters of development than other children do with the same problems but no dietary changes. This is especially in conjunction with the use of biodynamic craniosacral therapy because of the support for the suck-swallow-breathe reflex. I now feel that even my adult clients with TBI should be metabolically tested for food allergies. It simply speeds up the healing process in the brain and body.

Perhaps the most common problem I am presented with nowadays is infants with feeding issues. In my Volume Four, I created pediatric standards of practice. In that chapter, I discuss protocols for treatment and especially evaluating the suck-swallow-breathe reflex. I am very grateful to Alison K. Hazelbaker, PhD, for her work in integrating craniosacral therapy in the field of pediatrics. She wrote The Impact of Cranio-Sacral Therapy on Infant Sucking Dysfunction: A Pilot Study as her final thesis from her cranial training. Through her and the pediatric osteopaths, I learned to evaluate the suck-swallow-breathe reflex before working on the head. This is because the issues may be coming from the respiratory diaphragm as the esophagus passes through it and the intestinal tone in general.

Finally, over the past thirty years I have also maintained a private practice with adults. I gradually began working with adults who had experienced an MTBI and treated them primarily with craniosacral therapy and then biodynamic craniosacral therapy. MTBI stands for mild traumatic brain injury, the category concussions are placed in medically. Many adolescents and adults routinely experience mild, moderate, and severe concussions. Concussion experience is not limited to sports, but is certainly enhanced by sports such as hockey and football. As of this writing there are more than 3,000 former professional football players and their families suing the National Football League, claiming the league never warned the players about the potential long-term damage from concussions, which are common in football. I began working with concussed adults who had been in motor vehicle accidents or other types of accidents and had either experienced open-head injuries, in which the cerebral spinal fluid of the brain would leak out the nose or the ears, or closed-head injuries, typically known as a concussion or MTBI. I have almost always seen the healing response time of these clients improve.

I have also worked on many clients who had neurosurgery as children or adults and the improvement in the time of recovery is remarkable. I can say generally that all such head trauma clients of mine, whether from athletics or other types of trauma including surgery, have had a reduction in their headaches, followed by greater mental and emotional stability. Second, they experience relief from not only head pain but also neck pain associated with post-concussion trauma, which is discussed in current literature on the subject. Further results I see also include much greater self-regulation of emotion and thus indicating greater organization and integration through all levels of the brain. This includes better performance, whether it be school testing or athletics, and greater knowledge and sensitivity of one's own body and how to self-manage traumatic concussions in the future. This is true for infants and adults.

CHAPTER 17

Introduction to the Primary Period: Pre-Conception through the First Year of Postnatal Life

by Ann Diamond Weinstein, PhD

The following chapters are a collaborative effort with Michael Shea to provide the reader with a somatically sensitive introduction to the impacts of the prenatal and early postnatal period over the lifespan. By interspersing the material I have synthesized with somatic practices developed by Michael Shea, it is our intention to present this potentially activating content in a way that supports affect regulation and integration. It also provides practice in the development of an embodied quality of presence necessary to support healing of imprints and issues originating in the prenatal and early postnatal period. The definition that follows is an introduction to the material I have synthesized in these chapters. These chapters are, in part, my attempt to answer the question, What is prenatal and perinatal psychology?

Prenatal and perinatal psychology is the interdisciplinary study of the earliest periods in human development, including conception, time in the womb, experiences during and after birth, and experiences with caregivers and the family system through the first year following birth. Theory and research in embryology, epigenetics, evolutionary biology, psychophysiology, behavioral perinatology, neurobiology, attachment, and trauma provide the foundation for the exploration of *how* experiences during this critical development period impact an individual. Knowledge from these fields illuminate the physical, cognitive, social, and emotional impacts of our earliest experiences and how they form enduring response patterns that shape our development, behavior, and health over the lifespan. This definition combines concepts from the Association for Prenatal and Perinatal Psychology and Health (2009), McCarty (2000), Noble (1993), and Odent (2002).

The contributions of theorists, researchers, and clinicians in developmental psychology, affective neuroscience, attachment, and traumatology (Bowlby, 1988; Ainsworth, 1985; Beebe and Lachmann, 2002; Fonagy et al., 2002; Lyons-Ruth and Jacobovitz, 1999; Perry, 1999; Schore, 1994, 2001, 2002, 2003a, 2003b, 2012; Siegel, 2012a, 2012b; Stern, 2004; Tronick, 2007) demonstrate the critical importance of the quality of early *postnatal* dyadic interactions between infants and caregivers and the role these interactions have in shaping the development of the child. These early interactions, which affect the child's neurobiological development, are also understood to influence an individual's relationships over the lifespan.

Those of us who work in the field of prenatal and perinatal psychology suggest that there is crucial knowledge to be gained from the study of an even earlier period of human development—from conception through birth. A wealth of recent research demonstrates that our earliest experiences from the time of conception, time in the womb, and during birth may also resonate over our lifetime (Kaplan, Evans, and Monk, 2007; Khashan et al., 2009; Lupien et al., 2009; O'Connor et al., 2005; O'Connor et al., 2003; Sandman and Davis, 2012; Shonkoff, Boyce, and McEwen, 2009; Talge, Neal, and Glover, 2007; Van den Bergh and Marcoen, 2004; Van den Bergh et al., 2008).

It is clear we must focus our attention on the prenatal period to address environmental influences that can negatively affect the development and health of an individual throughout their life. Shonkoff points out one of the risks incurred by waiting until early childhood to intervene in adverse early environments: "For children in adverse environments, four years of inaction in the face of repeated threats to developing brain architecture is difficult to justify" (as cited in Schore, 2012, p. 12). He highlights the need for and benefit of working with women during pregnancy: "Advances in neuroscience suggest that interventions that enhance the mental health, executive function skills, and self-regulation capacities of vulnerable mothers, beginning as early as pregnancy, suggest promising strategies to protect the developing brains of their children" (p. 12).

I would suggest that in order to optimally protect and support the overall development of a human organism (not just the development of a prenate's or child's brain), the work with women Shonkoff describes above must begin prior to conception. In addition, if a woman has a partner who is present in her environment while her prenate is developing, they would benefit from the same supportive services. The benefits from these kinds of supportive services to a woman's relationship with her partner would also contribute to the optimal development of their child.

For practitioners working with women and their partners, an understanding of the quality of prenatal and early postnatal experiences and their potential impacts can inform their work with patients and increase opportunities for healing. This understanding also sheds light on important psychoeducational opportunities for practitioners in their communication with patients. Increasing patients' understanding of the benefits of cultivating nurturing environments for themselves and their prenates, and teaching them skills that enhance their capacity to do so, empowers them to contribute to the optimal development of their children.

Imprinting

Theory and research in multiple disciplines, including epigenetics, evolutionary biology, developmental psychology, quantum physics, and consciousness studies (among others) continue to expand our understanding of the nature of imprinting. There is controversy between these fields about the specific processes through which imprinting occurs. For the purposes of these chapters, I will acknowledge that imprinting occurs. The discussion of the controversy about *how* it occurs is beyond the scope of these chapters.

Women and men transition into parenthood carrying the imprints of their life experiences. They may enter parenthood intentionally or unintentionally, as biological parents, or with the help of donor eggs, sperm, and/or gestational carriers, or through the adoption or foster parenting of a child. Regardless of how an individual becomes a parent, science and medicine are now demonstrating how the conditions inside and outside women's bodies during the prenatal and early postnatal period profoundly affect their offspring's development, health, and behavior over the child's lifespan.

Evolutionary biology has shown us how the developing human organism, from the first weeks after conception through early infancy, "'reads' key characteristics of its environment and prepares to adapt to an external world that can vary dramatically in its levels of safety, sufficiency and peril" (Shonkoff, Boyce, and McEwen, 2009, p. 2257). This includes the adjustment of set points in key brain circuits.

Research and knowledge in all the disciplines mentioned above are converging to highlight the critical influence of the environment on many aspects of our development in the womb and the echoes of these environmental impacts over our lives.

Women and their partners' experiences of attempting to or actually conceiving a child, pregnancy, engaging a gestational carrier if one is unable to conceive and sustain a pregnancy, or adopting or foster parenting a child are shaped by their previous experiences, including those of trauma and loss. This includes the impacts and imprints of their own experiences of development in their mothers' wombs, of their own births, and their early interactions with their primary caregivers, whether these were their biological parents or others. Adolescents also become parents and carry the impacts and imprints of their past experiences into their experiences of conception, pregnancy, birth, and parenting. For ease of communication, I will refer to "women and their partners" here, but I am acknowledging the inclusion of adolescent girls and boys who become parents.

The imprints of our experiences are expressed in our bodies in states of health and disease, and through our behavior. The term "lived experience" refers to a view that acknowledges the multidimensional aspects of our experiences, the context within which our experiences occur and the meaning our experiences have in our lives. This includes our experience of space, time, our lived bodies, and our relationships. The term "lived body" refers to the subjective experience of our internal and external environment in all its aspects through our embodiment as human organisms. Our lived bodies allow us to perceive, interact with, and understand our world, and to make meaning of our experiences (Merleau-Ponty, 1958). Our experiences and the meaning they have in our embodied lives, in turn, shape our perceptions and future experiences. These include our earliest experiences in the womb and of birth.

Somatic Practice 1: Mindfulness of the Body

Take a moment to pause from the reading and orient to your body. Whether you are sitting or lying down, notice the weight of your body and the contact with the chair, couch, or bed. Really allow more contact with the surface of your body and the chair, couch, or bed. Scan your body starting at your feet and notice if your feet and legs feel relaxed. Adjust them as necessary. Next bring your attention to your pelvis and notice the contact your clothes are making with your skin. Now bring your attention to your trunk, sensing the front of your body and the back of your body from your shoulders to your pelvis. Now sense your shoulders, arms, and hands down to the fingertips. Adjust your body again as necessary for maximum comfort and ease. Now bring your attention to your head and neck. Allow a little bit of space between your teeth and close your eyes and allow them to get wider in a way that allows the eyes to drop back into their sockets. Now see if you can sense your entire body from the bottom of your feet to the top of your head. Take a deep breath and wait several minutes, being with the wholeness of your body before continuing to read.

Many individuals have experiences of trauma and violence before they attempt to or actually conceive, adopt, or foster parent a child. Recent research has shed light on the high incidence of violence and trauma experienced by women before and during the childbearing years and particularly trauma that involves the parts of their bodies involved in reproduction (Seng et al., 2001; Seng et al., 2002; Tjaden and Thoennes, 1998, 2000).

The imprints of experiences of violation are often manifested in women's lived bodies as traumatic stress symptoms (Gill, Szanton, and Page, 2005; Resnick et al., 1993; Tjaden and Thoennes, 1998, 2000) and may influence their experiences of conception, pregnancy, birth (Grimstad and Schei, 1999), and parenting (DiPietro, Costigan, and Pressman, 2002; Issokson, 2004; Kirkengen, 2010). These imprints may also influence women's experiences of medical care received at this time (Monahan and Forgash, 2000; Robohm and Buttenheim, 1996; Schachter, Stalker, and Teram, 2001; Seng et al., 2002).

Over the last several decades, the experiences of women and their partners of the conception, pregnancy, and birth of their children are increasingly shaped by assisted reproductive technology interventions used in treating those who face fertility challenges. The impacts of reproductive endocrinology treatment experiences on conditions inside and outside a woman's body that may influence an offspring's development, health, and behavior during the prenatal and postnatal period are only beginning to be explored.

The quality of care a woman receives during the pre-conception period, during her pregnancy, while she gives birth, and in the early postnatal period contributes to her experience and influences the conditions inside her body. These experiences, along with the imprints of a woman's earlier experiences, synergistically shape a woman's transition into motherhood, her child's growth, health, and behavior over the lifespan, and the crucial early attachment relationship that develops between them. The experiences of a woman's partner during the pre-conception through postnatal period converge with the imprints of their own earlier experiences and also shape their transition into parenthood.

The quality of the interactions between a woman and her partner during the pre-conception through early postnatal period affect their own and each other's psychophysiology, as well as that of their baby.

The vulnerability of the human organism during the prenatal period to the wide range of influences that leave long-term impacts on an individual has been well established (Nathanielsz, 1999; Thomson, 2007; Van den Bergh et al.,

2005; Verny and Weintraub, 2002). An understanding of *how* conditions inside and outside a woman's lived body may affect the development of her prenate (embryo and fetus), as well as knowledge of sensitive and critical periods in the prenatal development of the brain and autonomic nervous system, contribute to our understanding of the psychophysiology of an individual's later interpersonal interactions and the quality of his or her relationships.

It is my intention that the content presented in these chapters will enhance your understanding of the multidimensional and transgenerational impacts of these earliest experiences and thereby support your awareness of additional opportunities for healing, for both your patients and yourself.

Somatic Practice 2: Mindfulness of Breathing

Take a moment to orient to your body as you did in Somatic Practice 1. Now notice the quality of the air coming in through your nose or mouth. Simply pay attention to how air enters your body. After several breaths, notice how the air goes into your lungs and moves the lungs against the rib cage. Wait several breaths and notice how the breath moves into your abdomen. Can you sense your breath making contact with the sides, the back, and front of your abdomen? Wait several breaths and allow your breath to move into your pelvis. Notice if the breath can contact the sides of the hip bones, the back of the pelvis, and the front of the pelvis, close to your pubic bone. Wait several breaths and then synchronize your lungs, abdomen, and pelvis together.

Neuroception and Oxytocin

Neuroception and oxytocin play important roles in pre-conception, prenatal, and early postnatal experiences. It is important to understand the concept of neuroception and how it relates to the pre-conception, prenatal, and early postnatal period. One of the functions of a nervous system is to continuously evaluate the environment for risk. It is through our senses that we perceive our environment and our nervous system uses the information we take in to make these evaluations. This process occurs beneath the level of our conscious awareness. The concept of neuroception describes the neural circuits involved when our organism makes distinctions between environments that are safe, dangerous, or life threatening. As a species, we have a very long heritage of evaluating risk in the environment. The capacity to make these assessments evolved in primitive parts of the brain, which continue to perform these functions for us today. The perception of danger or life threat triggers a cascade of events in the brain and body that are expressed in different behaviors. It is important to note that the body and its sensory system usually initiates adaptive defensive behaviors such as fight-flight or freeze, before neural processing is finished.

One of the important adaptive defensive behaviors of mammals is called immobilization or, as referred to above, freezing. This is a very old, primitive type of defensive strategy in which body movement is inhibited, which reduces the metabolic load and thus minimizes the need for food. At the same time, endogenous opiates are released into the body, which raise the pain threshold of the body and create a type of numbing. These adaptive defensive behaviors are pervasive and also include immobilization for important prosocial activities such as conception, birth, breastfeeding, and attachment behaviors in general. When an individual perceives the environment as safe, these reproductive behaviors involve immobilization *without* fear. When they occur in an environment that is perceived as dangerous or life threatening, immobilization is coupled with fear and the changes in the body can be quite dramatic. An extremely slow heart rate, inhibited breathing, and low blood pressure are the physiological manifestations of immobilization involving fear.

Through the process of evolution, certain circuits in the brain originally involved in immobilization behaviors have also become involved in behaviors necessary to meet intimate social needs, as mentioned above. A unique neuropeptide—oxytocin—can influence the immobilization circuitry. Oxytocin is released during sexual intercourse, breastfeeding, birthing, certain forms of manual therapy, and other prosocial activities. It is important that an individual be able to perceive and experience safety in an environment, in order to support the release of oxytocin. Oxytocin is not released if our nervous system identifies the environment, including the people who are present, as dangerous. Neuroception of the environment as safe, dangerous, or life threatening may be triggered from signals in the external environment, but also from our internal environment, such as our experience of sickness, pain, or fever. Even a very flat facial affect in a person in an individual's environment can prompt a neuroception of danger and disrupt normal spontaneous interactions with others. It is quite well known that maternal depression and its effects on maternal affect in mother-child interactions cause serious brain changes in an infant and child and thus compromise long-term growth and development (Porges, 2004).

Oxytocin and Its Influence on Reproductive Processes and Parental Behavior

Porges mentions the role of oxytocin in reproductive behaviors and during activities that help establish social bonds. Uvnas-Moberg contrasts the role of oxytocin with vasopressin, another neuropeptide that is released when an individual's neuroception of the environment is that of danger and/or life threat. "Vasopressin is involved in behavior marked by defensiveness, boundary setting and aggression. Oxytocin instead produces behavior characterized by social interaction, friendliness and curiosity" (2003, p. 84).

Many interactions between women, their partners, their offspring, and their health and mental health care providers during the prenatal and perinatal period are shaped by the presence or absence of these hormones.

The following links take you to two very brief interviews on the role of oxytocin in reproductive processes and maternal behavior.

http://www.oneworldbirth.net/videos/when-and-how-is-oxytocin
-released-during-birth/

http://www.oneworldbirth.net/videos/michel-odent-on-the-love
-cocktails-in-birth/

The first link is to an interview with Kirsten Uvnas-Moberg, MD, a physiologist and researcher who has written a book called *The Oxytocin Factor*. In this very short video, she talks about the role and release of oxytocin during birth and breastfeeding.

The second link is to an interview with Michel Odent, MD, an obstetrician who has spent decades observing and attending births, researching the psychophysiology of reproductive processes, and evaluating the impacts of prenatal, birth, and early postnatal environments and experiences on women, their partners, and their offspring.

It is clear that the experiences of conception, pregnancy, birth, breastfeeding, and caregiving behaviors are facilitated by the release of oxytocin. The environment and context within which these experiences occur influence the effects of oxytocin. Uvnas-Moberg (2003) elaborates on this concept by explaining how the release of oxytocin during sexual relations is affected by the context in which sexual relations occur. "The more the encounter contains an element of tension and danger, the more it is influenced by oxytocin's sister substance, vasopressin, and so a stress reaction is produced" (p. 119). The author goes on to explain that sexual activity that involves pain or violence causes a stress reaction that "activates the aggression and defense mechanisms in the form of higher blood pressure, tightened muscles, and even reduced emotional responses and desensitization to touch" (p. 119).

Uvnas-Moberg's observations highlight the importance of considering how women's and men's past experiences affect their neuroception of the environment in which reproductive processes occur and the influence of their neuroception on the release of key hormones, which either facilitate or inhibit these processes.

Somatic Practice 3: Mindfulness of Happiness

Take a moment to practice mindfulness of body and breathing. After several breaths, notice what happens when you smile a little bit. Does this change the tone and texture of your body? When you are eating your next meal with someone you really like, notice how much you smile during the meal. Take the opportunity to smile frequently during the day. Even if it feels disingenuous to smile, try it anyway and see if it changes the sensation around the front of your body, especially your heart and rib cage. Notice any sensations of warmth while talking or being with another person during the day. See if you can allow the warmth that is free of any concepts to spread through your body and connect it to a smile.

Pregnancy, Affect Regulation, and Attachment

Through my experiences as a childbirth educator, birth doula, prenatal and perinatal researcher and specialist, and mother, I have come to understand the critical impact on women, their partners, and their offspring of their neuroception of safety, danger, or life threat in their internal and external environments. During the pre-conception through early postnatal period, the psychophysiological states evoked in a woman in reaction to her neuroception of safety, danger, or life threat have profound impact on how she experiences sexual activity, conception, pregnancy, labor, birth, bonding, breastfeeding or bottle feeding, and the behavior of her infant. These psychophysiological states also directly and indirectly affect the development, health, and behavior of her child, which, in turn, influences the quality of their attachment relationship.

Based on this introduction, I would like to highlight the relevance of the knowledge presented here for practitioners. As we know, the psychophysiological state of a health or mental health practitioner and the quality of care he or she provides has the potential to affect the psychophysiological state of the patient. In the case of a pregnant patient, the woman's body is the immediate environment within which her prenate is developing. Therefore, it would be prudent for practitioners who work with women and their partners who are going through the pre-conception through early postnatal period, to be especially aware of the fact that their behaviors in interactions with their patients have the potential to directly and/or indirectly affect a third being—*the developing prenate.*

In the early postnatal period, awareness of the *neonate* is equally important during patient-practitioner interactions, as the psychophysiological states they evoke may affect the newborn or infant who may be present during its parent's treatment session. It is also important to consider the impact of dysregulated states that may be activated in the patient in the aftermath of a treatment session and how these states might affect the patient's interactions with the baby.

As parents and researchers have long observed, prenates and neonates react to their environment, even if that reaction is one of shutting down in an environment that is experienced as overwhelming or aversive. It is now clear that prenates, in the environment of their mothers' wombs, and neonates and infants, in interactions with and in proximity to their primary caregivers, are affected by their caregivers' psychophysiological states.

Thomson (2007) acknowledges the fact that practitioners would benefit from understanding the impacts of maternal stress on the developing prenate because this knowledge can inform treatment decisions, especially when working with patients who are severely traumatized and dissociative (p. 85). Recent research on the effects of maternal prenatal stress on the fetus supports Thomson's suggestion for practitioners: "Ideally, therapeutic treatment should reduce the pregnant patient's physiological and psychological stress systems. Attention to resolving dissociative and trauma symptoms of the patient should not supersede the issues of regulation. Hopefully, interventions during this period can minimize negative effects on the prenate" (2007, p. 104).

Psychophysiology

By supporting enhanced psychophysiological regulation in pregnant patients, practitioners will be contributing to the healthy development of their patients' prenates, just as clinical experience and research have shown us the benefits of supporting parents' psychophysiological state regulation in their postnatal interactions with their babies.

It is my hope that the information I am presenting here will spark consideration of the relevance of this material to you as individuals, your experiences as practitioners, and the experiences of your patients. I suggest you hold curiosity about the psychophysiological states you observe in your patients when working with those who are facing pre-conception, pregnancy, and early postnatal challenges. Consider the possibility that these states may indicate activation that relates not only to your patients' current issues regarding these major life transitions, but may also reflect the activation of their own early imprints from their pre-conception through early postnatal development.

It might also be helpful to observe with curiosity your own psychophysiological states in interactions with patients and the relationship of these states to your own earliest experiences and imprints. In addition, I suggest you track your psychophysiological states while reading the material presented here, so you can pace yourself, resource yourself, and support self-regulation throughout this chapter. Prenatal and perinatal psychologists have found that this material can be activating and, at times, dysregulating. Pausing from time to time to focus on your own internal experience will provide space for self-care, enable you to better integrate the material, and perhaps deepen your understanding of your own earliest experiences.

As we prepare to explore the impact of a woman's environment on her prenate, I would like to raise another question, specifically for this audience to consider: What is the potential impact on a pregnant practitioner and her developing prenate of the psychophysiological states she may experience while working with patients? The ability to self-regulate while working with patients is especially important for pregnant practitioners and those attempting to conceive, to minimize the potential negative impacts of dysregulated psychophysiological states on themselves during the pre-conception period and their developing prenates over the course of their pregnancy.

In order to better understand the potential of a woman's environment to affect her developing prenate, including the environment of interpersonal therapeutic interactions, I will briefly summarize the development of the senses in the unborn child, some of the critical stages of prenatal brain and autonomic nervous system development, and the importance and impact of the timing of stressors from conception through the early postnatal period.

Somatic Practice 4: Mindfulness of Cardioception

Take a few moments to practice mindfulness of body and breath. Bring your attention to the center of your chest. Notice the movement of your respiratory diaphragm as you are breathing. Your heart rests on top of your respiratory diaphragm. Now see if you can sense the movement and activity of your heart without taking your pulse. Simply with your attention feel your heartbeat. Perhaps you feel a pulsation down through your arms. Or nothing at all. Then bring your attention to your breathing. As you inhale, the heart rate typically increases and as you exhale, your heart rate typically decreases. Spend some time noticing your breathing and its relationship with the pulsation of your heart. Allow the pulsation of your heart to spread and expand through your chest, abdomen, neck, and three dimensionally through your body. If you are still unable to sense the movement and activity of your heart, then when you wake up in the middle of the night to use the bathroom and return to bed, bring your attention to your heart as it will be easier to sense its movement then. Periodically, during the day, practice this mindfulness of heart and it will change your brain and body to peacefulness and equanimity.

Prenatal Development of the Senses

Our sensory receptors provide critical information to our nervous system to enable us to meet both internal and external challenges. The nervous system receives sensory feedback from two types of receptors. Interoceptors sense conditions in the body to support homeostasis. Porges (2011) defines homeostasis as "the autonomic state that fosters visceral needs in the absence of external challenge" (pp. 67–68); Fogel (2009) defines it as "a state of mental and physical health in which our cells are sufficiently nourished to maintain normal metabolism to preserve and grow body function" (p. 14). Exteroceptors sense conditions outside the body to deal with environmental (external) challenges.

Hearing

Hearing begins during the fifth week of gestation. The prenate actively hears before the end of the first trimester, but hearing continues to mature slowly until after the baby is born (Larsen, 2001). From 10 to 20 weeks gestation, along with the inner and outer ear structures, about 16,000 hair cells form (Thomson, 2004). By 4–5 months gestation, the eighth cranial nerve develops and carries auditory information from the ear to the brain. The most consistent sounds present in the embryo/fetal environment are the mother's heartbeat and her voice. By 23 weeks gestation, a fetus will both respond to sound and indicate sound preferences. By 26 weeks gestation, the fetus learns intonation, rhythm, and other speech patterns of the mother's voice, and by 34 weeks, the auditory threshold levels are similar to adult preferences.

A growing fetus develops selective preferences for particular sounds. The fetus registers the rhythm, volume, tempo, emotional quality of vocal tones, and sequences of its mother's speech. It is quite capable of discerning its mother's voice during the third trimester (Hartman and Zimmeroff, as cited in Foster and Verny, 2007, p. 273). The fetus habituates to sound and can respond with interest to outside noises. Of course, the most important sound to the fetus is that of its mother's voice. It brings pleasure to the fetus and thus the fetus begins a relationship and an interaction with her voice. It is also possible that loud noises can impair the hearing of a fetus (Elliot, 1999).

Vision

The earliest development of vision begins with the eyespots, which form around 28 days gestation (Tsiaris, 2002). Around 2 months gestation, the axonal connections form. Approximately 100 million neurons form the visual system between 14 and 28 weeks gestation, but these are not connected until later development. The fetus appears to see light through the mother's belly and the amniotic fluid during the last trimester. The vision system takes many years after birth to mature (Larsen, 2001).

Taste

Taste buds emerge on the tongue around 8 weeks gestation and by 13 weeks, these buds form in the mouth. By the fourth month gestation, the fetus can taste the amniotic fluid, which biases the fetus for future taste preferences (Hill et al., 2001). The fifth and ninth cranial nerves, trigeminal and glosso-pharyngeal nerves provide general sensory innervations to the tongue (Foster and Verny, 2007).

Smell (Olfactory)

The nostrils form around 7 weeks gestation (Larsen, 2001). The olfactory bulbs separate from the nasal cavity and the facial bones during the thirteenth week. At the end of the embryonic stage (8 weeks gestation) the olfactory sense is almost fully mature. By the end of the first trimester, the main olfactory subsystem is anatomically mature and actively performing as a sensory system.

Touch and Pressure (Tactile)

The tactile system is the earliest system to develop in utero. It is also the most mature sensory system at birth (Kandel, Schwartz, and Jessel, 2000, as cited in Foster and Verny, 2007). By 5 weeks, the embryo senses pressure to its lips and nose. Cutaneous sensory receptors appear in the fetus in the seventh week of gestation. At 9 weeks, the embryo's arms, chin, and eyelids also sense pressure. By 10 weeks, the legs sense pressure. At 14 weeks, most of the body responds to touch. Sensory receptors spread to all fetal cutaneous and mucosal surfaces by 20 weeks gestation. The last area in the body to develop a sense of tactile awareness is the back and top of the head, which does not develop until soon after birth. Elliot (1999) observes that this may help decrease the perception of pain during labor and birth.

The two major purposes of the tactile system are to provide protection and discrimination of input. Anand and Hickey (1987) explain that "pain pathways, as well as cortical and subcortical centers necessary for pain perception are well developed late in gestation, and the neurochemical systems now known to be associated with pain transmission and modulation are intact and functional." Anand (2005) notes: "Based on the available scientific evidence, we cannot dismiss the high likelihood of fetal pain perception before the third trimester of human gestation."

Proprioception

Proprioception is "the felt sense of the location and relative position of different parts of the body in relation to objects and individuals" (Fogel, 2009). It allows for a continuous internal awareness of body posture. Proprioceptors are found in the muscles, tendons, and joints. As they develop, so does proprioception. Tiny nerves carry messages that allow us to sense awareness of where our bodies are in space. This allows the coordination of movements. Proprioception also tells us about the position and movement of internal organs. Cells that line the gastric wall give sensory information to the brain when the stomach is full (Williamson and Anzalone, 2001).

Vestibular

The vestibular system helps the body respond to movement of the head and body in relation to gravity. It contributes to the sense of balance and equilibrium and a sense of where the body is, moving in space. "It provides us with a sense of center—in relationship to space, time, motion, depth, and self.… It is possibly the oldest and most primitive of the sensory systems. It functions largely below the level of our conscious awareness, yet our consciousness is affected greatly by it.… Differentiation of structures is apparent at 5 weeks gestation" (Weitensteiner, 2005). The vestibular system is located in the inner ear, in the bony skull near the hearing mechanism. Between 7 and 14 weeks, axonal fibers form the tiny hairs in the ears. These cilia support neuronal connections and provide movement information to the brain (Tsiaris, 2002). It is fully operational at 16 weeks post-conception. At 5 months gestation, the vestibular apparatus has reached its full size and shape (Weitensteiner, 2005). The rapid maturity of this system leaves it more vulnerable to damage than other sensory systems (Elliot, 1999).

Its early development results in its being more influential in organizing other sensory and motor abilities and influencing higher level emotional, relational and cognitive abilities (Weitensteiner, 2005).

Interoception

Porges (2011) defines interoception as "the ability to sense internal states and bodily processes." A large amount of sensory information is conveyed to the brain from numerous interoceptors that are located on the heart, stomach, liver, and other organs inside the body cavity. Interoception has both conscious and unconscious dimensions. On an unconscious level, "internal organs have sensors that send continuous information to brain structures, fostering stability (i.e., homeostasis) in internal physiology by rapidly adjusting to support specific motor behaviors and psychological processes. The internal sensations conveyed by these sensors provide information about physiological regulation" (Porges, 2011, pp. 76–77).

Fogel (2009) explains that interoception is involved in embodied self-awareness—"sensing our breathing, digestion, hunger, arousal, pain, emotion, fatigue" and the "body schema—an awareness of the movement and coordination between different parts of the body and between our body and the environment" (p. 11). Fogel notes that embodied self-awareness begins during the last two months of the third trimester of pregnancy. Fetal self-awareness involves both interoception and body schema. Fogel (2009) reports on dynamic 4-D ultrasound research films taken in the seventh month of gestation (Myowa-Yamakoshi and Takeshita, 2006). These films show the fetal mouth opening in anticipation, if the hand approaches the mouth. Fogel notes this as evidence that one part of the body recognizes its relation to another part.

We now have a brief outline of the development of sensory systems in the prenate. This knowledge challenges the myth that prenates *are not* having lived body experiences in their mothers' wombs and illuminates the need for practitioners to increase their understanding of human development during this time of unparalleled growth and increasing capacity for perception and interaction with the environment.

Somatic Practice 5: Mindfulness of the Senses

Take several minutes to orient to your body three dimensionally and your breathing. Notice your thoughts and the tempo of your thinking. Using your breath, every time you exhale, imagine your thoughts are actually flowing out of your body. After several minutes, bring your attention to your sense of hearing. What sounds can you actually hear in the room where you are located? See if you can specifically identify any particular sounds. Now move your hearing to outside into nature and, depending on where you are located, notice any sounds coming from outside. Now bring your attention to your eyes and your sense of seeing. Allow yourself to look out a window and simply let go of your attention to the objects in nature (or in the apartment building across the street). Wait a minute or two and close your eyes and bring your attention back to the space between your eyes. Wait a minute and open your eyes and let go of your attention once again to an object in nature outside the window. Repeat for a couple of minutes and then take a deep breath and relax.

Prenatal and Perinatal Pain Perception

Acknowledgment by the medical community of the capacity of prenates to experience their environment, including their capacity to perceive pain, has been a slow process. Until the late 1980s, the medical community believed that it was *unnecessary* to anesthetize premature and full-term infants who required major surgery, because these infants did not have the capacity to perceive pain. It was also believed that the anesthesia was too dangerous. As a result of these beliefs, premature and full-term newborns underwent major surgery unanesthetized. They were routinely given a form of curare to paralyze their muscles for surgery, rendering them incapable of movement, and also of expressions of pain and protest (Chamberlain, 1999).

At this time, Jill Lawson, a parent, became aware of the fact that her premature baby (and many others) had undergone major surgery without the benefit of anesthesia. In those years, this information was not usually given to parents whose babies were undergoing surgery. Lawson contacted the media and publicized this surgical practice and the poor outcomes for the many neonates who had these experiences (Chamberlain, 1999). The dissemination of this information, along with further research that revealed the capacity of premature babies and other neonates for pain perception, brought a change in medical practice. The administration of anesthesia was introduced into surgeries conducted on full-term newborns and premature babies. The research findings (Anand and Aynsley-Green, 1985; Anand, 1986; Anand and Hickey, 1987) demonstrated that infants perceive pain, need anesthesia, and tolerate it well, and suggested that neonates that had undergone surgery without the benefit of anesthesia may have been dying of metabolic and endocrine shock following these experiences.

Please keep in mind, individuals born prior to the mid-1980s (the youngest of whom are now in their early thirties) may have undergone major surgery as premature babies or full-term neonates without the benefit of anesthesia. The implicit imprints of these early overwhelming (and potentially traumatic) sensory experiences may be expressed in and resonate with current psychophysiological states.

Neonatal Assessment

Neurobehavioral and neurophysiological research has demonstrated that preterm babies are at greater risk for difficulties in social-emotional functioning and self-regulation at school age. Heidelise Als and her team have spent decades researching the impact on premature babies of their very early experiences in the neonatal intensive care unit and their subsequent development. In a recent study, Als, Duffy, McAnulty, Rivkin, and Vajapeyam (2004) investigated the impact of the *quality* of experience in the neonatal intensive care unit (NICU) on brain function and structure.

Als and her team had previously developed the Newborn Individualized Developmental Care and Assessment Program (NIDCAP). The development of the NIDCAP was based on the hypothesis that *environmental input may lead to altered pathway development due to unexpected and overwhelming sensory experience.* The researchers hypothesized that these unexpected and overwhelming sensory experiences may lead to deviant developmental functioning, especially of cortical association areas in the brain. The NIDCAP assesses neuro-organizational differences and disturbances in neonates and is used to both identify the individual needs of infants in the NICU and inform the quality of care provided to them to best support their development and capacity for regulation outside the womb.

In the research published in 2004, the NIDCAP was initiated with premature infants, 28–33 weeks gestation, within 72 hours of their admission to the intensive care unit. The results of this study by Als et al. (2004) demonstrated the effectiveness of the NIDCAP in enhancing brain function and structure in preterm babies and also provides further evidence that "the quality of experience before term may influence brain development significantly" (p. 846).

It is important to note, the capacity of a prenate to experience and react to its environment close to the end of a full-term pregnancy does not differ greatly from the capacity of a neonate to experience and react to its environment at and after birth. Thomson (2007) highlights the observation of DiPietro, Costigan, and Pressman (2002): "The postconceptual age at which birth normally occurs does not represent a significant transition in neurobehavioral development" (p. 1). Thomson elaborates:

> In other words, birth marks a change for respiratory functioning from fluid to oxygen, a more aerobic environment for brain development and increasingly more complex interpersonal sensory-affective engagements (Schore, 2001). But, it is only one developmental step amongst many that have already taken place. For the newborn, the seemingly new extrauterine experiences are more familiar than once thought. Preparation for extrauterine life is operational from embryonic through fetal development. (Thomson, 2007, p. 89)

In my view, it is imperative that practitioners in all fields who provide services to pregnant women and their partners acknowledge the artificial barrier that has been perceived to exist between prenatal and postnatal development and experience. This artificial barrier has veiled crucial aspects of human experience from the awareness of practitioners, prevented a deeper understanding of our development and behavior, and thus limited opportunities for healing in both patients and practitioners.

Somatic Practice 6: Mindfulness of Breathing

Repeat the practice of mindful breathing from Somatic Practice 2.

CHAPTER 18

Prenatal Autonomic Nervous System Development

by Ann Diamond Weinstein, PhD

Knowledge of prenatal development of the autonomic nervous system (ANS)—the system that is critical in regulating our psychophysiological state influenced by our neuroception of our internal and external environment—enhances our understanding of how the environment inside and outside a woman's body may affect the prenate during gestation, including the development and programming of its organs and systems. Kirby (2007) shows that when the heart starts beating at about 21 days post-fertilization, it is already being sensitized by a neurotransmitter of the parasympathetic nervous system (PNS). Then at 35 days post-fertilization the heart is sensitized by a neurotransmitter of the sympathetic nervous system (SNS). This back-and-forth pattern of development of the PNS and SNS branches of the autonomic nervous system continues through the entire time of pregnancy.

Porges (2011) explains that the ANS regulates homeostatic function and is composed of two subsystems, the parasympathetic (PNS) and sympathetic (SNS) nervous systems. "The PNS promotes functions associated with a growth and restorative system … [and is] concerned with the restoration and conservation of bodily energy and the resting of vital organs." Porges also describes the SNS, which "promotes increased metabolic output to deal with challenges from outside the body … [and] prepares the individual for the intense muscular activity required to protect and defend in response to external challenges" (p. 64).

In the human fetus, the development of the ANS mirrors the evolutionary development of this system in vertebrates. Porges notes: "The oldest circuits develop first and the newest circuit develops last, leaving it the most vulnerable to neural insult and the most sensitive to postpartum experience" (2011, p. 121).

Porges helps us understand the progression of development from the prenatal through postpartum period of the three major human adaptive behavioral strategies that are each supported by a distinct neural circuit involving the autonomic nervous system (ANS). These three adaptive defensive and social engagement behavioral strategies are:

- Immobilization—death feigning, whole-body freezing. Most mammals have the capacity to be immobilized. Immobilization is based on the dorsal motor nucleus of the tenth cranial nerve called the vagus. This nerve also regulates digestion and elimination in the gut tube and lowers heart rate.

- Mobilization—fight-flight behaviors. Depends on the sympathetic nervous system, which increases metabolic activity in the body by delivering more oxygen to the soft tissue system of the body by raising the heart rate and shunting blood from the core of the body to the extremities.

- Social communication or social engagement—facial expression, vocalization, listening. Depends on the newer, myelinated vagus coming from the nucleus ambiguous in the brain stem. Thus the vagus nerve originates in two different locations in the brain stem. The older system mentioned above and the newer system, which goes from the brain stem through the head and neck. The myelinated vagus supports calm states. It does this by constraining the influence of the sympathetic nervous system on the heart (Porges, 2004).

As described above, the oldest vertebrate autonomic system circuit is associated with immobilization or freezing behaviors. It is the earliest system to develop in utero, first appearing in the brain stem at 9 weeks gestation.

The sympathetic autonomic nervous system develops next. This system is associated with mobilization or fight-flight behaviors. Research in the prenatal development of the sympathetic nervous system is limited, but one study reported a link between fetal locomotor activity and increases in fetal heart rate between 16 and 20 weeks gestation. It is thought that increases in the fetal heart rate associated with fetal locomotor activity at this stage of gestation are due to, and evidence of, activity in the sympathetic nervous system. The likelihood that this behavior is evidence of sympathetic nervous system activity is also supported by the fact that the evolutionarily more advanced myelinated vagal circuit, a neural circuit that also affects heart rate, is not yet functional at this stage of gestation.

The unique features of the autonomic nervous system that support mammalian social behavior start to develop during the last trimester of fetal life. The functioning of this part of the autonomic nervous system is dependent upon myelination of neurons that begin at 23 weeks gestation, with the greatest increase occurring after 30 weeks gestation to approximately 6 months postpartum. Human infants are not born with a completely functioning myelinated vagal system. Their vagal system is only partially myelinated at birth (Porges, 2011, p. 128), but "sufficiently myelinated to allow the infant to signal a caregiver (by vocalizing or grimacing, for example) and to engage the social and nutrient aspects of the world (by gazing, smiling and sucking, for example)" (Porges, 2004, p. 22).

This information sparks curiosity about the *influence of experience* during the prenatal period on the development and programming of our ANS and thus our capacity for regulation and dysregulation over the lifespan. Based on Porges's work described above, several questions arise. First, what aspects of the prenate autonomic nervous system are functional at different points during gestation?

As noted above, in humans, up until 16 weeks gestation, only the oldest circuit in mammalian autonomic nervous system is developed. This may suggest that during this early period of gestation, the prenate's only defensive strategy option in reaction to what it experiences as aversive stimuli in the womb is immobilization or behavioral shutdown.

The research demonstrating evidence of sympathetic nervous system activity at 16–20 weeks gestation suggests that mobilization and fight-flight defensive behavioral strategies may be options for the prenate at this time, as it experiences its womb environment.

The most advanced neural circuit in the human ANS, the myelinated vagal system, develops from 23 weeks gestation through 6 months postpartum. This suggests that the capacity of this advanced neural circuit (when developed) to *inhibit* the excitatory influence of the sympathetic nervous system on the heart and metabolism, is *not* available to the prenate as it experiences its environment in the womb *until* the middle of the third trimester. One of the developmental benefits of a functional myelinated vagal system is that it expands our capacity to self-regulate and calm. This knowledge suggests that the adaptive behavioral strategies available to the prenate until the middle of the third trimester are limited to the earlier developing ANS neural circuits—initially shutdown behaviors and subsequently fight-flight behaviors.

In a description of the ANS circuits and the important contribution made by the myelinated vagal system to human social behavior after birth, Porges notes: "Without a functioning myelinated vagus, social behavior would be compromised, and more primitive defensive strategies, such as fight-or-flight mobilization … (mediated by the sympathetic nervous system) and shutdown behaviors (mediated by the unmyelinated vagal system) would be frequently expressed"

(2011, p. 126). Although Porges is not specifically referring to the prenatal period here, his statement supports the idea that the prenate's adaptive defensive strategies are limited by their gestational age and stage of development in utero.

The fact that the most advanced neural circuit is only partially myelinated and functional at birth has implications for the neonate's capacity for psycho-physiological regulation outside of the womb as well. If the prenate is born prematurely before 30 weeks gestation, it *will not* have the same adaptive resources provided by the partially functioning advanced neural circuit of the vagal system that would have developed, had the prenate been born at full term. Many premature babies are born before 30 weeks gestation and survive. Their behavior reflects the immaturity of their ANS system development.

In light of this information, it is important to consider the *quality of experience* of the woman and her prenate at any given time during gestation. As the mother's ANS shifts between regulated and dysregulated states while she interacts with her internal and external environment, we might ask, What is the functional capacity of her prenate's ANS at this point in its development? In other words, What adaptive physiological and behavioral strategies are available to the prenate as it experiences and reacts to the changing environment within its mother's womb over the course of the pregnancy?

Now that we know the prenate has the capacity for sensory experience, we can ask, *How* does the prenate *experience and react* to its environment at any given time during gestation and how can we observe their behavior? With the recent widespread use of ultrasound scans, observation of prenate behavior has become increasingly possible. One interesting study of prenate behavior was conducted by child psychotherapist and psychoanalyst Alessandra Piontelli (1992). In her book *From Fetus to Child,* she describes her observations of the ultrasound scans of eleven fetuses (three singletons and four sets of twins) several times over the course of their mothers' pregnancies.

Piontelli describes the fetuses' reactions to their womb environment and includes transcriptions of the conversations between the parents and the doctors during ultrasound examinations. These conversations are very instructive in terms of how the comments of the doctor about the behavior of the fetus(es) during the ultrasound affect the mother and her partner and how the behavior of the mother and her partner affect the behavior of the doctor.

The transcriptions reveal doctors' comments in which they share their interpretations of fetal behavior with the parents and attribute temperament styles to the prenate they project will continue after birth. They demonstrate no apparent regard for the fact that these statements might concern the mother and her partner and affect how they feel about their prenate in the present. Making negative temperament attributions to babies in the womb may also set up expectations for their behavior after birth that might affect parents' early interactions with their children and, in turn, their emerging attachment relationship. In addition, at times the practitioners' responses (and lack thereof) to the mother and her partner's questions during the exam reveal their impatience and lack of compassion, respect, and sensitivity for the patient, her partner, and her prenate. The lack of awareness on the part of the practitioners regarding the psychophysiological responses of these mothers, their partners, and their prenates to insensitive and disrespectful communications during this anxiously anticipated opportunity to "see" into the womb and connect reflect their lack of understanding about the implications and impact of prenatal experience on women, their partners, and their prenates, including those during treatment interactions.

Piontelli's research continued after the birth of the fetuses and through age four. During that period, she observed the children's development in their homes. Her observations and psychoanalysis of six children suggested to her that the children were deeply preoccupied with their experiences in the womb.

Other questions arise: What is the impact on the prenate's developing ANS of reactivity—particularly dysregulation—in its mother's ANS over the course of the pregnancy? How do the prenate's *patterns* of behavior and defensive strategies established in the womb shape the ongoing development and programming of their ANS and therefore the functioning of their ANS after birth and over their lifespan?

Paula Thomson's work sheds light on these questions. In her article, "Down Will Come Baby: Prenatal Stress, Primitive Defenses and Gestational Dysregulation" (2007), we gain insight into what she describes as "a prenatal relational model that outlines experience-dependent prenate development that is contingent on and concordant with maternal regulation and dysregulation. Not only anxiety, depression, and anger, but post-traumatic stress and dissociation in the mother may affect the neurobiology of the prenate" (Thomson, 2007, p. 85).

Behavioral Perinatology

DiPietro, Costigan, Nelson, Gurewitsch, and Laudenslager (DiPietro et al., 2008) note: "There are no direct neural connections between mother and fetus, but maternal experiences generate a cascade of physiological and neurochemical consequences that may alter the intrauterine milieu either directly or indirectly and thereby generate a fetal response" (p. 11).

Many contributions to our understanding of the maternal-prenate relationship have come from the field of behavioral perinatology—defined as "an interdisciplinary area of research that involves conceptualization of theoretical models and conduct of empirical studies of the dynamic time-, place-, and context-dependent interplay between biological and behavioral processes in fetal, neonatal, and infant life using an epigenetic framework of development" (Wadhwa et al., 2002, p. 150).

Research in behavioral perinatology has revealed a variety of short- and long-term impacts of maternal prenatal psychophysiological states, including stress, traumatic stress, anxiety, and depression on: (1) fetal development and behavior; (2) the risk for fetal intrauterine growth retardation; (3) premature birth; (4) the development of preeclampsia in women during pregnancy; (5) infant temperament; (6) infant cortisol levels; (7) negative behavioral reactivity in infancy; (8) intellectual and language functioning in toddlers; (9) emotional and cognitive problems in childhood; and (10) shortening of telomeres in DNA in young adults.

In the review article entitled "Impact of Maternal Stress, Depression and Anxiety on Fetal Neurobiobehavioral Development," Kinsella and Monk (2009) note that findings of the numerous studies they reviewed "are in line with the growing body of literature supporting the 'fetal origins hypothesis' that prenatal environmental exposures—including maternal psychologic state-based altera-tions in in utero physiology—can have sustained effects across the lifespan" (p. 425). For the purposes of this chapter, I will not focus on the long-term physi-cal health impacts of prenatal environmental exposures (cardiovascular disease, diabetes, hypertension, etc.) that have been demonstrated in many recent studies. Instead, I will focus on the neurobehavioral and mental health impacts of the maternal prenatal environment on the offspring. Kinsella and Monk point out that for many years there has been a focus on postnatal psychological distress, especially postpartum depression, but distressed psychological states, including depression, stress, and anxiety *do not occur more frequently or more severely after childbirth than during pregnancy* (p. 425). Vieten and Astin (2008) remind us of the work of Marcus, Flynn, Blow, and Barry (2003), and Flynn, Blow, and Marcus (2006) that suggest that pregnant women often do not receive screening, prevention, or treatment for their concerns related to their moods or experiences of stress (p. 67).

The following link will connect you to a brief clip from the film *Helping Children Heal: Trauma Brain and Relationship,* in which Bruce Perry describes how the maternal prenatal environment impacts the development and behavior of the prenate and neonate.

http://www.youtube.com/watch?v=AsCViRHzGHE

Much of the recent research suggests that the impacts of maternal prenatal stressors on their offspring are related to variations in the functioning of the maternal hypothalamic-pituitary-adrenal (HPA) axis. Recent research has illuminated the negative impact of maternal prenatal experiences of traumatic stress, chronic stress and common life stressors on offspring's neurodevelopment (Sandman and Davis, 2012; Talge, Neal, and Glover, 2007). The HPA is often considered to be the central regulatory system for psychologic distress (DiPietro et al., 2000).

Wadhwa and co-authors (2002) point out a significant observation related to the measures of stress that were most strongly associated with adverse outcomes: "Subjective measures of stress perception and appraisals are more strongly associated with adverse outcomes than measures of exposure to potentially stressful events or conditions" (p. 151). This illustrates the importance of gaining a deep understanding of women's perceptions of their experiences at this critical time in the prenatal development of their offspring, rather than just asking whether they have experienced specific events commonly identified as stressors.

Maternal Prenatal Anxiety, Depression, and Stress

Maternal prenatal anxiety and depression have also been shown to negatively affect women's offspring. Maternal anxiety and depression have been shown to "predict increased risk for neurodevelopmental disorders in children" and have also been associated with increased risk for future mental illness (Kinsella and Monk, 2009). The research suggests an association between prenatal anxiety and/or depression and: poor emotional adjustment in young children (O'Connor et al., 2003); HPA axis activation including attention deficit hyperactivity disorder symptoms in 8- to 9-year-olds (Van den Bergh and Marcoen, 2004); alterations in HPA axis activation in 4-month-olds (Kaplan, Evans, and Monk, 2007), as well as 10-year-olds (O'Connor et al., 2005); and 14- to 15-year-olds (Van den Bergh et al., 2008).

Research has revealed the relationship between cortisol levels and HPA activity associated with PTSD, depression, and experiences of stress (Lupien et al., 2009; Yehuda, 2002). Studies have also evaluated how much maternal cortisol passes through to the fetus. Studies demonstrate that 10–20 percent of maternal cortisol passes through to the fetus (Gitau et al., 1998; Glover et al., 2009). These findings suggest that at times of stress-induced activation of the maternal HPA axis, the level of cortisol that passes through to the prenate may be enough to exert long-term impacts on the prenate's developing brain (Kinsella and Monk, 2009, p. 435).

Tollenaar, Beijers, Jansen, Riksen-Walraven, and De Weerth (2011) describe three mechanisms through which prenatal maternal stress may affect fetal development. The first pathway, as suggested above, is through the dysregulation of maternal-fetal HPA axis and the passage of maternal cortisol across the blood-brain barrier of the fetus. The second pathway is based on the observation that prenatal maternal stress results in the reduction of the expression and activity of a particular enzyme produced in the placenta that normally regulates fetal exposure to maternal cortisol by changing it to its inactive form, cortisone. Reduction in the activity of this enzyme as a result of maternal stress allows higher cortisol concentrations to reach the fetus (Glover et al., 2009). The third pathway is based on research that suggests prenatal maternal stress reduces blood flow to the placenta through activation of the ANS and this leads to decreased availability of nutrients and oxygen to the fetus (Seckl, 2008). Kinsella and Monk (2009) note that two studies have been conducted on uterine artery blood flow and anxiety during pregnancy, and they have conflicting results—but measurements of uterine artery blood flow in each study were made at different times during pregnancy.

Thomson observes that these dysregulated maternal states during gestation affect the "structural-functional formations of the [prenate] LHPA axis [limbic hypothalamic-pituitary-adrenal axis] (Weinstock, 1997); the ANS (Coalson and Tomasek, 1992; Ng, 2000; Schweiger et al., 2004); the sensorimotor, vestibular, and proprioception systems (DiPietro et al., 2002); and the functional connectivity between limbic forebrain and midbrain/diencephalon regions (Shumake et al., 2004)" (Thomson, 2007, p. 90). In short, the prenate's experiences of dysregulated maternal psychophysiological states shape the establishment of their own either stable or unstable regulatory systems.

Davis and Sandman (2010) explain that during the prenatal period when fetal organs and systems are developing, they are vulnerable to both "organizing and disorganizing influences." These influences have "programming effects," which they describe as "the process by which a stimulus or insult during a vulnerable developmental period has long-lasting or permanent effect" (p. 131).

Thomson reminds us of the observations of Schore (1994) and Tucker (2001) that critical periods of accelerated growth that occur in various regions of the brain and autonomic nervous system render these regions vulnerable to excessive cell death. Thomson notes: "The entire gestational period is marked by multiple and overlapping neurobiological critical periods [and] can be considered a time of great prenate vulnerability" (2007, p. 90).

Somatic Practice 7: Mindfulness of Cardioception

Please practice mindfulness of cardioception, detailed in Somatic Practice 4.

CHAPTER 19

Impact of Maternal Psychophysiological States on the Development of the Prenate

by Ann Diamond Weinstein, PhD

A wealth of recent research in the fields of neurobiology, behavioral perinatology, and epigenetics has unveiled the relationship between maternal prenatal psychophysiological states and the development, behavior, and health of women's offspring over the course of their lifespan. I will provide a brief overview of some of the recent research that demonstrates this relationship.

Lupien and co-authors (2009) describe how stress hormones during the prenatal period affect brain structures involved in cognition and mental health. They emphasize the importance of timing and duration of exposure in the determination of specific effects on the brain, behavior, and cognition. The authors also acknowledge the role played by the interaction between gene effects and previous exposure to environmental adversity in determining specific impacts on brain structures, cognition, and mental health (p. 434).

These same authors provide an excellent summary of how the effects of stress (chronic, repeated exposure or single exposure to severe stress) at different stages in life "depend on the brain areas that are developing or declining at the time of the exposure" (p. 440). The authors describe the effects of stress on the brain during the prenatal period: "Stress in the prenatal period affects the development of many of the brain regions that are involved in regulating the hypothalamus-pituitary-adrenal (HPA) axis—that is, the hippocampus, the frontal cortex and the amygdala (programming effects)" (p. 440).

These authors also explain the relationship between early-life stress and reactivity to stress in adulthood:

Research now relates exposure to early-life stress with increased reactivity to stress and cognitive deficits in adulthood, indicating that the effects of stress at different periods of life interact. Stress triggers the activation of the hypothalamus-pituitary-adrenal (HPA) axis, culminating in the production of glucocorticoids by the adrenals. Receptors for these steroids are expressed throughout the brain; they can act as transcription factors and so regulate gene expression. Thus glucocorticoids can have potentially long-lasting effects on the functioning of the brain regions that regulate their release. (Lupien et al., 2009, p. 434)

The authors elaborate further on our psychophysiological reaction to a neuroception of threat and the role of the HPA axis in the stress system. (As mentioned above, HPA stands for the hypothalamic-pituitary-adrenal axis.) When the brain senses danger, a synchronized physiological response occurs between the autonomic nervous system, the neuroendocrine system, the neuroimmune system, and the metabolism of the body, down to a cellular level. The HPA axis or circuit is designed to shut off once the perceived stressor has been diminished. This allows the autonomic nervous system to return to a window of tolerance and optimal functioning. However, when the HPA axis is being triggered by the amygdala, which is the fear center of the brain, the stress response can be more intense and enduring. This is because the amygdala retains memory from preverbal development, as does the HPA axis, which begins to develop three weeks post-fertilization (Lupien et al., 2009).

Kinsella and Monk (2009) suggest the possibility of environmental imprinting, a process by which prenates are conditioned by stimuli in the prenatal environment so they will be better prepared for the postnatal environment. They suggest that fetal and neonate behavior may be the result of perception and learning in the womb. Research supports this suggestion, but I will not be covering that here.

Epigenetics

It is important that we understand the most recent thinking on the relationship between nature and nurture, or the impact of the environment on the expression of genes. This leads us to the field of epigenetics, which studies "the process in which experience alters the regulation of gene expression by way of changing the various molecules (histones and methyl groups) on the chromosome" (Siegel, 2012b, AI-30).

Bruce Perry provides an introduction:

Genes are merely chemicals. And without "experience"—with no context, no micro-environmental signals to guide their activation or deactivation—[they] create nothing. And "experiences" without a genomic matrix cannot create, regulate or replicate life of any form. The complex process of creating a human being—and humanity—requires both. (Perry, 2002, p. 81)

Meaney (2010) explains the role of epigenetics in human development based on recent research:

The recent integration of epigenetics into developmental psychobiology illustrates the processes by which environmental conditions in early life structurally alter DNA, providing a physical basis for the influence of the perinatal environmental signals on phenotype over the life of the individual. (Meaney, 2010, p. 41)

As Thomson notes, the interaction between genes and environment serves a purpose—it "specifically tailors the unborn for the world it is to enter" (Thomson, 2007, p. 90).

Bethany Hayes (2007) elaborates on this concept. She describes early development as an epigenetic process whereby the developing organism plays an active role in its own construction. The interactive process of development is affected by systems that are present during embryonic and fetal life to acquire information about the nature of the environment and to use this information to guide development.

Sandman and Davis (2012) note that the "human placenta is both a sensory and effector organ that incorporates and transduces information from its maternal host environment into the fetal developmental program." They further explain that detection of stress signals in the maternal environment by the "fetal/placental unit" alerts the fetus of a threat to survival. As a result, "the fetus adjusts its developmental trajectory and modifies its nervous system to ensure survival in a potentially hostile postpartum environment" (p. 446).

Research in epigenetics has largely been conducted on animals and reveals the transmission of environmental effects across generations over the animal's lifetime. A recent study conducted on humans, by Entringer, Epel, Kumsta, Lin, Heilhammer, et al. (2011) illuminates the impact of prenatal maternal psychophysiological states on the DNA of her offspring that is evidenced when the child reaches young adulthood. The study evaluated the relationship between maternal psychosocial stress exposure during pregnancy on telomeres, a DNA protein complex, in offspring at young adulthood. Telomeres are DNA-protein complexes that cap chromosomal ends and promote chromosomal stability. Telomere length is a marker of cellular aging in young adulthood; shorter telomere length is a sign of increased cellular aging (Entringer et al., 2011, pp. 13377–13378):

> [M]aternal psychosocial stress exposure during gestation is a significant predictor of the offspring's subsequent leukocyte telomere length…. This in turn suggests that the trajectory of cellular aging in humans may be influenced by stress in intrauterine life, thereby potentially increasing the susceptibility of prenatally stressed individuals for complex, common age-related diseases. (Entringer et al., 2011, p. 13378)

Davis and Sandman (2010) conducted research on the consequences of prenatal maternal stress for infant mental and motor development. They evaluated maternal cortisol and psychological state during pregnancy five times, and at 3, 6, and 12 months postpartum. Their findings highlight the importance of: (1) the timing of exposure to organizing and disorganizing influences, and (2) the developmental stage of organs systems in the determination of programming effects on the offspring. Their research revealed that exposure to elevated concentrations of cortisol early in gestation was associated with a slower rate of development over the first postnatal year and lower scores on the mental development index of the Bayley Scales of Infant Development (BSID) at 12 months. Interestingly, elevated levels of maternal cortisol late in pregnancy were associated with accelerated development over the first year and higher scores on the BSID (p. 131).

In 2011, Davis, Glynn, Wafarn, and Sandman's research provided evidence that prenatal "exposure to maternal cortisol and psychosocial stress exerts programming influences on the developing fetus with consequences for infant stress regulation" (p 119). The authors explain that their study demonstrates that:

> prenatal maternal stress and stress hormones alter the functioning of stress regulator systems in the offspring, independent of postpartum influences, and may be a potential mechanism for fetal programming of later psychiatric disorders. Although the observed associations are likely not explained by postnatal influences, it is highly likely that the prenatal and postnatal environment will jointly determine developmental trajectories (e.g., Bergman et al., 2008). (Davis et al., 2011, p. 127)

Primitive Reflexes

As you can see from the few studies on human mothers and their offspring mentioned above (there are many, many more), there is increasing evidence of the impacts of prenatal maternal psychophysiological states on the development and functioning of crucial systems in the offspring that are expressed over the offspring's lifetime.

Thomson (2007) suggests another way maternal stress can alter prenate neurobiological attachment and stress systems. One way is by shaping the development of prenate "fixed action patterns" that are "built from primitive defensive reflex activation" (p. 85). Thomson points out that these patterns bias the offspring's defensive, mating and caregiving behaviors "toward survival in a threatening world and may be more readily transmitted to subsequent generations" (p. 85).

Ogden, Minton, and Paine (2006) refer to Llinas's description of fixed action patterns as "sets of well defined motor patterns, ready made 'motor tapes' … that, when switched on, produce well-defined coordinated movements; the escape response" (Llinas, 2001, p. 133).

Thomson (2007) explains that prenates exhibit similar behavioral and physiological dysregulation while in the womb to traumatized premature babies in the neonatal intensive care unit (NICU). Close observation of premature babies in the neonatal intensive care unit has revealed the limited range of behavioral strategies that are available and functioning in the fetus earlier in prenatal development.

Thomson (2007) provides evidence that prenates' stress responses occur and are contingent on maternal stress. She directs our attention to the prenate's display of a nonverbal vocabulary (motor behavior) that portrays their distress. If we accept that nonverbal behavior in the context of the adult therapeutic relationship provides meaningful communication about an individual's state, perhaps we can begin to open to the possibility that the nonverbal behavior—the language of the prenate (and neonate)—also provides meaningful information about their state. Since sensory neurons differentiate beginning at 28 days postfertilization, even the embryo begins sensing and responding to its environment via a primitive nervous system. A resting heart rate for an embryo can be as high as 200 beats per minute, but will increase due to stress coming from the maternal environment. Stress states can also be recognized in the embryo and fetus by the presence of elevated neurotransmitters modulating stress, such as norepinephrine, cortisol and corticotropin releasing hormone. Patterns of greater physiological reactivity in the fetus may also appear to be prolonged states of stillness, disorganized movement patterns, facial grimacing and other signs of discomfort, as well as disruption in the sleep-wake cycle (Thomson, 2007).

Thomson hypothesizes that attachment behavior—particularly infant disorganized behavior—may have its origins in the prenatal period. This pattern of behavior may evolve from the development of primitive reflexes prenatally.

The basic organismic movement prenatally is to move toward nutrition and supportive behaviors and to withdraw from noxious stimuli. Since the prenate has limited ability to move its location to avoid danger, it must then use its biological systems to withdraw from the stimulus and inhibit the development of its sensorimotor systems. These type of "fixed action patterns" (Llinas, 2001) are deeply connected to the whole neuroendocrine immune axis that starts developing in an embryo when it is smaller than the fingernail on our little finger. It is well established that these complex physical and metabolic patterns can thwart normal development through the lifespan (Thomson, 2007).

Thomson emphasizes the principles of experience-dependent maturation and suggests that the effects of unresolved states of mind about trauma and/or loss in parents may not only be transmitted during infant caregiver interactions in the *postnatal* period (Hesse et al., 2003; Lyons-Ruth and Jacobvitz, 1999), but "may also be physiologically transmitted from the pregnant mother to the prenate" (Amiel-Tison et al., 2004; Huizink, Mulder, and Buitelaar, 2004, p. 87).

Unresolved Emotions

Unresolved states of mind about trauma and/or loss may follow reproductive experiences including spontaneous miscarriage, elective abortion, ectopic pregnancy (a life-threatening event where the embryo implants in the fallopian tube rather than the uterus, often requiring emergency surgery), stillbirth, as well as the birth of a premature baby and experiences of the baby's care in the neonatal intensive care unit.

Unresolved states of mind may also follow experiences related to reproductive endocrinology treatment for infertility including loss of eggs and embryos during in vitro fertilization treatment (IVF) and loss of one or more embryos or fetuses during a multiple pregnancy, through spontaneous miscarriage or elective pregnancy reduction procedures following IVF. There is a higher incidence of premature birth in women who undergo IVF treatment. Finally, these states of mind may also persist in parents who have suffered the loss of a child any time after its birth.

If you're interested in reading more about pregnancy reduction, the following link will take you to the *NY Times Magazine* article, August 14, 2011:

http://www.nytimes.com/2011/08/14/magazine/the-two-minus-one
-pregnancy.html?pagewanted=all

Gayle Peterson (1994) describes the impact on subsequent pregnancies of previous perinatal loss, especially in women who continue to suffer from PTSD. Peterson explains that women who have suffered previous perinatal loss experience additional emotional challenges in a new pregnancy. These include fear of another loss, "which has impact, not only on attachment to the unborn fetus, but also may precipitate heightened fear and panic states throughout pregnancy and into the labor process" (p. 149).

Peterson also points out that as these women approach a pregnancy that follows the pregnancy that was lost, they may re-experience feelings of attachment and loyalty to the lost child, which often makes it difficult for them to form an attachment to the next pregnancy. She notes that the disruption in bonding and attachment that can occur in these situations can have a "substantial impact on successive generations" (1994, p. 149).

Through her work counseling women in the prenatal and perinatal period, Peterson has observed: "Women who have absorbed the impact of their mother's unresolved prenatal loss during their own childhood are particularly vulnerable to high levels of anxiety and fear during pregnancy, childbirth and the ongoing maternal-child relationship" (p.150).

If we accept that unresolved states of mind about trauma and/or loss can be physiologically transmitted from the pregnant mother to the prenate, we might ask the following questions: How might a patient's own mother's unresolved states of trauma and/or loss have affected her during development in her mother's womb? How might these imprints be affecting experiences in the present of attempting to or actually conceiving her own child? How might these imprints affect her experience of being pregnant, giving birth, bonding, infant feeding, and the development of an attachment relationship with her own child? How might these imprints shape her neuroception?"

Gayle Peterson refers to the experience of women whose mothers suffered unresolved perinatal loss as "second generational unresolved grief." She observes that this issue is often unrecognized and therefore untreated. She suggests that, when a woman's mother suffered from unresolved perinatal grief during the time of the woman's conception, pregnancy, birth, and childhood, the woman herself may exhibit symptoms of survivor's guilt, which can be "identified in women who experienced a sense of responsibility to 'fill in for' or 'make up' the loss for their own mother" (1994, p. 150).

Peterson notes that women who have been affected by their mother's unresolved perinatal grief during their gestation and childhood are "particularly vulnerable to high levels of anxiety and fear during pregnancy, childbirth and the ongoing maternal-child relationship. These women tend toward significant expectations of loss in their own pregnancies, childbirths and parenthood" (1994, p. 150). If these maternal psychophysiological states are not addressed, the next generation may also suffer the impacts of unresolved grief.

Women may also experience unresolved states of mind about other traumatic events, including trauma that may follow conception resulting from a rape, or that occurs as a result of intimate partner violence and other abuse over the course of a woman's pregnancy. The psychophysiological states that follow these experiences are likely to affect her developing prenate.

CHAPTER 20

Consequences of Maternal Traumatic Stress Experience

by Ann Diamond Weinstein, PhD

The research of Yehuda, Engel, Brand, Seckl, Marcus, et al. (2005) demonstrates the transgenerational effects on the offspring of women with post-traumatic stress disorder (PTSD). The authors examined the relationship between maternal PTSD symptoms and salivary cortisol levels in infants of mothers directly exposed to the World Trade Center collapse on 9/11/2001 during their pregnancy. The study results support previous evidence of the importance of the timing of prenate exposure in determining postnatal effects. Lower cortisol levels were observed in both mothers and babies of mothers who developed PTSD in response to their experience of the WTC attacks, as compared with mothers who did not develop PTSD. Lower cortisol levels have been associated with PTSD and, in the acute aftermath of trauma, lower cortisol levels have also been associated with prior traumatization. Lower cortisol levels were most apparent in babies born to mothers with PTSD, who were exposed to the event in their third trimester of gestation (p. 4116).

Research by Khashan, McNamee, Abel, Mortensen, Kenny, Pederson, et al. (2009) demonstrates an association between maternal exposure to severe life events before conception and during the first trimester of pregnancy, and the risk of preterm birth, including instances when the exposure occurred six months prior to conception. They found an especially high risk of very preterm birth in women who experienced severe life events in older children in the first trimester. In addition, the authors found that women who had a previous baby born preterm and experienced severe life events in the six months before conception of the current pregnancy had a significantly increased incidence of preterm, very preterm, and extremely preterm birth in the current pregnancy (p. 6).

Bruce Perry sheds light on the long-term impact of maternal prenatal states on women's offspring. Perry has worked extensively with severely traumatized children and their parents. In a personal communication, Dr. Perry shared with me one of the unpublished observations from a study he and his team conducted, which focused on the impacts of prenatal drug exposure on children. Perry explained:

> [S]tress/distress/chaos/violence in the pregnant mother was more likely to be associated with poor outcomes than cocaine exposure… And we are finding very strong correlations between intrauterine distress/chaos/disruption and poor outcomes in the offspring—including all the way into young adult life. (personal communication, January 20, 2012)

Some of the stress and distress that women and their partners may experience during pregnancy may relate to feelings about the pregnancy itself. Women and their partners often face difficult decisions and ambivalent feelings in early pregnancy that may evoke a range of psychophysiological states that may imprint the experience and development of their prenate. If a woman attempts to terminate a pregnancy, but is unsuccessful, her baby, an "abortion survivor," may manifest long-term impacts of that imprinted experience in their health, development, and behavior. Babies that are given up for adoption carry the imprints of those early experiences (Karr-Morse and Wiley, 2012; Sonne, 2004; Verny and Weintraub, 2002).

The prenates who survive the prenatal death of their sibling(s) in utero (in the case of a multiple pregnancy), either through spontaneous miscarriage or elective pregnancy reduction following in vitro fertilization treatment (IVF), or the death of their sibling(s) (twin or triplet) in the NICU, also carry the imprints of these experiences. These imprints may be expressed in psychophysiological symptoms and states over the course of their lifetime.

Birth Processes and Trauma

There is now research that demonstrates the long-term impacts on offspring of their experiences during the birth process. Difficult births, pain-inflicting interventions (experienced by the baby) during birth, and neonatal experiences of pain have been correlated with self-destructive behaviors in adolescents, including suicide and drug abuse. Anand and Scalzo (2000) suggest that the imprints of traumatic birth experiences on the brain account for increasing rates of self-destructive behaviors in adolescents. An epidemiological study correlated the birth and death records of male victims of violent suicides—death by hanging, gun, jumping, or strangulation. The study found that most of the victims were born by forceps or vacuum extraction deliveries and in addition, experienced resuscitation and other pain-inflicting interventions at birth, compared to matched controls who died of other causes (as cited in Karr-Morse and Wiley, 2012).

Anand and Scalzo (2000) also reported on another study, in which a cluster of several factors were correlated with increased risk of suicide in adolescents. These included lack of care following birth, chronic maternal disease during pregnancy, and compromised breathing in the newborn. In addition to these factors, a correlation was made between sedatives given to mothers who didn't need them during birth and increased risk for subsequent drug abuse in the offspring. The authors explain: "The use of multiple doses of opiates, barbiturates and nitrous oxide during birth was linked to subsequent opiate or amphetamine addiction in adolescent children" (Anand and Scalzo, 2000, as cited in Karr-Morse and Wiley, 2012, p. 89). The study also revealed a stronger correlation between obstetric factors and later drug abuse in the offspring than between socioeconomic factors and addiction (also cited in Karr-Morse and Wiley, 2012, p. 89).

I do wonder how the researchers who conducted the study determined whether the women in the study "needed" the sedatives. I am curious about who made that assessment.

Penny Simkin, physical therapist, founder of Doulas of North America (DONA), doula trainer, birth doula, childbirth educator, and author, notes that pain in labor and birth, if it is overwhelming, becomes traumatic. The offspring of women who are psychophysiologically overwhelmed during labor and birth are affected by their mothers' experiences during that time, as well as their own experiences of uterine contractions and their passage through the birth canal. Traumatic births affect the quality of interactions between mothers and their babies immediately after birth and in the early postnatal period. These interactions may interfere with the establishment of a healthy early attachment relationship.

Peter Levine, developer of the Somatic Experiencing® approach to healing trauma, is the co-author, along with Maggie Kline, of *Trauma Through a Child's Eyes* (Levine and Kline, 2007). Levine and Kline provide a description of a child whose birth and early postnatal experiences were overwhelming and who suffered from the imprints of those experiences. The authors' description of the work with eight-year-old Devin illuminates the lived-body manifestations of prenatal and neonatal experiences, as well as the opportunities for healing that emerge from the expression of these experiences and an understanding of their meaning in play therapy. Devin presented with several diagnoses, including ADHD, auditory processing deficit, sensory integration dysfunction, and dyspraxia. His symptoms included hyperactivity, aggressive outbursts, focusing difficulties, and trouble completing assignments. Devin was also reported to be a daydreamer at school (a term often used by parents and teachers to describe a dissociative child) and had terrifying nightmares.

Levine and Kline recount the challenges and stressors that occurred during Devin's mother's pregnancy, difficult birth, and complicated early postnatal period:

> After taking a birth history, it was discovered that Maria, Devin's mom, had been on medication and bed rest since her twenty-first week of pregnancy to prevent preterm labor and premature birth. At thirty-seven weeks she went off meds, hoping to begin a natural labor. After Maria's water broke, her contractions were too weak to move the labor along so she was induced with Pitocin. Due to severe pain, she was given narcotics. There was concern about the low level of amniotic fluid, and Devin was under distress for a couple of hours before the medical staff discovered that the umbilical cord was wrapped around his neck three times. Suctioning was used, and he was blue at birth… Three weeks after his birth, Devin was hospitalized due to jaundice and high bilirubin levels. He was tested for a blood disorder. His mother described his condition as follows: "His red blood cells were bursting. He was diagnosed with hemolytic anemia. Weekly blood draws were taken, as Devin was held down screaming, to monitor his health."

It is important to consider the potential impacts on Devin of his mother's psychophysiological states during pregnancy, labor, birth, and the early postnatal period, as well as the stress and life threat Devin may have experienced directly throughout this period of time. It is likely that Devin's mother experienced a range of emotions including anxiety and/or fear about being able to sustain the pregnancy and avoid preterm labor or a premature birth. It is likely she also experienced great concern about the potential health problems and survival risk associated with premature babies.

Levine and Kline provide the therapist's report on play therapy sessions with Devin. This report illuminates the impact of his prenatal and early postnatal experiences and the way he expressed them through play in interactions with his therapist.

> Devin drew a rocket complete with rocket-launcher and trailer. "The astronaut," he explained, "was glued inside, and it would take ten seatbelts to make it safe, and he would have to wear two astronaut suits to come out because it's so cold out there."

He also drew the astronaut's lifeline, attaching it to the rocket. Next, he got our undivided attention when he announced, "The cord is the most important part." (Levine and Kline, 2007, p. 294)

Levine and Kline (2007) describe later play therapy sessions during which Devin demonstrated frustration and anger that was validated by the therapist. The therapist describes Devin's behavior during one session, when asked to choose something that might help him calm down after an angry outburst:

> Without wasting any time, he reached for the stack of pillows and began building a tunnel using the legs of a chair as a frame. Then he squeezed his body through it little by little. He turned himself around and proceeded with a little resistance on the top of his head. Remarkably, before he got all the way through he reached out for an electrical cord that was nearby and began wrapping it around his neck—just like the umbilical cord was wrapped! Gently he was assisted to unwrap it and continue his journey through the tunnel. After coming through the tunnel at his own pace, Devin crawled over to hug his mother, who was there to receive him... Maria reported that after that session, his frustration outbursts ended both at school and at home... After a four-month follow-up, Devin continued to cope with challenges free of tantrums, according to his mother. (Levine and Kline, 2007, p. 295)

Levine and Kline report that Devin continued to have difficulty regulating his behavior when stressed. They comment that Devin feels frightened to the point of terror when he is stressed. He experiences a sensation that he describes as "life or death." The authors note that this feeling is linked to holding in his breath and his belly. "All of his peculiar behaviors appear to be a courageous and ambitious attempt to guard against feeling the sensations of terror again that he presumably felt during and following his birth" (2007, pp. 295–296).

Parents and babies may also experience trauma when there is secrecy and shame around their conception, pregnancy, and birth, and when babies are given up for adoption soon after birth. Myriam Szejer, a child psychiatrist and psychoanalyst who practices on a maternity unit in France, has worked with these babies, some of whom have failure-to-thrive symptoms as newborns. Many women come to the hospital in which she works from other countries to have their babies when the circumstances around their conception and pregnancy are such that their own life is in danger and the option to terminate the pregnancy was unacceptable, unavailable, or dangerous. Some of these babies are given up by their parents as a result of these untenable circumstances and are cared for by the state or adopted.

Over the course of her clinical career, Dr. Szejer has come to understand the critical importance of *Talking to Babies: Healing with Words on a Maternity Ward* (the title of her book, 2005) in the very first days after birth. She has found it is especially helpful to talk to babies who are failing to thrive about the specific situations into which they have been born, including the problematic aspects of their histories, such as the death of a twin sibling or the death of a baby before them. She has found it is best if this can occur in the presence of their mothers and fathers. If this is not possible, it is still helpful to the baby for a respectful, compassionate other to explain to him or her the specific situations into which he or she has been born. In some instances, babies may exhibit symptoms of failing to thrive when they are being relinquished to the state for care with the hope someone will adopt them. Dr. Szejer has found it is crucial to their survival at times that they be told gently what is happening, who is caring for them, where they will be going, and who will be caring for them when they get there.

Women and their partners who themselves were given up by their biological parents and raised by adoptive or foster parents may face a range of psychophysiological states as they attempt to conceive and experience the pregnancy, birth, and early postnatal period of their own child. These states may also influence their offspring's development. Their own biological child may be the first and only blood relative with whom they've had a face-to-face relationship.

I would like to suggest that when we observe dyadic interactions between caregivers and their infants and/or children, either in person or on films of these interactions, we are observing the expressions—the manifestations of the imprints of the caregiver's and child's past experiences, *including each of their prenatal and birth experiences.* Given what we know today about the transgenerational transmission of dysregulated states, the origins of dysregulated, aggressive, and dissociated behavior in caregivers can often be found in the caregivers' own earliest experiences. Without knowing the full history, including the prenatal history of the caregiver, our understanding of the interaction we are witnessing may be limited.

Somatic Practice 8: Mindfulness of Transitions

Take several moments to practice mindfulness of your body and breathing. As you go through your day, it is full of many transitions. There are big transitions, such as getting up, getting dressed, having breakfast, going to work. What is your style of transition? Do you go fast or slow? Are you easily irritated or have no feelings at all about such a transition? Another big transition is going on a business or vacation trip. What is your style of packing your bag, getting to the airport, going through security, boarding a plane? Does your heart rate go up or down during that type of a transition? Are you impatient with security and gate agents? Or are you very patient and board the plane at the very last call? Being mindful of transitions and one's body and breath creates equanimity and peacefulness, unless, of course, your flight is cancelled. You can even bring attention to small transitions, like moving from your computer screen to the kitchen to have a break. It's all about style and seems to be imprinted from our conception and birth experiences.

Empathy

An essential aspect in witnessing these interactions is to hold compassion for the caregiver who may exhibit behaviors that are clearly dysregulating and misattuned to the child's needs, even though these misattunements may be activating to the observer and difficult to witness. One way to support this compassionate state is to remind ourselves that we don't know *what* the caregiver's earliest experiences were and, more important, *how* the impacts of those experiences have shaped their current behavior with their children. In fact, it is more than likely the caregivers themselves are not aware of the impacts of their own earliest experiences, or even the circumstances of their own conception, gestation, and birth. This contributes to the mystery surrounding their own psychophysiological programming that may be fueling their behavior and their experiences of dyadic interactions with their children.

How many of us have been offered the details of our conception, gestation, and birth? How many of us have asked our parents the details of these experiences? How many parents have secrets about these experiences and choose not to share them with us? How many of us have lost our parents and can no longer have a conversation with them about these experiences? Perhaps most important, how many of us live with an implicit sense, a shadow, of these experiences, but do not have explicit memory or narratives with which to connect them?

Research on Women's Experiences of Violence

The research literature on women's experiences of trauma demonstrates that a substantial number of women are survivors of violent experiences, in particular rape or sexual assault, child sexual and/or physical abuse, and partner violence. Many survivors suffer from traumatic stress symptoms, which result from a single or multiple traumatic events and can lead to the development of the chronic psychophysiological symptoms of PTSD for years following these experiences. Traumatic stress symptoms are one aspect of the lived body's expression of past trauma. The imprints or inscriptions (Kirkengen, 2001) of traumatic experiences are embodied and often manifested in the health of the individual as adaptations and/or disturbances in psychophysiological processes, systems, and behavior.

Research demonstrates that the physiological systems in the body that are affected by trauma, in particular, the neuroendocrine, immunological, and vasomotor systems, also play crucial roles in conception and the ability to sustain a pregnancy (Cwikel, Gidron, and Sheiner, 2004; Dobson et al., 2003; Ferin, 1990; Gallinelli et al., 2001; Norwitz, DSchust, and Fisher, 2001; Uvnäs-Moberg, 2003).

The majority of women who have been victims of violence were exposed to trauma *well before or during their childbearing years and many to trauma that breached their body boundaries and involved the parts of their bodies involved in reproductive processes.*

The following statistics give you a sense of the prevalence of these experiences in women's lives prior to or during the period in which they attempt to or actually conceive, are pregnant, give birth, and begin to establish their postnatal relationship with their babies.

Plichta and Falik (2001) report on the Commonwealth Fund's 1998 Survey of Women's Health, which projected that more than "four out of ten women in the U.S. are likely to have experienced one or more forms of violence including child abuse (17.8 percent), physical assault (19.1 percent), rape (20.4 percent), and intimate partner violence (34.6 percent)" (p. 244).

Kilpatrick, Edmunds, and Seymour (1992) reported on the National Women's Study, which found that "one out of every eight adult women, or at least 12.1 million American women, has been the victim of forcible rape sometime in her lifetime" (p. 2). This study also revealed that age at the time of rape as reported by the women surveyed was less than 11 years old in 29.2 percent, 11–17 years old in 32.3 percent, 18–24 years old in 22.2 percent, and 25–29 years old in 7.1 percent (p. 3).

In a study of the prevalence of adult sexual assault in a general population sample conducted by Elliot, Mok, and Briere (2004), 22 percent of the 472 female participants reported experiences of adult sexual assault. Fifty-nine percent of the women who reported experiences of adult sexual assault also reported experiences of childhood sexual abuse (p. 203). In a study of the prevalence of self-reported childhood physical and sexual abuse in a general population sample (Briere and Elliot, 2003), 32.3 percent of the women participants reported "childhood experiences that satisfied the criteria for sexual abuse" and 19.5

percent of the women participants reported experiences that "met criteria for physical abuse" (p. 1205).

Tjaden and Thoennes (2000) reported on the prevalence of male-to-female intimate partner violence (IPV) as measured by the National Violence Against Women Survey. Survey data included the lifetime incidence of intimate partner violence. Among the women respondents, 4.5 percent "reported being raped by a current or former marital/opposite sex cohabitating partner at some point in their lifetime … 20.4 percent of the women reported being physically assaulted by a current or former marital/opposite-sex cohabitating partner at some time in their lifetime" (p. 151).

Studies vary widely in their findings of the prevalence of intimate partner violence during pregnancy, depending on the specificity of the assessment tool and whether verbal abuse as well as physical abuse is included. One U.S. study (Bailey and Daugherty, 2007) that used a detailed and behaviorally specific tool (the Conflict Tactics Scale) found that "81 percent of prenatal patients at a family practice clinic reported some type of IPV during pregnancy; 28 percent reported physical IPV, and 20 percent reported sexual violence" (as cited in Bailey, 2010, p. 185).

A cohort of woman who have experienced trauma may currently experience, have experienced in the past, or will experience symptoms of post-traumatic stress disorder. Knowledge of the prevalence of violence against women and the psychophysiological impacts associated with it enhance our understanding of the challenges a substantial number of women face during the pre-conception through early postnatal period.

Estimates of the prevalence of lifetime PTSD among women of all ages range from 10.4 percent to 12.3 percent, with rates of 25–50 percent among women exposed to abuse or assault trauma (Seng et al., 2001). Kilpatrick et al. (1992) note: "Almost one-third (31 percent) of all rape victims developed PTSD sometime in their lifetimes" (p. 7). In another study, Kilpatrick et al. (1989) noted that of women who experienced completed rape, perceived life threat, and injury, almost 80 percent developed PTSD (as cited in Resnick et al., 1993, p. 984).

Health Impacts of Past Experiences of Trauma

These statistics demonstrate *that* there is a relationship between adverse experience and health, but, as Anna Luise Kirkengen, MD, PhD, illuminates in her groundbreaking book *The Lived Experience of Violation: How Abused Children Become Unhealthy Adults* (2010), the exploration of *how* such experience, particularly violation and trauma, has been inscribed into the lived body may reveal the meaning the experience has for the individual. Recognition of the lived-body expression of that "incarnate experience" (Kirkengen, 2008) and its meaning may expand opportunities for healing.

Kirkengen reminds us of the value of holding presence with and witnessing an individual's lived-body expression of traumatic experiences, especially experiences of "shaken embodiment" (Behnke, 2003), no matter when, over their lifetime, the experiences occurred. Kirkengen (2001) explains:

> It is thus our task as phenomenologists [I would suggest health and mental health care practitioners as well] to learn to *hear* the silent sounds of the body passed over in silence, to listen instead of shouting it down—particularly when this body is "mutely testifying" to unspeakable violations that have been "socially silenced." (as cited in Behnke, 2003, p. 8)

Kirkengen's work (2010) suggests that it is essential that we consider *how* these experiences of trauma and violence may be expressed in women's behavior and health during the pre-conception through early postnatal period. It is crucial that we understand *how* a woman's reproductive experiences at this time, including normal lived body experiences of pregnancy can activate previously abated traumatic stress symptoms, exacerbate existing traumatic stress symptoms or trigger new ones. It is critical that we appreciate *how* the inscriptions of these experiences and their expression in women's lived bodies may affect women's offspring from the prenatal period through the establishment of their early attachment relationship.

In the work of Wadhwa, Glynn, Hobel, Garite, Porto, et al. (2002) and Wadhwa (2005), we are reminded of the impact of the womb environment on the earliest programming of psychophysiological systems and processes. The authors explain that fetal organ systems and physiological processes are programmed in utero, including neuro-immuno-endocrinological and vasomotor processes *involved in both stress/trauma reactions and reproductive processes.* This work highlights the fact that the reproductive processes of the *prenate* are also programmed in utero and shaped by the womb environment. This is an additional concern associated with the impact of women's experiences during pregnancy.

In a recent study, Seng et al. (2010) found that "post-traumatic stress disorder is more prevalent in perinatal rather than general samples of women (6–8 percent versus 4–5 percent)" (p. 176). The authors suggest that "psychological aspects of pregnancy may increase vulnerability to PTSD, particularly when PTSD is the result of childhood sexual abuse trauma, intrafamilial abuse, previous pregnancy loss, prior traumatic birth, or when pregnancy is the result of sexual assault" (p. 177).

Seng et al. (2010) explain that psychological and physical processes associated with pregnancy are potentially triggering for past or recent trauma survivors, especially those who experienced sexual trauma. The psychological process of preparing for motherhood and developing an attachment to the prenate can be triggering for these women. The normal increase in breast sensitivity that develops early in pregnancy, as well as the experience of fetal movement can also be triggering. The labor, especially medicalized labor, may activate or exacerbate traumatic stress symptoms in trauma survivors.

The authors note that, despite the limited availability of prospective evidence:

> Investigations conducted postpartum have correlated pre-existing PTSD with experiencing birth as a traumatic event and have identified potential triggers; pain, feelings of powerlessness, negative interactions with health care providers, unmet expectations for labor, and medical interventions. (Seng et al., 2010, p. 177)

In women who have had in the past, or currently have traumatic stress symptoms, the normal physical changes of pregnancy may also affect their experience of PTSD symptoms. During pregnancy, women may experience increased heart and respiratory rates, shortness of breath, and nausea, which might feel similar to physical sensations associated with anxiety. Women may mistake the normal somatic changes of pregnancy with physical sensations associated with PTSD hyperarousal, and thereby trigger the cycle of hypervigilance, re-experiencing, and numbing (Seng et al., 2010).

Seng et al. also describe some of the extensive neuroendocrine changes during pregnancy that may affect the expression of PTSD symptoms. Pregnancy is associated with changes in the hypothalamic-pituitary-ovarian (HPO) axis, especially increases in plasma concentrations of progesterone and estrogen, which affect mood and cognition.

There are also changes during pregnancy in the HPA axis, among which are increases in plasma cortisol, the stress hormone. It is possible that the hormonal changes during pregnancy in both the HPA and HPO axes could affect the expression of PTSD symptoms by increasing the frequency and emotional intensity of traumatic memories, which then affect mood, motivation, social cognition, sleep, and concentration (Seng et al., 2010).

Somatic Practice 9: Mindfulness of Resilience

Take several moments to practice mindfulness of body and breathing. Resilience is a calm and peaceful state of mind that returns quickly after a stressor or upsetting experience. In your day or week, there are always stressful experiences. How willing are you to move more quickly toward a calm state of mind after a stressful experience? Do you feel you have no control over how you get back to a calm state of mind? Resilience is the hard work of self-regulation and noticing the choices you have during stressful events or, at the very least, noticing the choices you have as soon as the stressful event ends. Be willing to practice mindfulness of body and breathing during and after stressful events and make a commitment to becoming more resilient with such mindfulness.

When Survivors Give Birth

Penny Simkin and Phyllis Klaus (2004) have written an outstanding book on childhood sexual abuse entitled *When Survivors Give Birth*. The authors explain that although there aren't national statistics on the rate of childhood sexual abuse, the estimated incidence based on a number of recent studies is between 25 and 40 percent of girls and 20 and 25 percent of boys. Most perpetrators are male (10 males to 1 female). In more than 80 percent of the cases, the perpetrator is known to the child.

Simkin and Klaus point out that in the case of childhood sexual abuse, children often have few survival mechanisms available other than dissociation and loss of memory. They emphasize that the loss of memory of the abuse does not eliminate the pain; rather, "the pain finds its expression in indirect ways, through sexual behavior, physical or somatic manifestations, and psychosocial and mental health disturbances" (p. 22).

When Survivors Give Birth provides practitioners with an understanding of the range of psychophysiological behaviors that may be experienced by women in the pre-conception period, during pregnancy, birth, and postpartum that may indicate a past history of abuse, whether or not a woman has conscious recall of those experiences. Women who do have conscious recall of these experiences may choose not to share this information with practitioners. Whether or not a practitioner is aware of the connection between a woman's past experiences of childhood sexual abuse and her current psychophysiological dysregulation is not as important as the exploration of the woman's unique needs as she moves through this life transition. Helping a woman find ways to express and meet her needs, and assisting a woman in the development of internal and external resources that she can access as she faces challenges that may arise during pregnancy, birth, and the early postnatal period will support her prenate's development and reduce her chances of having a traumatic birth. Helping a woman take steps to reduce the potential for a traumatic birth may support the possibility of a positive birth experience. Imagine, for a moment, the difference between the quality of early maternal-infant interactions when a woman is experiencing new or recently exacerbated traumatic stress symptoms (including dissociative behaviors) as she interacts with her baby in the days following its birth, and the quality of interactions when she is free from traumatic stress symptoms after experiencing the birth of her baby as empowering and perhaps even healing.

Simkin and Klaus remind us that "it is most upsetting for a woman to discover or relive past trauma at a time when she would like to prepare to welcome a new baby" (p. 34). They also shed light on: (1) the possibility that pregnancy and childbirth may represent a challenge to *every* survivor, and (2) how a woman experiences her personal relationships and the quality of care she receives from professional caregivers at this time can make the difference between the confirmation of her self-worth and retraumatization (p. 34).

Simkin and Klaus include quotes and descriptions of some of the feelings of survivors of childhood sexual abuse during pregnancy. One woman expressed the following:

> From the moment of Joseph's conception I felt victimized—my body overtaken yet again, and when I learned the baby was a boy, just the thought of it was frightening—I didn't like the idea of a penis growing inside of me. (p. 33)

Another woman's doctor referred her to psychotherapy when she became ill while expecting her first baby and the treatment was unsuccessful, as related by Simkin and Klaus:

> Betty became severely ill and dehydrated with hyperemesis gravidarum (almost constant vomiting) and required hospitalization. After appropriate but unsuccessful medical treatment, her doctor recognized the possibility of an emotional link, and referred Betty for psychotherapy. Betty soon discovered she harbored a hidden fear that if her baby were a girl, the baby would not be safe. She realized that she was projecting some of her own prior lack of safety during childhood onto her unborn baby. This seemed to be causing the nausea and vomiting—which evoked memories of the nausea and vomiting she experienced after oral sexual abuse by her grandfather. Once this connection was made, she could "separate" the baby she was carrying from herself as a child in the past and the vomiting ceased. She learned to imagine a safe place where her baby would be protected from

harm. (Her safe place was in the arms of a guardian angel.) She also learned a method of mentally "containing" her abuse experiences to keep them from surfacing. (pp. 37–38)

Simkin and Klaus describe the experiences of another survivor whose sexual abuse began when she was a baby:

Emma was surprised to hear that other pregnant women talk with excitement about their unborn babies. She found the fetal movements annoying and even painful. She often had negative images and disturbing thoughts about the fetus. The thought of breastfeeding was abhorrent to her. She couldn't picture herself sharing her breasts. She worried that if the baby were a boy these feelings would be even worse. Emma needed help to bond prenatally with her baby. In exploring these disturbing thoughts with her therapist, she began to understand that she associated her negative feelings about the fetus with past abuse by her father, which began when she was a baby. Her feelings of being taken over as a baby were recreated when she felt taken over by her fetus. It was important for her to learn to visualize her fetus as a separate little being, independent from her abuse memories. This helped her to feel closer to her baby. (pp. 38–39)

Another survivor idealized her baby:

Holly saw her unborn baby as the saving hope of her unhappy life. She felt trapped in a loveless marriage, unable to turn to her husband for nurturing. She had enormous difficulty being intimate, tried to avoid sexual relations, and had numerous physical complaints. She had been sexually abused by a stepbrother throughout her teenage years and saw herself as having no power and little worth. She expected this baby to be her friend, someone to love her and to give her life meaning.

She was unconsciously displacing onto the baby her need to be taken care of and to be given what she had not received as a child. Being able to talk about some of these expectations in therapy helped her understand that they were unrealistic. She began to distinguish her own needs from what her baby would need, to recognize that she had the ability to assume the caretaking role with the infant. (pp. 39–40)

Discussion

During pregnancy and birth, many abuse survivors face issues related to control, helplessness, exposure of their bodies, restraints, immobilization, trust in their bodies, trust of strangers and authority figures, pain and especially genital pain, penetration of their bodies, and discomfort with new situations.

Medical examinations and procedures, doctor-patient interactions involved in gynecological and obstetrical care, and reproductive endocrinology treatment for infertility may activate the autonomic nervous systems of women. For women with trauma histories or current traumatic stress symptoms, settings and procedures that require them to remain immobile in vulnerable body positions can remind them of past trauma and elicit fight/flight/freeze responses (Hilden et al., 2003; Robohm and Buttenheim, 1996; Weitlauf et al., 2008). One such position is the position required during pelvic examinations, in which women lie on their backs with their feet in stirrups and knees separated while they are in close contact with medical providers. A woman's experience of the quality of care she receives greatly affects her psychophysiological state while she's attempting to conceive and during pregnancy, birth, and the early postnatal period. All women would benefit from receiving care provided with sensitivity. Supporting women in seeking out practitioners who have the capacity to provide sensitive care may be critical in preventing retraumitization of trauma survivors.

Impact of Practitioners' History of Trauma on Patient Care

When practitioners (health or mental health) themselves have a history of past trauma, they may be triggered by their patients' discussions of their abuse experiences or their behavior when their memories are triggered. If the caregiver provides prenatal, birth, and postpartum care to women and their partners, their behaviors in interactions with their patients may be shaped by their unresolved issues relating to their past trauma. This behavior may affect their patients' felt sense of safety, their psychophysiology, and treatment outcomes. Simkin and Klaus share the experiences of a female family doctor who attended births:

> Sherril, a family doctor, shared her story with us. As a family doctor who attended births, she had an unusually high rate of Cesarean sections—44 percent. She started psychotherapy to cope with other troubling events in her life. During therapy, she realized the association of her childhood abuse history with her absolute fear of and avoidance of any aspect of birth that represented pain to the genital area. She also recognized that she might have transmitted this anxiety and fear to her patients. As her awareness grew and her healing took place, she became able to help them have more trust and confidence in their bodies. Her Cesarean rate dropped dramatically to 19 percent. As Sherril began to trust the birth process herself, she could

separate her past tension and fear related to her own bodily pain from the present reality of normalcy for most of her pregnant clients. (Simkin and Klaus, 2004, p. 141)

Sherril's story provides an example of how the imprints of health care providers' own experiences (from conception to the present) can affect interactions with their patients. Their unresolved issues relating to trauma and loss can be played out in interactions with their patients and affect the quality of care they provide, their treatment decisions, and treatment outcomes for their patients, including their offspring. It is likely that health care practitioners who choose to provide care to women, their partners, and their offspring during their experiences of pre-conception, pregnancy, birth, and the early postpartum period are not aware of how their own imprints from their prior experiences of trauma and loss effect their interactions, their patients' experiences of care, and their treatment outcomes.

The following link will take you to a one-minute interview with renowned midwife Ina May Gaskin talking about the impact of birth attendants' fear on women in labor:

http://www.oneworldbirth.net/videos/the-problem/ina-may-gaskin-on -fear

The next link will take you to a video interview with Ray Castellino, an experienced clinician who works closely with midwife Mary Jackson supporting women, their partners, and their babies before, during, and after birth. Castellino discusses the importance of the "rhythm" or "tempo" a practitioner brings to interactions with a pregnant woman and her prenate, and the woman's partner, and the necessity for practitioners to heal themselves in order to best help their patients.

http://www.youtube.com/watch?v=VyWgc5qUYuw&feature=related

Women's experiences of the quality of care they receive during this time are remembered for a long time to come. Simkin found that women continue to vividly remember their feelings about their first childbirth experience for decades to come. In a study of women's immediate written descriptions of their first childbirths compared with descriptions written many years later, Simkin and Klaus found that both positive and negative memories were "accurate, vivid and still laden with emotions, including pride in themselves, enhanced self-esteem, joy, love or anger, sadness and remorse" (2004, p. 60). Phyllis and Marshall Klaus and John Kennell remind us that "the nurturing a woman receives during this vulnerable time can influence how she nurtures and feels about her infant" (as cited in Simkin and Klaus, 2004, p. 60). It is important to consider the impact and meaning of a woman's experiences during conception, pregnancy, and birth in order to understand how they shape her early interactions with her baby and lay the foundation for their attachment relationship.

CHAPTER 21

Assisted Reproductive Technologies

by Ann Diamond Weinstein, PhD

This chapter is about women's experiences of reproductive endocrinology treatment for infertility. It sheds light on the impacts of these experiences on women's lives. The use of assisted reproductive technologies (ART) is growing worldwide. ART includes all reproductive endocrinology treatments that involve the handling of eggs and/or embryos, including in vitro fertilization-embryo transfer (IVF-ET) and frozen embryo transfer (FET). ART also includes procedures used in oocyte (egg) donation and "gestational carriers"—instances where a woman volunteers to carry a pregnancy for another woman who is unable to conceive and/or carry a pregnancy to term (SART, 2008, para. 1). During IVF-ET, the oocytes and sperm are combined in a culture dish in the laboratory. Fertilization and very early embryo development occur outside the body, rather than in the fallopian tube. Once early embryo development is recognized, the embryos are transferred into the uterus (SART, 2008, para. 2). The first live human birth following IVF was reported in 1978, in England. The technology continues to develop and be introduced into current medical practice.

Research in reproductive endocrinology has begun to reveal the negative impact of stress on fertility, including stress resulting from the infertility treatment process itself (Boivin and Schmidt, 2005; Cwikel, Gidron, and Sheiner, 2004; Eugster et al., 2004). Studies have also indicated that stress and negative psychological states adversely affect infertility treatment outcomes (Boivin and Schmidt, 2005; Kloneff-Cohen et al., 2001).

Limited research has been done on the long-term impacts on women and their offspring of this groundbreaking medical-technological approach to human conception. One reason is it has been a relatively short period of time since its widespread introduction into medical practice. Another reason is that advances in other areas of diagnostic and medical technology that have expanded research and knowledge in related fields (embryology, epigenetics, neurobiology, psychoneuroendocrinology, immunology) have paralleled the development of assisted reproductive technologies and only recently have made it possible to evaluate the subtler impacts of this approach to conception. Recent knowledge in epigenetics raises many questions about the potential transgenerational impacts of assisted reproductive technologies since this medical technology is manipulating the environment of conception, thus contributing to the "environment" part of the "Genes × Environment" equation. Recent studies have begun to shed light on some epigenetic impacts of IVF treatment. More research is needed on the impacts of IVF on the long-term health and behavior of children conceived through this process and on their reproductive experiences as adults of the conception, pregnancy, birth, and early parenting of their own children.

Impact and Meaning

A particular area of interest of mine has been the exploration of the experience, impact, and meaning of assisted reproductive technologies in women's lives. My doctoral research (Weinstein, 2010), entitled "The Experiences of Women Who Received Reproductive Endocrinology Treatment for Infertility," was a qualitative, phenomenological study in which I conducted in-depth, face-to-face interviews with women who reported traumatic stress and/or dissociative symptoms during and following infertility treatment. The women were in treatment from ten months to eight years, during which time they experienced a wide variety of reproductive endocrinology treatments and outcomes. The participants ranged in age from thirty-two to fifty-three.

Six themes emerged from the transcripts of the interviews that synthesize the multidimensional aspects of the participants' experiences of treatment. I will briefly summarize the themes.

The participants described cycles of a wide range of rapidly shifting emotions while receiving reproductive endocrinology treatment. The array of feelings described by the participants encompassed the full spectrum of human emotions—hope, joy, disappointment, desperation, frustration, anger, shame, sadness, and grief.

Theme 1, The Emotional Roller Coaster: Cycles of Treatment Evoke a Range of Intense and Shifting Emotions Challenging the Women's Capacity to Cope, illuminates the participants' experiences trying to cope with frequently changing and, at times, conflicting emotions that were repeatedly evoked over the course of menstrual and treatment cycles.

Pam, one of the research participants, shared her experience of the emotional roller coaster. She expressed her feelings at the beginning of an IVF cycle:

Well, you know, obviously I'm gonna get pregnant. I have a whole SWAT team of doctors working on me. They certainly know what to do. I'm on this magical medication, Clomid, which fixes whatever's wrong with my ovaries and causes my eggs to be fabulous.

She then explained that the most "traumatic" moments she experienced were following each unsuccessful treatment cycle: "I was convinced I was going to die. I would … cut off a limb … I would sell my soul to the devil to be pregnant at this point."

Theme 2, *Protecting Oneself from Painful Emotions and Physical Challenges Through Compartmentalization, Disconnection, and Dissociation*, elucidates the protective mechanisms the participants described using in the face of the physical and emotional stress/trauma of repeated treatment cycles and their outcomes. Participants expressed feelings of disconnection during the treatment and one participant expressed feelings of disconnection after successful treatment and the birth of her baby.

Lilah, a participant who had a child and was undergoing treatment to conceive a second child described her feelings during a treatment cycle:

I'm just like a drone sitting in the corner. I'm not part of the conversation. I'm not a part of the room. I'm in my own little place. I just physically am there, but my mind's not…. Not really wanting to be there, but having to be there, and just, so going into myself.

Zoe, another participant, shared her feelings following successful IVF treatment and the birth of her baby:

I think when you feel like it's a gift, then you go to this place where you aren't sure if in fact you are entitled to it…. That feeds the feeling of being somewhat disconnected, because if you don't quite feel entitled to this gift, then … it's easy to avoid bonding … and bonding is hard, especially if you don't feel … it's something you deserve.

Theme 3, *The Lived-Body Experience of Treatment Evokes Feelings that Range from Trust and Safety to Fear and Threat*, provides an in-depth understanding of the women's experiences of the physical aspects of the treatment they received. Women reported having body-memories of exams and procedures long after they occurred.

Lilah described her experience:

I can remember the *feeling* of him [the doctor] putting the speculum inside me. Like I can actually feel it, like it didn't go away. It didn't leave … my vagina remembers exactly how it felt when he was putting that speculum in me. And like it's gonna cringe if I ever have to go back to him and have it done again, because I'm anticipating what it's gonna feel like, because I remember exactly how it felt.

Theme 4, Changes in Appearance and Internal Sensations Evoke Negative Emotions Toward a Body that Feels Unfamiliar and is Viewed as "Uncooperative," elucidates another aspect of the mind-body impact of the women's treatment experiences. The women described how their attention oscillated between three aspects of their mind-body experience: (1) a focus on internal body sensations for clues to whether or not they had conceived, and if so, ongoing signs of early pregnancy; (2) a focus on changes in their external appearance resulting from reactions to treatment medications and procedures; and (3) an awareness of how the changes they sensed in their bodies affected their experiences moving in space. The women described feelings of unfamiliarity with their bodies as they experienced their bodies' reactions to the treatment, which made it easier for them to see their bodies as separate, uncooperative, and the source of their disappointment and frustration.

Pam described her feelings about her body after repeated unsuccessful IVF treatment cycles:

[My body] wouldn't cooperate. It wouldn't do what I would tell it to do. It wouldn't get pregnant when I wanted it to…. It becomes your enemy. It becomes your obstacle…. You get really, really pissed off with your own body because I feel like I have these unborn children and my body is killing them off for some reason. My body won't accept them [the embryos] back…. When the embryos are transferred back in, my evil, horrible uterus kills them and I don't know why. And I try to talk to my uterus about that. It doesn't respond. It doesn't answer.

Theme 5, Layers of Loss Unnamed and Unprocessed Contribute to the Burden of Cumulative Unresolved Grief, sheds light on aspects of loss described by the participants. This theme acknowledges the losses participants carried into and through reproductive endocrinology treatment and illuminates how multiple cyclical losses endured over repeated unsuccessful treatment cycles with little time or context for processing, compounded previous losses and created a reservoir of unresolved grief.

Pearl, another study participant, described her feelings after the loss at twenty weeks of a fetus conceived during reproductive endocrinology treatment:

We'd lost our baby in May and we had a concert that was in July or August and I had planned my maternity outfit that I was gonna wear to this concert. And I was so excited, I bought it extra big.... So then I go … to get dressed for this concert and I couldn't get dressed, because I couldn't put on anything but that maternity outfit and I didn't need that maternity outfit.... And I'm in my room and I'm just bawling my eyes out and I can't, I can't get dressed.... And I know for me now, part of my fear of conceiving is the fear of losing another one. So then I've been working on that … healing the trauma of the last loss and forming the belief that that was that and the next one will be different.

Theme 6, The Quality of Care Received from Health Care Providers Affects Women's Experiences of Treatment, focuses on the quality of care women experienced while they were undergoing treatment and the factors that they felt affected their experiences of the interpersonal and technical aspects of the care received. The theme also includes the participants' insights into the quality of care that would have supported more positive lived experiences of treatment. Multiple factors contributed to the women's experiences of the care they received. Two factors emphasized by the women were: (1) the health care provider's capacity to be present and engaged in a caring and respectful way during appointments, and (2) the health care provider's technical skills and sensitivity to how the quality of physical care affected the women's physical experiences of treatment, especially their experiences of pain.

Pearl described a very positive experience of care with one doctor: "[He's] right there listening, eye contact, heart facing you, like very much engaged with you as a human being." She saw another doctor during and IVF cycle with whom she had a very different experience:

I had no choice but to somehow force myself to let him *shove* it [the speculum] into me … otherwise I would have taken all those drugs and made all those follicles for nothing. So this was a critical juncture.... I just let it hurt.... You know you don't want to piss him off either … you're in this very vulnerable place.... I could have said to him, "Stop fucking hurting me and what are you doing?" but then I run the risk of pissing off the doctor who's … the one holding the catheter with my precious embryos in them, you know, it's like you can't piss off the guy who's doing that.

Pam thought back on her experiences in treatment and shared this: "The best description is I really don't think that they [the health care providers] see you as a person. They don't see you as a living, breathing human being who's experiencing a stressful process."

A deep exploration of Pam's experiences may be found in the chapter "Pam's Themes," which I contributed to Michael Shea's *Biodynamic Craniosacral Therapy,* Volume Three (2010).

Somatic Practice 10: Mindfulness of Breathing

Practice mindfulness of body and breathing for as long as you need right now.

Insights Gained

I will expand here on a few of the insights I gained from listening to the women's experiences and analyzing the transcripts of their interviews. The experiences shared by the participants revealed the many sacrifices each woman made at great cost to her physical, emotional, and spiritual well-being to endure the fertility journey and reproductive endocrinology treatment. Their experiences, at times, pushed them to the edge of and, at times, beyond their "affective window of tolerance" (Siegel, 1999, p. 253; Ogden, Minton, and Paine, 2006, pp. 26–27), causing them to have difficulty integrating their mind-body experiences throughout the process.

Lived-body experiences of treatment triggered or threatened to trigger past unresolved trauma in some women, including prenatal and perinatal trauma, developmental trauma, experiences of loss, abuse, neglect, and abandonment, transgenerational trauma, previous reproductive losses, and other childhood and adult trauma. For some women, the reproductive endocrinology treatment exams, tests, and procedures themselves created highly stressful and even traumatic experiences, which also pushed them beyond the edge of their window of tolerance.

Recurrent dysregulated states of mind along with their psychophysiological effects were precipitated by repeated and cyclical negative experiences throughout the fertility journey and reproductive endocrinology treatment process. Women attempted to cope with these overwhelming experiences by disconnecting mind from body and compartmentalizing these experiences within different self-states (Bromberg, 1998) in their minds, using the most basic defensive adaptations evoked by perceived threat to their mind-body survival, including dissociation and depersonalization. These defenses were engaged by the women in the service of allowing the treatment, with all its physical and emotional stressors, to be performed on and in their bodies through interpersonal interactions with medical providers in order to fulfill a persistent, compelling longing—an instinctual biological drive to reproduce and create a child.

The women were confronted with a mind-body, psycho-neuro-immuno-endocrinological dilemma—a conflict arising at the interface of the fundamentally aggressive and intrusive reproductive technologies and the species-specific evolutionary process of reproduction passed down through the generations. This process is currently understood to be best supported by a feeling of safety at all levels of mind and body (Porges, 2001). The women often faced tension and competition between two of the most basic human instincts—to survive in the face of a felt sense of threat and to reproduce. This conflict that was created in a woman's body-brain-mind often demanded engagement of the most basic protective defense mechanisms. The employment of these defense mechanisms, in turn, evoked the body-brain-mind reactions and conditions that hindered the integration of these experiences and supported the development of, or exacerbation of, existing traumatic stress symptoms.

Given the relatively short period of time since the widespread use of in vitro fertilization and other assisted reproductive technologies in the treatment of infertility, we do not have research on the impact of this treatment on the reproductive experiences of women and men who were themselves conceived through these processes. This research would depend on these individuals having this information about their own conceptions. There is so much we do not yet know about the long-term effects of these processes.

You may be asking how the experiences of women who receive reproductive endocrinology treatment for infertility relate to the experiences of other women who do not undergo this treatment. I'd like to point out here that a similar conflict may also be present in pregnant and birthing women who have *not* gone through infertility treatment. We must consider that all women carry the imprints of their life experiences from their own conception to their attempts to conceive, their pregnancy with, and birth of their child. Their neuroception of the care they receive during pregnancy and birth may evoke a felt sense of danger and/or life threat while, at the same time, they feel they need to rely on the assistance of care providers to birth their baby. Some women feel they need to be "good patients" in order to elicit from the provider the assistance they believe they need.

Whether their past experiences of trauma predispose them to retraumatization in the environments within which they receive care, or the current circumstances of their pregnancy and birth and the care they receive overwhelm them, women employ defense mechanisms to protect themselves and their babies. These defense mechanisms, as described above, hinder the integration of these experiences and thus put women at risk for developing traumatic stress symptoms, including dissociative symptoms, chronic PTSD, and postpartum depression. The work of prenatal and perinatal psychologists, infant mental health clinicians and attachment researchers has revealed the impact of these states on women's early interactions with their infants and the establishment of their attachment relationship.

Double Bind

Bromberg (1998) contributes to our understanding of the dilemma—the double bind faced by women who have suffered early interpersonal trauma in relationships with caregivers or peers. The double bind often arises in women's experiences of the care they receive and their interactions with practitioners during the pre-conception period, pregnancy, birth, and the early postnatal period.

> What of situations where there are competing algorithms at the same moment? What of a moment when your mother bounds toward you with fangs bared? Or a moment when your father approaches with penis bared? Or … where your peer group suddenly becomes a pack of hyenas, stripping *you* bare while you are still alive? The algorithm of fight, flight, or hiding pertains only to escape from predators. What does someone (particularly a child) do when there is another strong algorithm operating, such as "obedience to a parent or an adult" or "love of one's caretaker" or "being accepted by one's peers"? This is the situation, I suggest, that, at least from an evolutionary standpoint, defines the meaning of trauma, and may explain why natural selection seems to have endowed the human mind with a Darwinian algorithm that helps us cope with trauma by providing what Putnam (1992) called, "the escape when there is no escape" (p. 104)—the mechanism of dissociation. (Bromberg, 1998, p. 243)

Bromberg's explanation of the process by which an individual resorts to dissociation as a survival adaptation can help us understand the dissociative behaviors of women who experience "competing algorithms" while undergoing reproductive health experiences:

> When drastically incompatible emotions or perceptions are required to be cognitively processed within the same relationship and such processing is adaptationally beyond the capacity of the individual to contain this disjunction within a unitary self-experience, one of the competing algorithms is hypnoidally denied access to consciousness to preserve sanity and survival. When ordinary adaptational adjustment to the task at hand is not possible, dissociation comes into play. The experience that is causing the incompatible perception and emotion is "unhooked" from the cognitive

processing system and remains raw data that is cognitively unsymbolized within that particular self-other representation except as a survival reaction. (Bromberg, 1998, p. 243)

Understanding how dissociative behaviors are evoked in some women, when faced with "incompatible emotions or perceptions" during and following experiences of conception, pregnancy, birth, and the early postnatal period, highlights the importance of helping women safely process and heal from the experiences that evoked these dissociative reactions at the appropriate time.

With the awareness that reproductive processes are best supported by a feeling of safety, practitioners can inquire about and learn to recognize the expression of safety in a woman's lived body, through the quality of her voice, her words, and her nonverbal behavior. This awareness can help practitioners adjust their behavior in interactions with their patients to support their experience of safety in the treatment environment.

If we provide women with the opportunity to share, in their own way, what they are comfortable sharing, and what is important to them about their experiences, we can begin to hear them—their voices, their pain, their suffering, their strength, their hope, their confusion, their desperation, and their triumphs. If we bring compassionate hearts to our interactions with them, we learn so much more than the statistical research demonstrates. We understand, not only *that* they had been affected by their experiences, but *how*.

Somatic Practice 11: Mindfulness of Wholeness

Take a few moments to practice mindfulness of body and breathing. After several minutes bring your attention to the space immediately around your body. This region 15–20 inches off of the body forms an envelope in which the fear centers of the brain continually monitor. Allow yourself to become consciously aware of this area. Imagine that you are breathing in and out of the space around your body.

After several minutes, bring your attention to the room you are in. Notice the walls in front and in back of you. Notice the ceiling above you and the floor below you. Take several moments as if your lungs were filling the room with your breath.

After several minutes, bring your attention to the area around the building you are in. Visualize what is in front of the building extending out to the horizon and do the same for the back of the building. Then sense the space above the building all the way up to where the sky turns blue.

Now bring your attention after several minutes down into the earth below you, at least a mile or two. After several minutes, allow yourself to have your attention evenly suspended between your body, the space around your body, the room you are in, and the entire natural world outside the building. Breathe in and out of that whole space.

Expectations and Discussion

I'd like to note here another common experience that occurs in the aftermath of difficult or traumatic experiences during pre-conception, conception, pregnancy, and birth, when the outcome is a healthy baby. Women and their partners are often told by well-meaning care providers, family, and friends that all that matters is the end result, the fact that "you have a healthy baby." This communicates an expectation that having a healthy baby mitigates the impacts on women and their partners, of trauma experienced during these periods. Comments such as these indicate a failure to recognize and appreciate the psychophysiological inscriptions left by the overwhelming quality of these experiences.

Once again, I remind you that in these instances, there are three survivors—the woman, her partner, and the baby. The baby was a prenate who had its own experience of events that its mother and her partner experienced as traumatizing. Prenates' behaviors in utero and after birth may express how they were affected by those experiences. A woman's partner may be traumatized by these experiences, particularly those in which he or she perceives the life of the childbearing partner and/or the prenate or neonate to be in danger or threatened—those experiences in which the partner feels helpless to reduce or alleviate the partner's or baby's expressions of pain and suffering.

The research presented earlier regarding the relationship between a woman's prenatal (even pre-conception) psychophysiological states and the health, development, and behavior of her offspring raises many questions about how practitioners can support families in healing the impacts of their *experiences* of pre-conception, infertility treatment, pregnancy, birth, and the early postnatal period.

What are the safest, most effective ways to support women and their partners through these life transitions and, at times, challenging experiences? Will the therapeutic treatment approach chosen by a practitioner move a woman and her partner (if she has one) toward psychophysiological regulation? If the chosen treatment further dysregulates a woman and her partner, how will it affect her reproductive physiology and, potentially, the outcome of reproductive endocrinology treatment she may be receiving simultaneously? How will it affect her pregnancy? How will it affect the development of her prenate? If a woman is pregnant, or becomes pregnant as a result of, or coincidentally after terminating reproductive endocrinology treatment, what therapeutic and psychoeducational experiences will expand her ability to access internal and external resources to support self-care and self-regulation thereby supporting her developing prenate?

In the next chapter, I will explore some of the implications for practitioners of the material I've presented and recent studies that focus on treatment modalities that have been used with pregnant women and their outcomes.

CHAPTER 22

Implications for Practitioners

by Ann Diamond Weinstein, PhD

I would like you to consider the following questions as you read this chapter: What are the implications of the preceding chapters for practitioners? How can practitioners best support women, their partners, and their offspring before, during, and after their experiences of conception, pregnancy, birth, and the early postnatal period?

First, I'd like to outline several overarching implications for the field that emerge from the material I've presented. The research and knowledge presented here highlight the need for:

- Education of women and their partners about the importance and potential positive impact of addressing and healing issues of unresolved trauma *before* they attempt to conceive

- Screening of women and their partners for psychophysiological states, including depression, anxiety, traumatic stress, and dissociation that may affect them and their offspring during attempts to conceive, pregnancy, birth, and their early postnatal experiences

- Services and resources that support and enhance psychophysiological regulation in women and their partners, especially for those who exhibit symptoms of unresolved issues, stress, traumatic stress, and other negative psychophysiological states during the pre-conception, prenatal, and early postnatal period

- Services and resources for women, their partners, and their children that support healing of the impacts of their experiences of conception, pregnancy, birth, and the early postnatal period whenever the lived body manifestations of these experiences become evident—in the days, weeks, months, or years after they occur

223

Therapeutic Interventions

Based on the abundance of emerging research demonstrating the impact of maternal prenatal states on the development, health, and behavior of offspring over the lifespan, it is important to consider how therapeutic interventions during pregnancy may affect both the woman and her prenate. Since therapeutic interventions may trigger or exacerbate maternal state dysregulation, and thereby influence the development and programming of the prenate's organs and systems with potential lifelong impacts, careful consideration must be given to treatment options when working with pregnant women.

A number of recent studies have explored the effects of different therapeutic interventions on pregnant women. Only one study monitored fetal responses during the intervention (DiPietro et al., 2008). If a study demonstrates a positive impact of an intervention on a pregnant woman, but does not evaluate fetal responses, birth outcomes, or neonatal behavior, we are missing information that may have important implications for the choice of treatment options.

Careful observation of each pregnant woman's nonverbal behavioral indicators of her psychophysiological state may assist practitioners in choosing treatment interventions and tracking patients' reactions to them. Babette Rothschild provides a list of noticeable signs of ANS activation. She explains that when the sympathetic branch of the ANS is activated during "positive and negative stress states," including "sexual climax, rage, desperation, terror, anxiety/panic, trauma," the following signs can be observed: faster respiration, quicker pulse, dilated pupils, pale skin color, increased sweating, and cold and/or clammy skin. When the parasympathetic branch of the ANS is activated during "rest and relaxation, sexual arousal, happiness, anger, grief, sadness," these signs can be observed: slower, deeper respiration, slower pulse, constricted pupils, flushed skin color, and dry, usually warm skin to touch (Rothschild, 2000, p. 48).

Porges (2004) describes observable indicators of neural regulation of the muscles of the face and head that influence an individual's neuroception of the engagement behaviors of others. The observation of these behaviors can assist a practitioner in understanding whether a patient is experiencing a felt sense of safety, danger, or life threat. In a situation where people's neuroception of the environment (external or internal) is one of safety, they "make eye contact, vocalize with an appealing inflection and rhythm, display contingent facial expressions, and modulate the middle-ear muscles to distinguish the human voice from background sounds more effectively." In a situation where people's neuroception of the environment (external or internal) is one of danger or life threat, "the eyelids droop, the voice loses inflection, positive facial expressions dwindle, awareness of the sound of the human voice becomes less acute, and sensitivity to others' social engagement behaviors decreases" (p. 22).

Recent research has been conducted on the effects of the following three treatment approaches on pregnant women: a mindfulness-based intervention (Vieten and Astin, 2008); massage therapy (Field, Diego, and Hernandez-Reif, 2010); and induced guided imagery relaxation (DiPietro et al., 2008). Case vignettes of psychodynamic psychotherapy treatment with two pregnant patients have been reported by Bergner, Monk, and Werner (2008).

In a pilot study conducted by Vieten and Astin (2008), an eight-week mindfulness-based intervention was used with pregnant women to test its effects on stress and mood during the pregnancy and in the early postpartum period. The authors collected measures of perceived stress, positive and negative affect, depressed and anxious mood, and affect regulation prior to, immediately following, and three months after the intervention in the postpartum period. Mothers who received the intervention showed significantly reduced anxiety and negative affect during the third trimester in comparison to those who did not receive the intervention. As Vieten and Astin point out, "the brief and non-pharmaceutical nature of this intervention makes it a promising candidate for use during pregnancy" (p. 67). It would be interesting to assess fetal responses to a mindfulness-based intervention in pregnant women.

In a recent article reporting on their research, Field, Diego, and Hernandez-Reif (2010) review the negative effects of prenatal depression and cortisol on fetal growth, prematurity, and low birthweight. The authors report on their recent studies of the effects of prenatal massage therapy provided by the women's partners, and massage therapy combined with group interpersonal psychotherapy from 20 weeks until the end of the pregnancy. Field et al. (2010) report that prenatal depression, elevated cortisol, prematurity, low birthweight, and postpartum depression were reduced by prenatal massage therapy provided by the women's partners. Massage therapy combined with group interpersonal psychotherapy was also effective for reducing depression and cortisol levels.

Field, Figueiredo, Hernandez-Reif, Diego, Deeds, and Ascencio (2008) also assessed the effects on the *partners* of the women, who provided the massage. They found that partners who massaged pregnant women versus the control group partners reported less depressed mood, anxiety, and anger across the time they were providing the massage therapy. In addition, scores on a relationship questionnaire that the authors developed for the study improved more for the women and the partners in the massage group (Figueiredo et al., 2008).

DiPietro, Costigan, Nelson, Gurewitsch, and Laudenslager (2008) conducted a unique study in which they evaluated fetal responses to induced maternal relaxation using an 18-minute guided imagery relaxation manipulation during the thirty-second week of pregnancy. Other studies have evaluated fetal heart rate responses to maternal anxiety and stress (Monk et al., 2000). This study by DiPetro et al. (2008) sheds light on the effects of a positive manipulation and further illuminates the "concordant and contingent relationship" (Thomson, 2007), between maternal psychophysiological state and fetal physiological markers. It suggests the benefits for mother and prenate, of the use of guided imagery relaxation during pregnancy.

Bergner et al. (2008) describe the use of psychodynamic psychotherapy "when problematic aspects of women's representational world lead to negative or dysregulated affect.… This kind of therapeutic intervention aims to achieve mood improvement, address a woman's emerging relationship with her baby, and potentially, influence the course of fetal development" (p. 399). In two case vignettes, Bergner et al. report positive effects of the psychodynamic treatment intervention on the patients' moods and their relationships with their baby. It is unclear how the practitioner(s) who treated the pregnant women was assessing their shifting psychophysiological states during and after the intervention. As noted above, tracking of the noticeable signs of pregnant women's psychophysiological states during treatment interactions can shed some light on the potential regulating/dysregulating impact of the treatment interaction on both the woman and, most important, her prenate.

Somatic Practice 12: Mindfulness of Wholeness

Take time to practice mindfulness of wholeness, as detailed in the preceding chapter.

Neurosequential Model and Rhythmic Experience

In a recent presentation, Bruce Perry discussed the "neurosequential model of therapeutics" (NMT). Perry and his team developed this model in an effort to find more effective ways to work with children who experienced chaos, threat, traumatic stress, abuse, and neglect. Perry acknowledges the importance and impact of experiences that occur as early as the prenatal period (as noted earlier, in personal communication, January 20, 2012).

As we know, early adverse experiences alter the developing brain and result in negative functional effects. Perry suggests that therapeutic experiences can allow for "healing, recovery, and restoration of healthy function" in individuals who've had these experiences, but "the nature, pattern, timing, and duration of therapeutic experiences are very crucial in determining whether a 'therapy' is genuinely therapeutic" (Perry, 2006, p. 27).

Although an in-depth discussion of the complexity and richness of the work of Perry and his team is beyond the scope of this chapter, one aspect of the NMT model inspired me to contact Dr. Perry about the applicability of that aspect of the NMT approach to work with pregnant women, their partners, and their prenates. I will share his answer with you, but first, I will lay the groundwork for understanding his answer from his previous work.

In earlier work, Perry (2006) explains:

The stress response systems originate in the lower parts of the brain and help regulate and organize higher parts of the brain; if they are poorly organized or regulated themselves, they dysregulate and disorganize higher parts of the brain. Traumatic stress will result in patterned, repetitive neuronal activation in a distributed and diverse set of brain systems. Trauma can have an impact on functions mediated by the cortex (e.g., cognition), the limbic system (e.g., affect regulation), the diencephalon (e.g., fine motor regulation, startle response), and the brainstem (e.g., heart rate, blood pressure regulation). *The key to therapeutic intervention is to remember that the stress response systems originate in the brainstem and diencephalon.* As long as these systems are poorly regulated and dysfunctional, they will disrupt and dysregulate higher parts of the brain.... All the best cognitive-behavioral, insight-oriented, or even affect-based interventions will fail if the brain stem is poorly regulated.... Alternative brainstem-modulating interventions are beginning to emerge—or rather, are being rediscovered and appreciated for their fundamental therapeutic value. Music and movement activities that provide patterned repetitive, rhythmic stimulation of the brainstem are very successful in helping modulate brainstem dysregulation.... Several therapeutic approaches, including eye movement desensitization and reprocessing (EMDR), involve patterned rhythmic activation of the brainstem as part of the intervention. We have hypothesized that EMDR is effective because it can short-circuit the chain of traumatic memory that follow a specific traumatic event by tapping into a much more powerful brainstem—diencephalon memory—the association created in utero. Powerful associations are made during the prenatal development of the brainstem and diencephalon between rhythmic, auditory, tactile, and motor activity at 80 beats per minute (i.e., the maternal heart rate heard and felt in utero) and the neural activation mediating the sensation of being warm, satiated, safe, and soothed. EMDR, dancing, drumming, music, and patterned massage can all quiet the brainstem through rhythmic activity that provides brainstem stimulation at 80 beats per minute or subrhythms (40, 60) of this primary "soothing" pattern (Perry, 2002). Such patterned, repetitive, rhythmic activity has always been a central element of healing and grief rituals in aboriginal cultures. The use of music and movement interventions with traumatized children has been very promising (e.g., Miranda et al., 1999, pp. 39–40)

In thinking about Perry's presentation, I became curious if he thought pregnant women and their partners might benefit from patterned, rhythmic, repetitive movement to modulate and heal their own brain stem dysregulation before conception and/or during pregnancy, and thus benefit the development of their prenates. Here is Bruce Perry's answer: "I absolutely do believe that providing pregnant mothers (couples) with nurturing, regulating and physiologically rhythmic input will impact—in a positive way—the developing fetus" (personal communication, January 20, 2012).

In a webinar presented by The National Institute for the Clinical Application of Behavioral Medicine (June 6, 2012), Bessel van der Kolk also commented on the importance of rhythmic experiences in the treatment of traumatic stress. He noted that trauma survivors often lose their sense of "interpersonal rhythms" and suggested that rhythmic dance, drumming, and safe group dance can be helpful in reestablishing this connection. van der Kolk also commented that positive emotions and intense vitality affects beneficially affect health. Rhythmic group experiences may support the experience of positive emotions and intense vitality affects.

Although van der Kolk was not talking about the prenatal and early postnatal period in relation to these treatment suggestions, rhythmic experiences can be offered to pregnant women and their partners, especially those who have experienced traumatic stress. Perhaps rhythmic experiences during pregnancy may enhance the sensitivity of parents and their babies to "interpersonal rhythms," positively affect their interactions before and after birth, and support compassionate connections.

It is interesting to note that decades ago, Michel Odent, MD (1984) described the benefits he felt pregnant women and their prenates could experience from participating in a weekly singing and dancing group at the hospital where he practiced. Practitioners and patients participated together and were led by a woman who accompanied the group on piano. Odent noted that her quality of presence evoked a sense of community in the group. He commented: "Singing encourages women to feel comfortable, unself-conscious and expansive—to experience and release the whole range of emotions.... But above all, it is a pleasure to sing and dance. And pleasure must not be underrated; it can only enhance pregnancy" (pp. 27–28).

I would suggest that the practitioners who participated in the singing and dancing group may have experienced the same benefits as the pregnant women. Perhaps rhythmic group experiences for practitioners could enhance their sensitivity to "interpersonal rhythms" with their patients.

Stephen Porges also describes the potential benefits of music and singing. He provides an explanation of why listening to melodies, vocal music, and singing can be used by individuals to stimulate their social engagement system. This system, when engaged, supports our receptivity to connection with others, as well as health and healing processes (Porges, 2011, p. 295). It can be activated or deactivated in practitioner-patient interactions depending on the patient's neuroception of safety in the internal and/or external environment of the treatment setting. It is possible that van der Kolk's (2012) comment on the ability (or lack thereof in those who suffer from traumatic stress) to be sensitive to the "interpersonal rhythms" of others can be understood in the context of the physiological changes associated with activation or deactivation of the social engagement system described by Porges (2011). This system controls muscles in the middle ear (to enhance our ability to extract vocalizations from background noises) and laryngeal and pharyngeal muscles to regulate intonation of vocalizations. Stimulation of the social engagement system usually occurs in face-to-face interactions where an individual experiences a neuroception of safety.

Porges notes that there are two ways that listening to vocal music and singing can also provide stimulation to the social engagement system, *without* the usual requirement of face-to-face interactions and reciprocity. This is particularly important when working with individuals who have experienced trauma, who may experience face-to-face interactions as threatening, and their neuroception in face-to-face environments is one of danger and/or life threat.

The first way that vocal melodic music provides a portal to the social engagement system is through the stimulation of the middle ear muscles. Listening to melodic vocal music that stimulates these muscles in the same way they are stimulated during face-to-face interactions in the context of a neuroception of safety allows individuals who suffer from traumatic stress to exercise this part of their social engagement system. They can experience the same benefits from this physiological auditory shift, without the usual requirement of face-to-face reciprocity and a feeling of safety to occur (Porges, 2011, p. 252).

The second way music provides a portal to the social engagement system is through the use of the breath during singing. Singing requires changes in breathing that include long exhalations. Inhaling and exhaling affects our heart rate in different ways. Breathing "gates" the influence of the mylenated vagus on the heart. When we inhale, the influence of the vagus nerve on our heart is diminished and our heart rate increases. When we exhale, the influence of the vagus nerve our heart is increased and our heart rate decreases. Long exhales evoke a feeling of calmness and a neuroception of safety, which lead to activation of the social engagement system, receptivity to connection with others, and states that support health and healing (Porges, 2011, p. 254).

Energy Psychology

Patterned, rhythmic, repetitive movements are also incorporated in energy psychology modalities. Recent research and clinical experience from the field of energy psychology shed light on additional interventions that may support psychophysiological regulation (the reduction of hyperarousal and hypoarousal) during the pre-conception, prenatal, and early postnatal period. Energy psychology "integrates established clinical principles with methods derived from healing traditions of Eastern cultures.… Energy psychology utilizes cognitive operations such as imaginal exposure to traumatic memories or visualization of optimal performance scenarios—combined with physical interventions derived from acupuncture, yoga and related systems—for inducing psychological change.… This combination purportedly brings about, with unusual speed and precision, therapeutic shifts in affective, cognitive, and behavioral patterns that underlie a range of psychological concerns" (Feinstein, 2010). Energy psychology tools have been used to help individuals shift constricting core beliefs that emerged from experiences originating in the prenatal and early postnatal period (McCarty, 2011).

Research including randomized controlled studies on the effects of energy psychology modalities have begun to be published and practitioners in this field have shared extensive clinical and anecdotal experience on the application of this approach in psychotherapy. For more information on these modalities, the recent research on its effectiveness and explanations of proposed mechanisms of action, access the article by Feinstein (2010) entitled "Rapid Treatment of PTSD: Why Psychological Exposure with Acupoint Tapping May Be Effective," available at http://www.apa.org/journals.

The chapter content here has provided a foundation upon which to understand the importance of the work prenatal and perinatal practitioners do with adults and children, including prenates and neonates. This young field grew from the clinical experience of practitioners and the experiences of the individuals and families who worked with them. The research in neurobiology, psychology, behavioral perinatology, and epigenetics only recently confirmed much of what practitioners in this field have learned through their clinical experience over the past several decades.

It is possible you may also have had interactions with patients in which implicit recall of their earliest experiences emerged, whether or not you and/or the patient were consciously aware in that moment of the source of these psychophysiological states—of the emotions, behaviors, perceptions, and bodily sensations that they experienced.

Cellular Imprinting

Work in the field of psycho-neuro-immuno-endocrinology helps us understand how experiences may be biochemically stored and held in our bodies. The work of Bruce Lipton (2005) and Candace Pert (1997) shed light on how our experiences are imprinted at the cellular level, which provides one lens through which we may understand how individuals may be able to access their earliest experiences. Verny and Weintraub (2002) explain:

> Before we had brains or even bodies, we consisted of nothing more than a cell. First an egg and a sperm that merged to form a single cell, and then a collection of cells dividing again and again. The biochemical "experience" of those early cells forms the first precursors of memory—not memory as we think of it in our present-day lives, but an ancient cellular memory from a time when, chrysalis-like, we had a different form. (p. 155)

Verny and Weintraub (2002) remind us of the observations of cellular biologist Bruce Lipton that shed light on the phenomenon of cellular memory. Lipton notes that cells read their environment, assess information, and then select appropriate responses to maintain their survival (p. 156). The immune system provides an example of cellular memory. Our immune defenses are activated through cells that recognize and *remember* infectious invaders. Candace Pert's work provides an understanding of the fact that "the nervous, endocrine, and immune systems are functionally integrated in what look like a psychoimmunoendocrine network" (as cited in Verny and Weintraub, 2002, p. 158). The existence of this network enables us to understand the fact that the strength of our immune response (a process we often conceive to be a function of our physical body) can be influenced by emotions that are evoked with the recall of memories in our mind.

Verny and Weintraub mention another system in the body that operates with "information substances" known as ligands. Ligands include transmitters, peptides, hormones, and other factors that circulate through the body and brain. Pert describes the way ligands communicate with cells:

> Though a key fitting into a lock is the standard image, a more dynamic description of this process might be two voices—ligand and receptor—striking the same note and producing a vibration that rings a doorbell to open the doorway to the cell.… A chain reaction of biochemical events is initiated.… These minute physiological phenomena at the cellular level can translate to large changes in behavior, physical activity, even mood. (as cited in Verny and Weintraub, 2002, p. 158)

Neuroscientists now widely accept that the ligand system involves multiple types of cells throughout the body, from the gut, to the spleen, to the heart. These cells produce a flow of ligands that travel in the extracellular fluid and communicate feeling, mood, and memory to all regions of the body and the emotional centers of the brain. Pert and her team found that receptors for ligands were densest in the limbic system, but were also spread throughout the body. This supports our latest understanding of ourselves as a single interactive network—body-brain-mind. In addition, this knowledge illuminates a new understanding of where in our bodies intelligence and memory are located—not just in the brain, but throughout the body (Verny and Weintraub, 2002).

This knowledge has implications for prenatal and perinatal psychology. It enhances our understanding of the clinical experiences of practitioners in the field. Verny and Weintraub explain:

> We do not need fully developed central nervous systems or brains to receive, store, and process information. Information substances from the mother, be they stress-related cortisol or feel-good endorphins, enter the baby's blood system affecting receptors at every stage of development, no matter how early in life. Before our children have even rudimentary brains, they are gathering, within the cells of their bodies, their first memories. Our earliest memories are not conscious, nor even unconscious in the standard sense … we record the experience and history of our lives in our cells. (2002, pp. 159–160)

Implicit Memory

Prenatal, birth, and early postnatal experiences are recorded in implicit memory. Siegel (2012b, AI-30) notes that implicit memory:

> … involves parts of the brain that do not require conscious, focal attention during encoding or retrieval. Perceptions, emotions, bodily sensations, and behavioral response patterns are layers of implicit processing. Mental models (schema or generalizations of repeated experiences) and priming (getting ready to respond) are basic components.

When implicit memory is retrieved, it lacks the feeling of something that has been "recalled" and individuals may not even be aware that the feelings they are having during the retrieval of the memory are being generated from something from the past. They experience the implicit memory as emotions, behaviors ("fixed action patterns"), perceptions, and bodily sensations.

Jenny Wade (1998) brings another perspective to prenatal and birth memories. She reviews clinical research conducted by Chamberlain (1990, 1998), Cheek (1986, 1992) and Wambach (1981) on prenatal and birth memories, in the context of theories of memory and neurological research. The data from this research on prenatal and birth memories, along with recent research that demonstrates that prenates have a greater capacity to perceive and react to their environment in utero and learn from their experiences in the womb than previously thought, challenge the fields of medicine and psychology to consider newer theories of memory that can account for these findings.

Wade (1998) speaks of three schools of memory theory:

> … that can be grouped according to the location of memory in the body: local (in identifiable structures); non-local (associated with identifiable body structures, but not necessarily reducible to them); and completely non-physical, or transcendent.

She notes that research on memory suggests that "consciousness may not be dependent on the central nervous system, or even on the body."

Wade presents regression data supported by independent findings from fetal observation that can only be accounted for if one is "to accept that a physically transcendent source of consciousness—or at the very least, one that functions outside any known physiological processes—exists as a source of memory." She notes that the research she presents is "strictly limited to the most conservative proofs in the empirical tradition—memories of non subjective events that could be validated by independent, third-party observations."

Wade explains that based on the regression data and the three theories of memory mentioned above, there appear to be two sources of memory from prenatal and birth experiences: "Verbatim transcripts and veridical memories showing complex mentation and extrasensory knowledge suggest a non-physical source of fetal consciousness interacting with a physically-based source, a finding congruent with current neurological theory" (Wade, 1998).

Conclusion

Whatever our individual beliefs are about the location of memory and consciousness and their relationship, we can hold curiosity about whether prenatal and perinatal experience may have contributed to an individual's issue. This curiosity may be informed by an individual's description of his or her problem as a longstanding one, an issue that has existed for as long as they can remember. When this is reported, prenatal and perinatal psychologists suspect the possibility that the issue has an early trauma embedded within it, one that may have occurred during prenatal, birth, or early postnatal experiences, one that may be processed and healed by accessing the associated implicit imprints. Emphasis is placed on individuals being conscious and aware of their internal states, as well as knowing how to best create their own sense of safety as they explore these early experiences.

For decades, practitioners in the field of prenatal and perinatal psychology have been supporting the exploration and expression of our earliest experiences in their work with infants, children and adults. Individuals are offered a quality of presence that supports a felt sense of safety and the experience of being heard and seen. The individual's experiences are acknowledged and honored. Understanding is gained about how these experiences have affected the individual, shaped their way of being in the world, and the meaning these experiences have had in the individual's life. New opportunities for healing emerge.

Several clinicians in the field of prenatal and perinatal psychology have shared their experiences working with individuals and families (infants, children, and adults) whose symptoms and issues resonate with experiential imprints originating in the prenatal and perinatal period. This following list mentions the pioneering work of only some of the clinicians who have contributed to the field. Their work provides a window into their approaches to working with the impacts of prenatal and perinatal experiences: Thomas Verny (Verny and Kelly, 1981; Verny and Weintraub, 2002), David Chamberlain (1990, 1998), David Cheek (Rossi and Cheek, 1988), William Emerson (1997, 2000), Stan Grof (1975, 1985), Barbara Findeisen (2001), Phyllis Klaus and Penny Simkin (Simkin and

Klaus, 2004), Ray Castellino (1995, 2000), Wendy Anne McCarty (2000, 2002, 2004, 2008), Gayle Peterson (1994), and Bobbi Jo Lyman (2007).

The following link will connect you to a brief video clip from a wonderful film entitled *The Psychology of Birth: Invitation to Intimacy,* which includes a segment with David Chamberlain, early pioneer, clinician, researcher and prolific author in prenatal and perinatal psychology and Barbara Findeisen, prenatal and birth psychotherapist and author.

http://www.youtube.com/watch?v=cf9WipMBAio

Another link, below, will connect you to a video of Ray Castellino discussing the importance of talking to prenates and providing them with information about what is going to happen. Castellino speaks from decades of experience helping families heal from difficult and traumatic birth and early postnatal experiences.

http://www.youtube.com/watch?v=sxHkLIKx4Bw&feature=related

In an effort to reach clinicians and clients who are interested in understanding more about how to work with prenatal and birth memories in adults, Bobbi Jo Lyman (2007) wrote a workbook and practice manual entitled *Prenatal and Birth Memories: Working with Your Earliest Experiences to Help Your Life Today.* Lyman shared her own journey and that of a client with whom she worked to provide the reader with step-by-step examples of her approach to the process.

As so many clinicians and researchers have attempted to articulate using different language, the *quality of presence* that enables a healing connection with an "other" is perhaps the most essential aspect of person-to-person therapeutic interactions. The research and the experiences of individuals presented here emphasize the crucial need for practitioners to bring careful awareness to the quality of presence they embody in interactions with women, their partners, and their offspring, from pre-conception through the early postnatal period.

Our medical-technological approach to conception, pregnancy, birth, and the early postnatal period has supported the creation of a "dissociative cocoon" (Bromberg, 1998, 2006) that has left many caregivers, and at times, women and their partners, blind to the impact of the *quality of these experiences.* Often, in their aftermath, the expressions of these experiences in the lived bodies of women, their partners, their offspring, and their caregivers "mutely testify" (Kirkengen, 2001) to how they have been affected.

The *quality of experience* that would be most beneficial to the health and development of women, their partners, and their offspring during this critical time is perhaps best facilitated by a *quality of presence* that supports a felt sense of safety, similar to the one that supports healing in psychotherapeutic interactions.

And, to come full circle, a compassionate presence at a rhythm and proximity that supports a felt sense of safety is essential in supporting the exploration and healing of prenatal, birth, and early postnatal experiences. We can only begin to "hear the silent sounds" (Kirkengen, 2001) of these imprints if we open our minds to the likelihood that they exist and have meaning.

I will leave you with this thought: If the need for healing from the imprints of pre-conception, prenatal, birth, and early postnatal experiences is not recognized, and the process of doing so is not facilitated and supported, the impacts of these experiences may be left unresolved and may be passed on to generations to come in ways we have yet to understand, appreciate, and predict.

Please … pay attention.

Glossary

Affect regulation: "The mechanisms by which emotion and its expression are modulated. Allan Schore's regulation framework focuses on the importance of attachment relationships in shaping the important prefrontal circuitry [of the brain] involved in affect regulation early in life" (Siegel, 2012b, AI-3).

Epigenetics: This field studies "the process in which experience alters the regulation of gene expression by way of changing the various molecules (histones and methyl groups) on the chromosome" (Siegel, 2012b, AI-30). More simply put, epigenetics explores the relationship between nature and nurture, or the impact of the environment on the expression of genes.

Implicit memory: "Involves parts of the brain that do not require conscious, focal attention during encoding or retrieval. Perceptions, emotions, bodily sensations, and behavioral response patterns are layers of implicit processing. Mental models (schema or generalizations of repeated experiences) and priming (getting ready to respond) are basic components" (Siegel, 2012b, AI-38). When implicit memory is retrieved, it lacks the feeling of something that has been "recalled" and the individual may not even be aware that the feelings they are having during the retrieval of the memory are being generated from something from the past. They experience the implicit memory as emotions, behaviors ("fixed action patterns"), perceptions, and bodily sensations (Siegel, 2012b, AI-38).

Additional Resources

Here are some additional brief videos and an audio podcast that I recommend.

Monty Python: The Meaning of Life (Birth): This video may make you laugh, but sadly, it is not that far off from the experiences of some women, their babies and their partners of hospital birth. http://www.dailymotion.com/video/x1sh3y_monty-python-the-meaning-of-life-bi_fun

Sheila Kitzinger on fear in childbirth: http://www.oneworldbirth.net/videos/the-problem/sheila-kitzinger-on-fear-in-childbirth/

Michel Odent on birth and the neocortex: The importance of the environment in supporting the normal birth process. http://www.youtube.com/watch?v=KiPd8N19a8k

Penny Simkin on early sexual abuse and its impact on women's experiences of breastfeeding. http://breastfeeding.blog.motherwear.com/2009/03/podcast-early-sexual-abuse-and-breastfeeding-with-penny-simkin.html

The Association for Prenatal and Perinatal Psychology and Health: www.birthspsychology.com If you choose to become a member, you have online access to the *Journal of Prenatal and Perinatal Psychology and Health*—an abundance of articles.

The following website contains free access to the Primal Health Research database which explores correlations between the "primal period" (from conception until the first birthday) and health in later life. http://www.birthworks.org/site/primal-health-research.html

CHAPTER 23

Prenatal Craniosacral Therapy

by Valerie Cora

This chapter is about working with women who are pregnant or who have just had their baby. Photographs are included to help the reader translate this information into clinical practice. Working with a pregnant mom requires a few considerations for both the mother-to-be and the practitioner. A lot of questions have come up in the craniosacral therapy profession about pregnancy and how we work with pregnant women. I will provide some basic information that is vital to know about each trimester of working safely with a pregnant woman. Most of this has to do with proper positioning of the mom on a massage table. Although craniosacral therapy does not have to be performed on a massage table, it is very practical to use one to provide the utmost comfort for the expectant mom.

First Trimester: Week 0 to Week 13

When working with a woman during this period any position on the table is acceptable, including:

- Supine, with or without a knee bolster, if it is comfortable for the mom

- Prone, with or without an ankle bolster, if it is comfortable for the mom. A pillow for her head may be used and a towel might be needed under the shoulders and clavicles to adjust for breast tenderness.

- Semireclining, using cushions, pillows, or tilt table with a knee bolster. Although it is not necessary during the first trimester to maintain a 45-degree angle of semirecline, it is good practice as it will become necessary during the second trimester.

- Sidelying, using pillows for support of the legs and a pillow for her head (described in more detail below, for the second trimester)

• Seated, in a chair or on a couch, depending on client comfort

Second Trimester: Week 14 to Week 26

Working with a woman during this period requires some special considerations.

Prone is not recommended from this point onward; this includes not using any body cushions with belly and breast cut-outs. There is much debate over the use of cushions and tables with cut-outs. The consensus of the leading educators in pregnancy massage across the country is to avoid this position. Lying prone after week 14 may increase the strain of the uterine ligaments because the mom's belly is too small for the opening, or it increases intrauterine pressure because the mom's belly is too big for the opening, or it is simply unappealing for a mom to lie on top of her baby.

Supine is acceptable from week 14 to week 22 in a modified position. The use of a pregnancy pillow (Figure 23.1) under the right hip will move the fetus off the mother's vena cava, preventing possible supine hypotensive syndrome. A pillow that is not tapered or a folded bath towel will work as well, but may not be as comfortable for the mother. If at any time the mother describes feeling nausea, dizziness, or lightheadedness, immediately turn her onto her left side. Any such symptoms will subside instantly.

Supine is not recommended after 22 weeks except for short periods of time (2 to 5 minutes) with a hip pillow. This timeline does not fit well into the biodynamic model of craniosacral therapy because of the amount of time spent in each hand position, which usually exceeds 2–5 minutes.

Semireclining is a great option for the second and third trimester table positioning. There are many wedge pillows available today that can be used to bolster the mom in this position if the practitioner does not have an adjustable table (Figure 23.2). The wedge should be at least 12 inches high with additional cushioning up to 24 inches high as needed. The optimal angle for the mother-to-be in is at least 45 degrees up to 75 degrees. This depends upon her comfort. It will also be necessary to use a knee bolster.

Sidelying is the best option for the second and third trimester. This position is typically how the mom sleeps every night. With proper bolstering it will provide the best opportunity for the mother to settle as well as allow the most access for the practitioner's hand positions. Ideally, a full body pillow should be used along with a head pillow. The body pillow will provide the best support if it is medium firm to firm. The head pillow should be as thick as necessary to keep the mother's cervical spine in alignment with her thoracic spine (Figure 23.3).

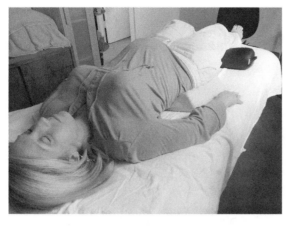

Figure 23.1. Modified supine position for mother in the first trimester.

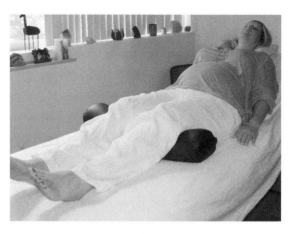

Figure 23.2. Mother semireclining.

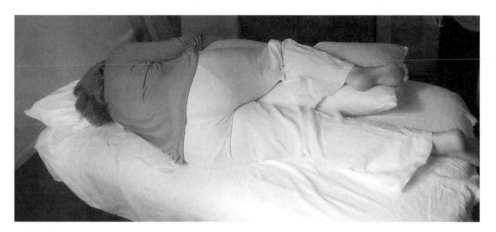

Figure 23.3. Mother sidelying.

Third Trimester: Week 27 to Week 40+

Semireclining, sidelying, and seated are the acceptable positions for the last trimester. All of the considerations mentioned for the second trimester also apply here. There are a few general considerations to keep in mind. Some obstetricians will instruct their patients to never lie on their backs or to only lie on their left sides. Practitioners must ethically honor these requirements without fail during the duration of treatments.

Many practitioners work with a table height of 30 inches or more. It may be necessary to keep a foot stool in the treatment room to accommodate a mother getting on and off the massage table. Pregnant women in second and third trimesters may have to get up during the session to use the restroom, so a foot stool should be easily accessible.

Extra Comfort Measures

There are a few comfort measures a practitioner can take in addition to safe bolstering:

- Using a small wedge pillow under the woman's axillary area in sidelying (Figure 23.4) can relieve shoulder pressure and numbness in the arm and hand during the treatment.

- Using a small wedge pillow under the woman's belly in sidelying (Figure 23.5) can relieve some of the pressure a mother may feel in her sacrum while lying on her side.

- When supporting a woman in sidelying with a full body pillow, it is good to make sure her top leg and foot are completely on the pillow to allow for the best circulation while on her side. The bottom leg should be completely out from under the pillow for the same reason (Figure 23.6).

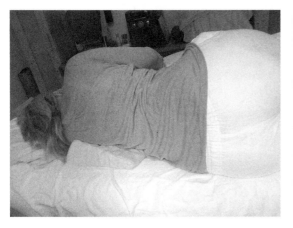

Figure 23.4. Shoulder support, mother sidelying.

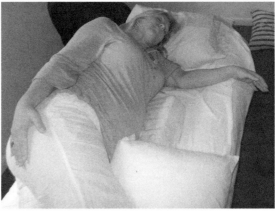

Figure 23.5. Baby support, mother sidelying.

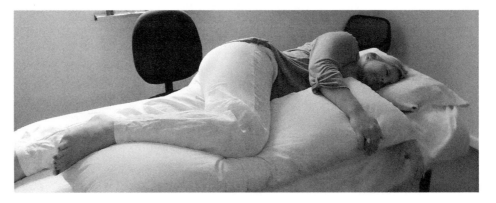

Figure 23.6. Full body pillow, mother sidelying.

Now that the pregnant client is completely comfortable, it is necessary for the practitioner to be completely comfortable as well. The practitioner's own body mechanics and ergonomics around the table are every bit as important as the comfort of the client. Using pillows and other props to support the practitioner's arms and hands are vital for sensing stillness in a session. Having a chair that is adjustable for multiple positions is also important. Keep in mind that a pregnant woman, especially in third trimester, may not be able to stay in any one position for too long. Later in this chapter will be some examples of practitioner support while working.

Discussion

There are many benefits of manual therapy for mothers-to-be and for their babies-to-be. Just as there are special considerations for positioning per trimester, there are also considerations emotionally and physiologically for the mother and her child in each trimester. Unpublished research in Germany indicates that human bodies are 92 percent fluid and maintain that amount proportionally through the lifespan starting after conception. Biodynamic craniosacral therapists work primarily with fluid movement in the body, so when working with a pregnant woman practitioners are touching 92 percent of the body as compared to 8 percent for manual therapists who work exclusively with soft tissue. This becomes more significant for the mother-to-be as her fluid body increases in volume as much as 50 percent by her thirty-sixth week of pregnancy.

In the first trimester the mother's body has so much to manage. The endocrine glands accelerate the release of several hormones. These hormonal changes stimulate multiple physiological changes. This in turn often increases emotional stress, especially during the time of discovery of the pregnancy (when a woman misses her menses). With her body working so hard metabolically, the mother may experience extreme fatigue and anxiety. She may experience bouts of nausea throughout the day for weeks on end. Biodynamic craniosacral therapy sessions during this time provide a vital touch to integrate psychological, physiological, and spiritual balance in her fluid body, as she adapts to the demands of pregnancy. Recent research has proven the value of craniosacral therapy for pregnant moms with pelvic pain (in press). One can infer that this therapy would be excellent for pregnancy in general.

In her second trimester the mother-to-be will have gained weight. As her body prepares for birth she may experience loose ligaments, have back and pelvic pain, have increased digestive distress, and feel the discomforts of slow circulation. On a more positive note, she may also feel the first strong movements of her baby in her womb. She becomes more sensitive to her inner body. Biodynamic craniosacral therapy during this time supports her inner resources for health. A biodynamic session can create the space for a mother to get in touch with her body and her baby. In the stillness of a session the common aches and pains of structural change can reorganize via the organization of fluid movement.

As she transitions into her third trimester it is once again a time of mixed emotions. The reality of birth brings anticipation and anxiety. Her fluid body is approximately 30 percent greater by this time, creating edema especially at the end of the day. As her uterus prepares for birth she may experience Braxton-Hicks contractions. Physiologically her digestion, elimination, and respiration are stressed as they are compressed by the growing baby. Often during biodynamic sessions in the third trimester, mothers become more verbal, expressing concerns and fears about the transition to motherhood. Holding her with compassion and empathy can help her with this process. Stillness and the slow tempo of Primary Respiration in the fluid body enhance empathy and compassion. Working with the pelvis can ease structural pain as has now been demonstrated in the research mentioned above. Working with her heart and liver relieve the discomforts of heartburn, indigestion, and shortness of breath.

The following sections discuss specific handholds in client positions.

Sidelying

When working in sidelying use the props and bolsters discussed above. If you do not have these props, get them. It is best not to work with a pregnant woman without proper support.

The Primitive Streak

The superior hand makes contact at C3. The inferior hand makes contact at the base of the sacrum, thumb at the base and one or two fingers at the coccyx (Figure 23.7). It is important to support your arms in this position. This is typically my first position when working in sidelying. It is easy to settle as a practitioner and easy for clients to settle as they are in a position that promotes deep relaxation. Often if the fetus is parallel to the mother's spine, you can sense a powerful expression of the midline of both the mother and baby. This hand position can also be used with mother and infant with the same intention (Figure 23.8).

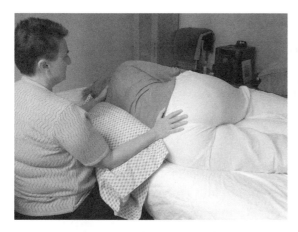

Figure 23.7. Pietà, mother sidelying.

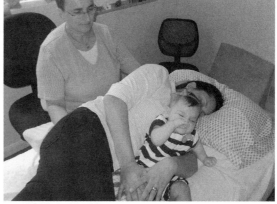

Figure 23.8. Pietà, mother with baby.

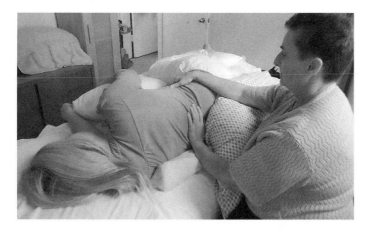

Figure 23.9. Feminine midline, mother sidelying.

The Bubble of Love

The top hand makes contact at the level of the umbilicus posteriorly. The bottom hand makes contact at the umbilicus anteriorly. Using a pillow I rest this arm on the mother's hip and the pillow (Figure 23.9). Whenever making contact with a mother's belly, first ask permission. I also ask the fetus for permission. If for any reason I have to take my hand away, I ask for permission each time I return to her belly. From this position I am able to hold the mother and infant as one fluid being. I am able to observe Primary Respiration from the feminine midline (the umbilicus).

Semireclining

When working with pregnant women in this position the 45- to 75-degree angle is very important. When working with a mom and infant, however, an incline will be more comfortable for the mom to hold her baby, but the angle is not as important in postpartum work.

Pietà

The superior hand (toward the head) is placed first at the shoulder. The inferior hand is placed under the thigh, wherever your hands can reach with comfort (Figure 23.10). As with all sessions it is from here that we can witness the whole, and come into relationship with the fluid body. When working with a mother and infant I modify this position. The baby is face down, heart to heart with the mother. I place my superior hand under the mother between the shoulder blades. I am able to sense the mother and infant hearts as one (Figure 23.11).

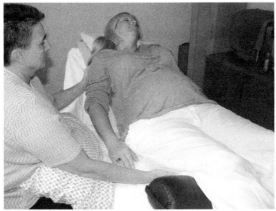

Figure 23.10. Pietà, mother semireclining.

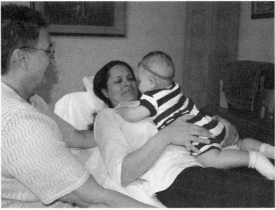

Figure 23.11. Pietà, mother and child semireclining.

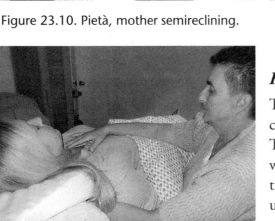

Figure 23.12. Feminine heart, mother semireclining.

Heart Fulcrum

The hand toward the head is placed under the client with the thumb at the base of the neck. The hand toward the feet is placed softly on the woman's chest, just below the clavicles, fingertips and thumb straddling the sternum (Figure 23.12). That arm is supported by a pillow placed on top of the client. Wait a few minutes for your body to settle before checking in for the client's comfort. This is working with the heart from the feminine midline.

Umbilicus (Bubble of Love)

This hand position is the same as in sidelying. The bottom hand slides under the mother and straddles the spine at the level of her umbilicus. The top hand rests on either side of the belly button (Figure 23.13). This is not a precise hand contact because you need to modify your hands based on the size of mother's abdomen. Softly cup the top hand so contact is with the fingertips and the thenar area of the palm.

This can also be done with mother and infant postpartum. When the baby is lying belly to belly with her mother the top hand is placed on the back of the infant (Figure 23.14). I am not too particular with hand position here. I usually place my hand just above the iliac crest, but anywhere the baby lets me touch is good for me.

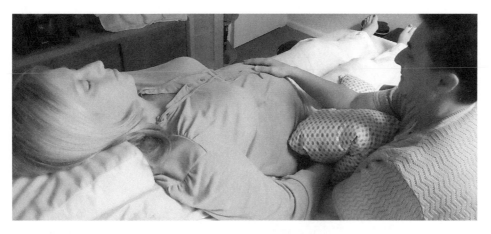

Figure 23.13. Feminine midline, mother semireclining.

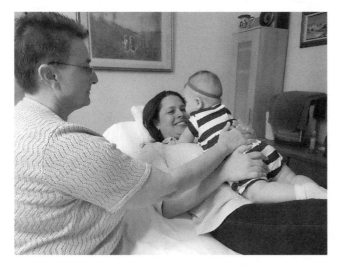

Figure 23.14. Feminine midline,
mother and baby semireclining.

Other Positions and Transitions

There are many ways to accommodate a pregnant woman or a mother and infant. Holding your attention on Primary Respiration, the sacred space and nature allows for the use of several hand positions.

The Head

In the first trimester the head is easy to work with. I typically use hand positions that have my hands lateral to the midline like the inferior lateral angle of the parietal bone (ILA) or a modified Becker hold. (Michael's Volume Four has a complete description of the hand positions.) If I move to the midline I like the occipital hold (Figure 23.15) or the atlanto-occipital hold. When working with a woman in second or third trimester, I will work with her head in transition. For example, after 22 weeks when moving from sidelying to semireclining I will work with more lateral hand positions after getting her settled in her 45- to 75-degree position. When working with a second trimester woman when moving from one side to the other I will pause in the modified supine position to work with her head and then complete the transition to the other side.

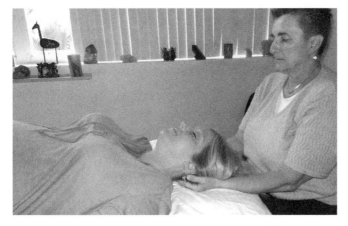

Figure 23.15. AO joint, mother in modified supine.

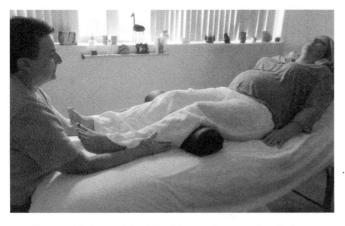

Figure 23.16. Midcalf hold, mother semireclining.

The Feet

With pregnant women I prefer to finish the session at the feet rather than the sacrum. This is because there is so much going on at the sacrum it can be challenging to remain spacious and move attention out to the horizon and back. I use a different hand position at the feet as well, staying lateral of the midline. I place my hands at the level of the calf, engaging them on the lateral borders or underneath them (Figure 23.16). This allows the mother to feel her three dimensionality as most of her attention during this time is held on her own pregnancy midline (vagina).

Seated

Often a practitioner may have to work with a pregnant woman or mother and infant without a massage table. Making yourself and the woman very comfortable would be the primary goal here. When seated on a couch I find the most comfortable contact is one hand behind the mother's back at a level that is comfortable for both of us. If she is holding her baby I may make contact with the infant's back (Figure 23.17). If a mother needs to breastfeed during her session I modify my hand position for the infant to just off the head (Figure 23.18). Primary Respiration is my only intention when working with a mother and baby.

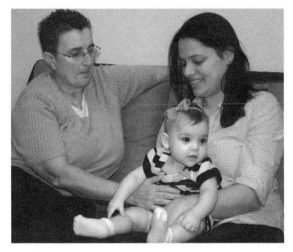 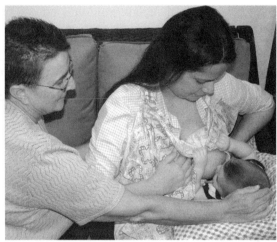

Figure 23.17. Feminine midline, mother and child seated.

Figure 23.18. Feminine midline, holding space while breastfeeding.

Postpartum Work

During the postpartum period (sometimes called the fourth trimester) the attention a mother received during her pregnancy is transferred to her new baby. This is a time of great change for both mother and child. It is important that mom receives time just for her. Biodynamic sessions for mom during this time create the opportunity for reorganization of her spine, pelvis, and the muscles that worked so hard in the previous nine months. Other issues that may be present are birth experiences that did not go as planned or physical trauma during stage 2 labor. The endocrine system shuts off the release of several hormones as soon as labor is over. This change can increase emotional stress once again.

It is also an excellent time to work with the mother and the baby. Biodynamic craniosacral therapy with the mother and her child can increase bonding and support better breastfeeding by facilitation of the latch and sucking reflex. Sessions can also be done with the father if he is available. Dads need a lot of support as well. The practitioner's spacious attention to the mother enhances the reorganization of her cranium and pelvic structures. Frequently the mother will be holding her baby during a session. The growth and development of the infant's heart, lungs, and digestive system are facilitated through the sustained direct skin contact with the mother during sessions. It is vital that the practitioner supports both mother and child as one, maintaining a witness presence during the treatment when another caregiver is unavailable to hold the baby.

Biodynamic craniosacral therapy hand positions with a pregnant woman can be duplicated with mother and infant. The first consideration I pay attention to when determining hand positions is, Can I maintain sustained contact comfortably, and then am I able to get a sense of the whole with this position?

Biodynamic craniosacral therapy can facilitate a woman's health during the childbearing year and postpartum period. It can ease the discomforts of the physiological and musculoskeletal changes during these times. Develop a sense of awareness of the interconnected relationship that is going on between the mother and her embryo, fetus, and infant with slowness and stillness.

CHAPTER 24

Biodynamic Treatment Methods for the Baby in NICU (Neonatal Intensive Care Unit)

by Phyllis Aries, MA, BCST, OTR

Dedication and Gratitude

Please know that I experience words as pale echoes of my vibrant feelings, while I reflect on my desire to express gratitude.

I dedicate these two chapters to my parents. My mom's generous, clever, and fun-loving spirit has nurtured my essence and taught me to understand love. My memories of my dad are rich, with his inventive nature and warmhearted humor thriving in a stream of creative energy, giving to the world with the ease and grace of feathers in a light wind.

I'm thankful for the profound and masterful teachings of Michael Shea, magnifying the potential of life's positive forces, while weaving knowledge and understanding with the power of the heart.

I'm grateful for my husband Robert's gentle stream of support, along with his skill and perseverance in managing the challenges of photography and the tangles of technology. I recognize the value of my daughter Olivia's lively contributions and insightful observations. I am grateful to my sister Susan for her expression of the word *sisterhood* in every sphere of my life. I am thankful for my brother Steve's love.

I am impressed with the NICU babies, creating avenues for this deep healing work to support others. As they convey their needs and preferences so sweetly, the net of trauma unravels, and health emerges as a strength within freedom.

I am grateful to the NICU staff for expressing genuine curiosity and encouragement, and broadening my understanding of babies through open conversations, illuminating both converging and opposing perspectives.

I'm thankful to all of the babies, children, families, and adults featured here for the magnitude of their generosity and warmhearted spirit lacing the photography experiences, with each image unfolding as a unique treasured gift.

I value the strength, heartfelt empathy, and enduring support of my supervisor, Janine Kahan McLear, as she affirms the nature of this work with wisdom and humor, and smoothes the path for progress.

I'm grateful to Judith Anderson for her generous spirit and wealth of knowledge, contributing to my understanding of nonviolent communication, and creating a practice group full of meaningful connection and love.

I'm happy that the bridges leading me to this work have brought me a cherished friend, Ilene Sperling. I'm grateful for her kindness, clarity, and use of humor, as our closeness brightens my heart.

I honor the richness and inspiration in the work of Heidelise Als, Jane Carreiro, David Cameron Gikandi, Stephen Porges, Marshall Rosenberg, Allan Schore, and Daniel Siegel.

Introduction

Embracing the baby's NICU experience through the biodynamic process creates a unique connection to well-being and fosters innate health. These NICU handholds have evolved as congruent matches to experiences encountered by the NICU babies. The handhold descriptions are designed to convey information through a sequence of photographs and text.

Each treatment technique described here features a photograph that demonstrates the method with a baby. The written explanation typically contains three parts, with an occasional additional one or two parts. The first part outlines the position for baby and then therapist. The second part in the text identifies usual therapeutic indications in relation to the baby's NICU experiences, diagnoses, or characteristics. A third part reviews structural changes and therapeutic processes frequently expressed during treatment. Extra written sections may specify treatment options, involving alternative positions for the baby and/or therapist. Also, additional sections may suggest subtleties in the quality of the technique, beneficial in orienting or shaping the unified connection.

Most of the treatment techniques include photographs demonstrating a mommy and baby or daddy and baby handhold adaptation. All handholds contain photographic examples of handhold adaptations for working with adults.

In two handholds (Mama Bear's Care and the Ahh), the description is organized with three variations outlined individually. For example, Mama Bear's Care comprises the options of Mama Bear's Soothing Surroundings, Mama Bear's Protection from Pain, and Bathing in Mama Bear's Love. Also, one photographic series illustrates the possibility of blending two handholds, with a mommy and baby photo progression combining Friends with Holding Love. Last, the handhold called the Hula Hoop is adapted into a treatment sequence named Little Hula Hoops, where a parent is supported while comforting baby in an isolette.

Several clinical processes are described. The subtleties in the sensations experienced during these processes may be more easily recognized through a few expanded explanations. *Pulsing* is a rhythmic motion characterized by a downward and forward direction, reversing into an upward and backward motion. Pulsing may be experienced in varied forms: localized pulsing, slow pulsing, and broad unified pulsing. With *localized pulsing* present in a smaller area (e.g., in baby's fluid body), I often use telescoping to widen and settle into a broadened treatment space. *Slow pulsing* frequently appears as a portion of the merged treatment process, while *broad unified pulsing* is sensed as large, deep, and profound, encompassing the space in and around the baby and therapist. During broad unified pulsing, I tend to soften my presence, frequently quieting my own breath and remaining physically still, thereby permitting the baby's full expression of its unique therapeutic process. Typically, a beautiful stillness or decompression follows broad unified pulsing. *Descending* is a term used to signify the experience of a weighty, slow, and wide downward motion throughout the treatment space. The surrounding area often shifts to a darker and more dense consistency. As this downward motion progresses, I tend to use telescoping, and expand the treatment space, while remaining open to transitions in the treatment process.

Though these handholds and treatment techniques are aligned with NICU babies, many of these methods are beneficial in the treatment of full-term and older babies without hospital experiences, as well as adults. All treatment techniques are based on the therapist's ability to perceive Primary Respiration or stillness in himself or herself and then with the baby.

Floating Air Balloons: Lifting the Intubation Sensation

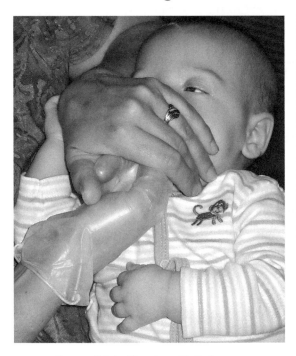

Figure 24.1. Floating Air Balloons.

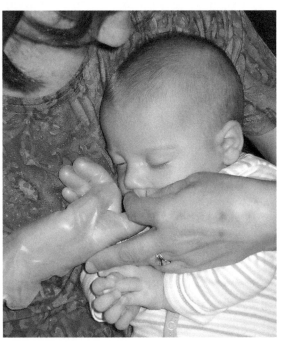

Figure 24.2. Floating Air Balloons, alternative handhold—anterior maxilla.

Position

Baby: Support baby in semireclined sitting, supine, or sidelying on therapist's lap, or comfortable surface; use blanket rolls to fully support baby. Position baby facing you.

Therapist's right hand: Place gloved index finger along midline of palate with palm facing upward (Figure 24.1).

Therapist's left hand: Place palm facing down and fingers held together gently, cupping left hand over right hand; place medial and ventral aspects of palm and little finger along baby's zygomatic, maxilla, and nasal bones; maintain gentle cupped hand position spanning inferiorly overlying right hand.

Alternative position for therapist's left hand: Place pads of thumb and index finger inferior and lateral to nares overlying anterior maxilla (Figure 24.2).

Additional alternative positions for the therapist's hands:

Right hand: Thumb pad lightly contacts right lateral aspect of the hyoid bone; index or long finger pad lightly contacts left lateral aspect of the hyoid.

Right hand: Palm is facing down onto baby's upper chest overlying trachea or sternum.

Left hand: Palm is facing downward, and thumb is supporting pacifier on baby's mouth; palm and fingers are cupped with fingers held together gently. Base of palm and finger pads are draped along lateral aspects of baby's head and may contact superior mandible, maxilla, zygomatic, temporal, sphenoid, or frontal bones.

Therapeutic Indications

Following intubation.

High arched palate.

Oral-motor uncoordination following intubation.

Structural Changes and Therapeutic Processes

Lateral expansion through the palate or maxilla.

Softening through the oral and/or pharyngeal tissues.

Improved oral-motor suction pressures.

Increased organization and comfort with oral-motor functions.

Pulsing with heat release through contact areas.

Cessation of sucking with quieting of body movements.

Deepening/descending.

Deep rest.

Adult Handhold Adaptations

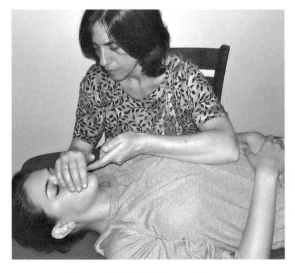

Figure 24.3. Palate midline.

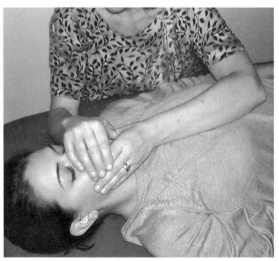

Figure 24.4. Maxilla.

Unsnapping the Baby's CPAP Cap (CPAP: Continuous Positive Airway Pressure)

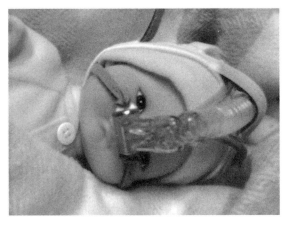

Figure 24.5. Doll with CPAP support, anterior view.

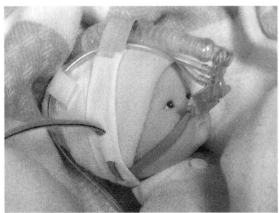

Figure 24.6. Doll with CPAP support, lateral view.

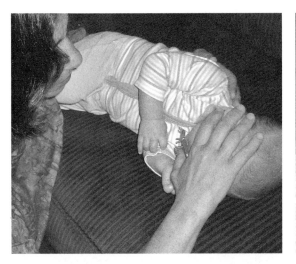

Figure 24.7. Unsnapping the baby's CPAP cap.

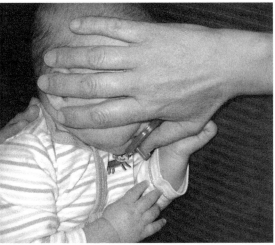

Figure 24.8. Unsnapping the baby's CPAP cap, thumb supporting pacifier.

The use of a doll in Figures 24.5 and 24.6 illustrates the placement of the CPAP apparatus. Viewing the position of the hat, straps, and nasal piece further clarifies the baby's experience, and intent of the treatment methods to complement the benefits of receiving oxygen support.

Position (Figure 24.7)

Support baby in sidelying on your lap or comfortable surface. If needed, use blanket rolls to fully support baby in sidelying. Position the baby so that he or she is facing you.

Your hand overlying the baby's face is held in a soft open position, creating the sense of a broad and unified connection with the baby's skin. Your hand may be experienced as a warm weighty blanket, comforting the baby in the knowing that no one will be asking anything of him or her; all is done, and there is endless time to rest.

With the baby in left sidelying, you use your right hand on the baby's head. With the baby in right sidelying, you use your left hand on the baby's head. Your hand position may need to be adjusted in relation to the baby's head size.

Place your thumb or palm in front of the baby's mouth. The thumb or palm may aid the baby in stabilizing the pacifier (Figure 24.8). If preferred, you may use the gloved index finger (of the opposite hand) in the baby's mouth.

Your thumb lies adjacent to the baby's nose (possibly in relation to the maxilla and nasal bones). The distal palm or fingers may align with the mandible, vomer, ethmoid, maxilla, zygomatic, sphenoid, frontal, temporal, or parietal bones.

Therapeutic Indications

Prior CPAP experience with prongs and/or mask design.

Following noxious tactile experiences, especially along the face and head.

Following stressful medical care.

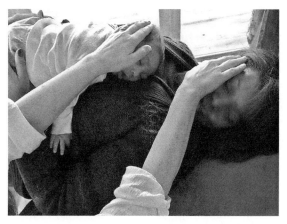

Figure 24.9. Unsnapping the baby's CPAP cap, mommy and baby.

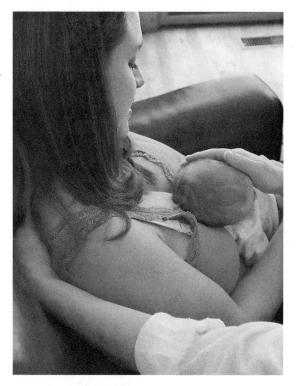

Figure 24.10. Unsnapping the baby's CPAP cap, mommy and baby in alternative sitting position.

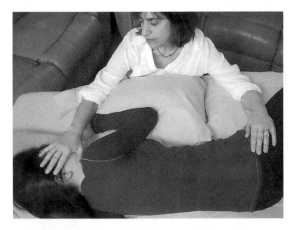

Figure 24.11. Unsnapping the baby's CPAP cap, adult handhold adaptation.

Therapeutic Processes and Structural Changes

Cessation of sucking with deepening/descending.

Broad unified pulsing.

Decompression and softening through structures.

Disorganization resolving into settling, and then stillness.

Deep rest.

Sense of profound peace.

Removing the Baby's Nose Warmer: Easing Off the CPAP Prongs and Mask (The Part of CPAP Positioned on Nose)

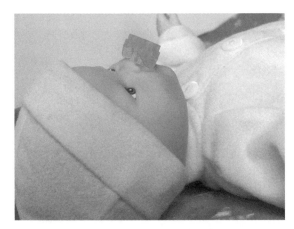

Figure 24.12. Doll with CPAP prongs.

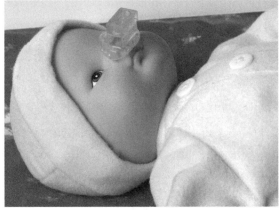

Figure 24.13. Doll with CPAP mask.

The use of a doll in Figures 24.12 and 24.13 is designed to broaden the understanding of the baby's experience, while visualizing the angles of pressure applied through the application of the CPAP prongs and mask.

Position

Baby is supported on comfortable surface, or your lap in supine or sidelying.

To optimize positive responses with this hand placement, complete the initial stages of treatment, allowing the baby time to ease into a deep restful state.

Following CPAP prongs

Your dominant hand is positioned with index finger pad on dorsal aspect of nasal bone, while thumb and long finger are placed adjacent to alar sidewall (lateral to nares and along maxilla, as shown in Figure 24.14).

Your nondominant hand supports along the baby's cervical spine and occiput, or cervical spine and shoulders.

Options for Treating Following CPAP Prongs

Therapist's dominant hand: If compression is sensed with contact, position your thumb and digits approximately 1 inch off of the baby's nasal bone and maxilla; Slowly ease onto surface of nasal bone and ascending process of maxilla (Figure 24.15).

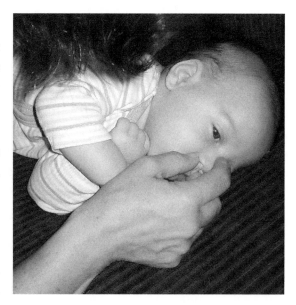

Figure 24.14. Removing the baby's nose warmer, easing off the CPAP prongs and mask.

Therapist's dominant hand: Place index finger on dorsal aspect of nasal bone, and position thumb and long finger approximately one-half inch inferior to nares (the openings to the nostrils) off skin surface.

Therapist's dominant hand: Start off the skin surface and slowly position your index finger on dorsal aspect of nasal bone, and place thumb and long finger pads along lateral aspects of columella and philtrum. The columella is the fleshy external end of the nasal septum seen as a strip of skin between the nostrils. The philtrum is the medial cleft located between the inferior aspect of the nose and the superior aspect of the upper lip (Figure 24.16).

Therapist's nondominant hand: Position gloved index finger pad in oral cavity along palate, or support pacifier for intra-oral connection.

Following CPAP Mask

Therapist's dominant hand: Position index finger pad on root of nose (most depressed aspect of nose located between orbits), with thumb and long finger adjacent to alar sidewall, lateral to nares and along maxilla (see Figure 24.24).

Therapist's nondominant hand: Supports along cervical spine and occiput, or cervical spine and shoulders.

Options for Treating Following CPAP Mask

Therapist's dominant hand: Handhold may gradually shift from off skin surface to position of contact. Index finger on root of nose, with thumb and long finger along ascending process of maxilla (Figures 24.17 and 24.18).

Therapist's dominant hand: Place index on root, with thumb and long finger pads along lateral aspects of columella and philtrum (Figure 24.19).

Therapeutic Indications

Following CPAP or nasal canula.

Following feedings through nasogastric tube.

Following suctioning or repogle (repogle is a soft plastic tube inserted into the baby's nose or mouth for continuous suctioning of excess secretions).

Following ear, nose, and throat examinations.

Structural Changes and Therapeutic Processes

Comfort or softening of facial expression, and/or a peaceful resting state.

Disorganization resolving into reorganization, and settling of facial, pharyngeal, and cranial structures.

Localized or broad unified pulsing or stillness.

Removing the Baby's Nose Warmer

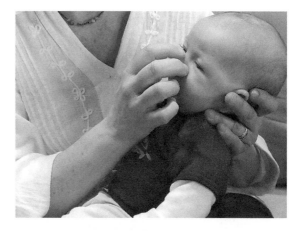

Figure 24.15. Nasal bone and ascending process of maxilla.

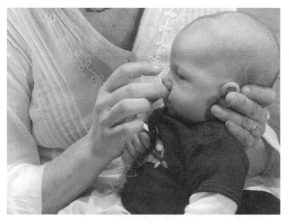

Figure 24.16. Nasal bone, off skin surface, columella, and philtrum.

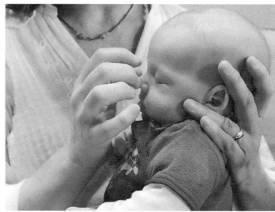

Figure 24.17. Root and maxilla, off skin surface.

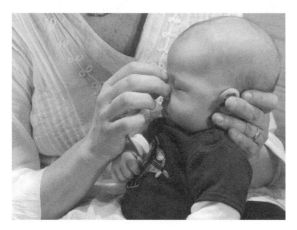

Figure 24.18. Root and ascending process of maxilla.

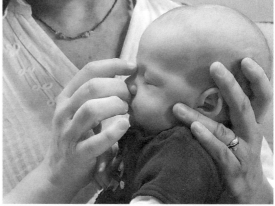

Figure 24.19. Root, columella, and philtrum.

Removing the Baby's Nose Warmer: Mommy and Baby

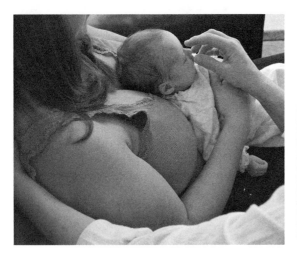

Figure 24.20. Off skin surface, nasal bone and maxilla.

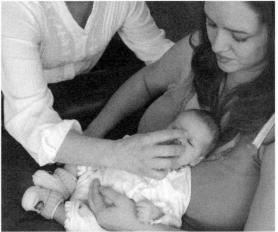

Figure 24.21. Root, maxilla, and alar sidewall.

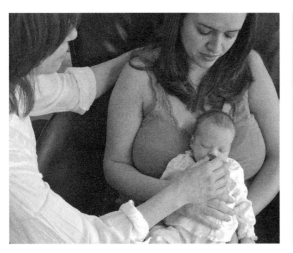

Figure 24.22. Maxilla and nares, anterior view.

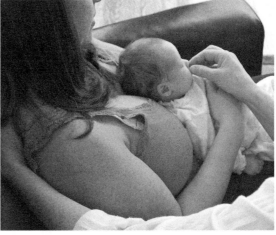

Figure 24.23. Maxilla and nares, lateral view.

Removing the Baby's Nose Warmer: Adult Handhold Adaptations

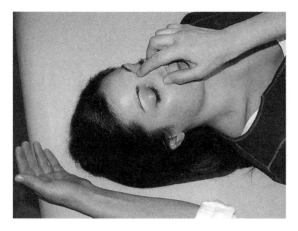

Figure 24.24. Root and alar sidewall.

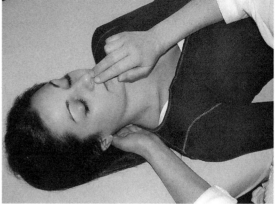

Figure 24.25. Philtrum.

Grandma's Chicken Soup: The Immune Booster

This hand position is named in honor of my mother for her warm loving heart, softness in nurturing inner strength, and amazingly yummy chicken soup!

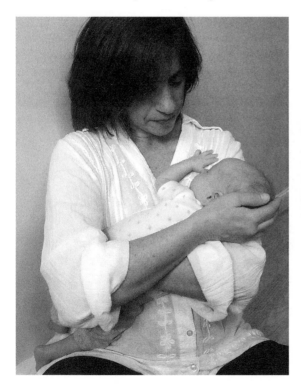

Figure 24.26. Grandma's Chicken Soup: The Immune Booster.

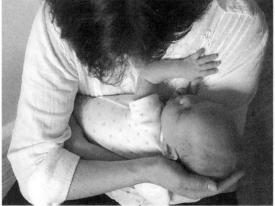

Figure 24.27. Grandma's Chicken Soup, top view.

Position (Figure 24.26)

Baby: Held facing you, diagonally on your chest and abdomen. The baby's head approximates your upper left chest, and feet are positioned along your lower right abdomen, with adaptations to match the baby's size. Support the baby's upper body for a heart-to-heart connection, and guide the baby's chest and lower body toward neutral alignment through the spine. It is beneficial for you to be sitting in a reclined position to increase the baby's comfort and distribution of weight.

Therapist's left hand: Support the posterior aspect of the baby's pelvis, cupping the sacrum, with a relaxed and expansive hand.

Therapist's right arm (Figure 24.27): If possible, position your right elbow over your left hand, approximating this position as the baby's size permits. The elbow maintains an open and expansive sense, while adding a soft grounding component. A downward projection through the baby's feet may be offered in the treatment as desired.

Allow the ulnar aspect of your right forearm to gently cradle and support the baby's right side along the length of his or her body. Within the baby's comfort, lengthen and align the baby's spine.

Your right hand may encircle the baby's shoulders and head for comfort, according to the size ratio and optimal support.

Therapeutic Indications

Medical disturbances associated with compromises in immunity.

Stressful experiences related to medical, physical, or emotional conditions.

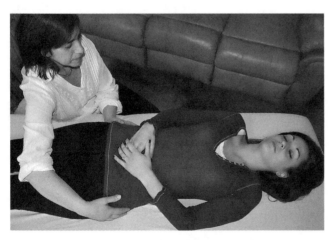

Figure 24.28. Grandma's Chicken Soup, adult handhold adaptation.

Structural Changes and Therapeutic Processes

Broad decompression through pelvis.

Expression of upward flow.

Wide expansive lateral decompression.

Deep stillness and sense of peace.

The GIG (Grounding into Gravity)

This handhold is named in honor of my husband Robert for the sense of deep peace I experience in the presence of our love, and his astounding musical talent!

Position (Figure 24.29)

Baby: Prone on a comfortable supportive surface.

Therapist: Connect with baby using soft palms along the thoracic and pelvic areas. Maintain uniform contact through the palms for an even weight distribution. A sense of trust and security is experienced, while relying on the earth for support. Acceptance of the earth's gravitational support is felt through the heart, and welcomed in the physical being.

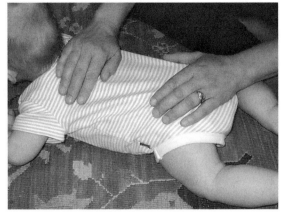

Figure 24.29. The GIG
(Grounding into Gravity).

Therapeutic Indications

Difficult delivery.

Hospitalizations or medical care.

Compromised family involvement and/or adoption.

Limited sensory system regulation.

Structural Changes and Therapeutic Processes

Therapist shifts to a sense of trust and security within stillness or Primary Respiration.

Therapist connects with the heart in relation to accepting the earth's support.

Therapist maintains an open connection (frequent cycles of attunement) with the baby.

Baby softens and relaxes into supporting surface.

Broad decompression or unified deep stillness.

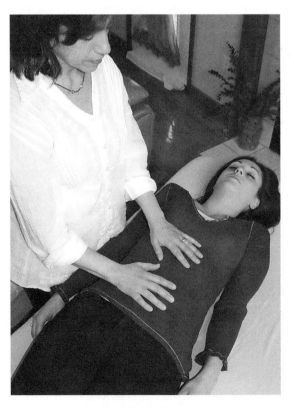

Figure 24.30. The GIG,
adult handhold adaptation.

The Hammock Hold

Position (Figure 24.31)

Baby: Sitting semireclined on your lap.

Therapist's left arm: Cradling baby against your body and inner aspect of left arm.

Therapist's left hand: Supports left side of baby's pelvis, with your thumb or thenar eminence positioned anteriorly, palm along lateral aspect of pelvis, and digits extending under baby.

Therapist's right hand: Thumb along right side of baby's diaphragm, palm over anterior aspect of diaphragm, and digits extending along left side of diaphragm.

Options for right hand:

Gloved index finger in baby's mouth, or index supporting pacifier in baby's mouth and other digits along mandible (Figure 24.32).

Shifted superiorly, spanning lungs and thoracic cavity (Figure 24.33).

Spanning diaphragm, abdominal viscera, and pelvis (Figure 24.34).

Shifted to left side of baby's chest overlying heart (Figure 24.35).

Palm supporting sacrum.

Therapeutic Indications

Painful facial expressions, painful crying, irritability.

Hyper-responsive sensory systems.

Scapular elevation and/or medial compression through thoracic cavity.

Sense of dense or taut connections (e.g., heart and diaphragm).

Disorganized respiration and/or increased respiratory work effort.

Tachycardia.

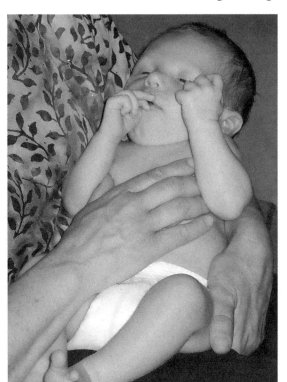

Figure 24.31. The hammock hold.

Therapeutic Processes and Structural Changes

Transition to quiet state, deep rest.

Higher threshold for challenging environmental conditions and sensory system regulation.

Breathing stabilization with slowing of respiration.

Work of breath diminishes.

Heart rate orients to comfortable ranges (pre-term infant heart rate 140–160; full-term infant heart rate 100–160, with 80–100 functional if asleep).

Softening or melting through dense or taut areas.

Vertical decompression with lengthening.

Sense of trust and safety in the world.

Decompression with expansion through the thoracic cavity.

Alternative Handholds

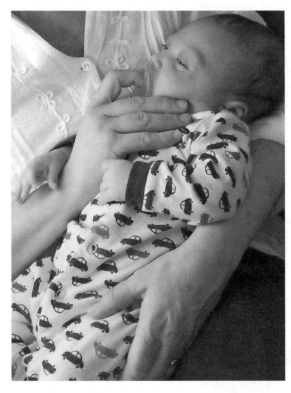

Figure 24.32. Right hand over mandible, intra-oral treatment through pacifier.

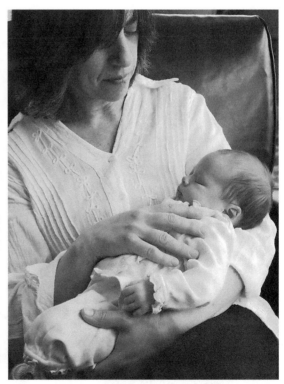

Figure 24.33. Right hand overlying lungs.

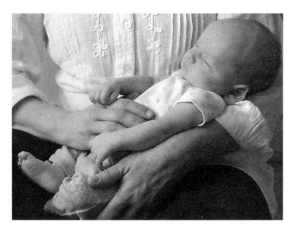

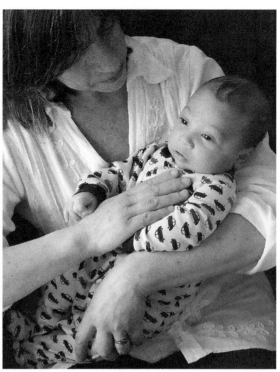

Figure 24.34. Right hand overlying diaphragm, abdominal viscera, and pelvis.

Figure 24.35. Right hand over heart.

Adult Handhold Adaptations

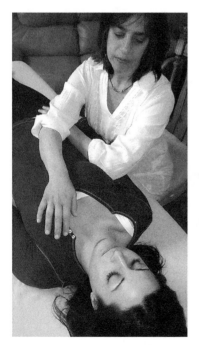

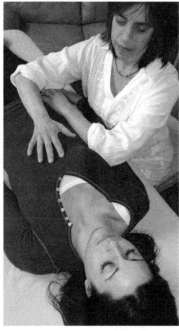

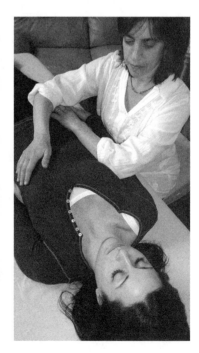

Figure 24.36. Heart.　　　　Figure 24.37. Diaphragm.　　　　Figure 24.38. Stomach.

Flower Power: Baby's Breath

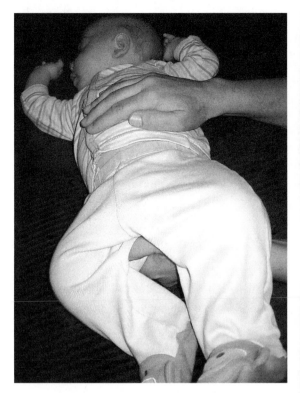

Figure 24.39. Sacrum and diaphragm.

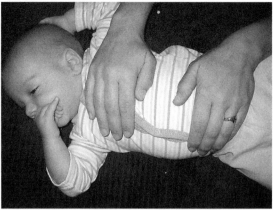

Figure 24.40. Overlying thoracic and abdominal chambers.

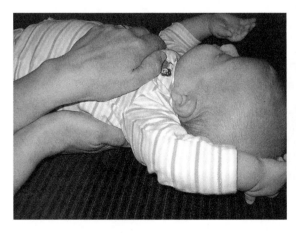

Figure 24.41. Ventral and dorsal lungs and trachea.

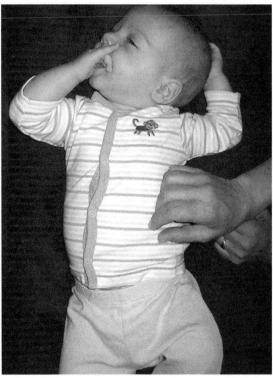

Figure 24.42. Feather-light thumb and index pad.

Position

Baby: Any comfortable position on your lap, or supported in blanket rolls. Supine position may be easier for two of the handholds: (1) Figure 24.40, showing overlying thoracic and abdominal chambers, and (2) Figure 24.42, showing feather-light thumb and index pad contact.

Therapist: It may be beneficial to observe the baby's respiration, maintaining a sense of acceptance while using distant telescoping.

You may initiate treatment by creating security and grounding with a gentle sacral hold. This connection brings a sense of safety, and positive responses to the handholds supporting respiration, lungs, and diaphragm.

Four Positions

Sacrum and diaphragm (Figure 24.39): Therapist modifies the amount and distribution of pressure in connection with the diaphragm.

Overlying thoracic and abdominal chambers (Figure 24.40): Therapist may use telescoping (cycle of attunement) to support a balance in thoracic and abdominal cavity pressures.

Ventral and dorsal lungs and trachea (Figure 24.41): Therapist's attention to the softness of palms, and the use of distant telescoping, may be beneficial.

Feather-light thumb and index finger pad (Figure 24.42): Therapist creates a sense of connecting with a small window in relation to the diaphragm, and the totality of the respiratory system.

Therapeutic Indications

Current or prior oxygen support, including intubation, CPAP, and nasal canula.

Diagnosis of respiratory distress syndrome, bronchopulmonary dysplasia, atelectasis, aspiration and cardiac difficulties.

Tachypnea, increased work of breathing, frequent catch-breaths, shallow breaths, irregular respiration with breath holding.

Shifts in respiratory function mirror endurance or postural limitations.

Head and body movements reflect respiration.

Therapeutic Processes and Structural Changes

Initial hesitation and then gradual deepening.

Broad unified pulsing.

Period of disorganization followed by reorganization and settling.

Deep, full inspiration in conjunction with lateral decompression.

Shifts in respiration characterized by smoothness, regulated rate, and oxygen saturation.

Generalized restful state and comfort in relation to respiration.

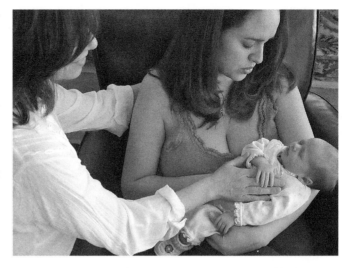

Figure 24.43. Flower Power, mommy and baby.

Adult Handhold Adaptations

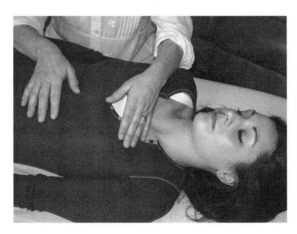

Figure 24.44. Diaphragm and lungs.

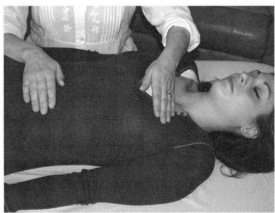

Figure 24.45. Abdominal and thoracic chambers.

Holding Love: Hugging Baby's Heart

Position (Figure 24.46)

Baby: Therapist is sitting in a reclined position and holding the baby in an upright position. Baby is facing you and supported against your chest for a heart-to-heart position.

Therapist's right hand: Supports baby's lower body.

Therapist's left hand: Mold hand along baby's posterior and lateral chest on the left side, supporting a heart-to-heart connection.

Position Options:

Baby may be in any comfortable position on your lap or supportive surface with blanket rolls forming nest. Baby's left side is closest to you.

Your hands are cupped above and below the left side of the baby's chest/heart.

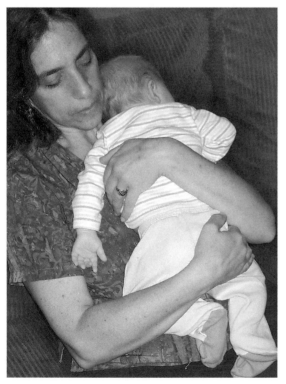

Figure 24.46. Holding Love:
Hugging Baby's Heart.

Therapeutic Indications

Hyper-responsiveness through sensory systems.

Irritability and/or physical discomfort.

Compromised sleep patterns.

Family visits infrequently.

Tachycardia and/or tachypnea.

Delays in feeding related to behavioral disorganization.

Cardiac diagnoses.

Structural Changes and Therapeutic Processes

Transition to quiet alert or restful state.

Sleep, deep rest, sense of peacefulness.

Softening through musculature, quiet body.

Slowing of heart rate and/or respiratory rate.

Improved state regulation and organization for feeding functions.

Deepening/descending.

Isolated deep, full breaths.

Broad slow pulsing.

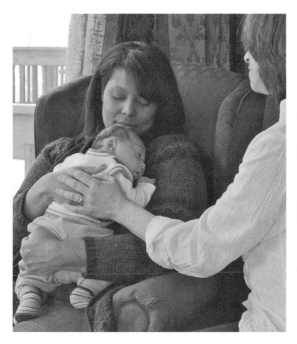

Figure 24.47. Holding Love, mommy and baby.

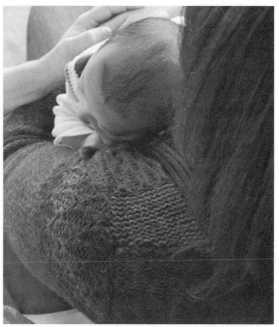

Figure 24.48. Holding Love, mommy and baby, posterior aspect of heart.

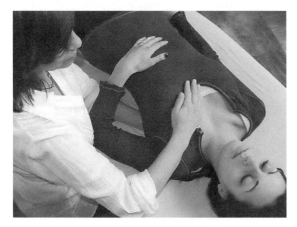

Figure 24.49. Holding Love, adult handhold adaptation.

Friends: Holding Hands

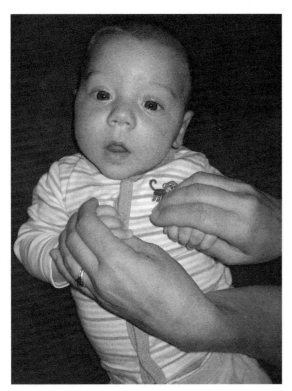

Figure 24.50. Friends: Holding Hands.

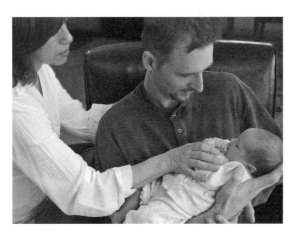

Figure 24.51. Friends: Holding Hands, daddy and baby.

Position

Baby: Any position is possible, though sidelying or supine may be optimal for connecting with the baby while holding hands.

Therapist: All forms of holding either one or both hands are used, though it may be easiest for you to place the thumb or index finger into the baby's palm from the ulnar aspect (Figure 24.50).

Soften your finger and create a sense of closeness experienced with the comfort of friendship.

If the baby appears fearful, gentle cupping over the baby's hand may be used to initiate treatment, shifting gradually to a soft skin contact.

Position Adaptations

Baby holds your finger, while you use a gloved digit or secure the pacifier in the baby's mouth.

Useful for combining with Friends: Holding Hands. Extend a finger toward the baby's hand, allowing the baby to hold it, while connecting with a sense of comfort and security. Other handholds that combine well: Floating Air Balloons, Unsnapping the CPAP Cap, the Candy Cane, the Cooo, the OASIS.

Therapeutic Indications

Hospitalizations or medical care: Arms secured to diminish unsafe movements during caregiving experiences including: IV (intravenous) placement, intubation, nasogastric tube placement, and eye exam.

Challenging attachment situations and/or adoption.

Traumatic birth.

Tightness through shoulder girdle, intercostal musculature, or upper extremities in relation to respiratory/digestive difficulties, or increased muscle tone.

Brachial plexus injury.

Structural Changes and Therapeutic Processes

Baby's initial tightness of grasp or fearful facial expression ease into softness.

Restful state.

Broad unified pulsing.

Deepening/descending.

Relaxation and lengthening through tight musculature.

Slowing of respiration.

Mommy and Baby

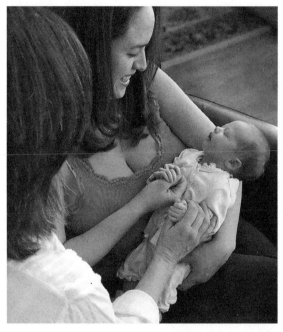

Figure 24.52. Anterior view.

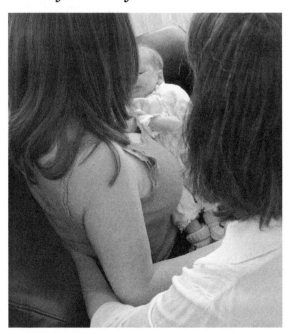

Figure 24.53. Posterior view.

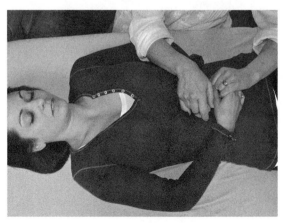

Figure 24.54. Friends: Holding Hands, adult handhold adaptation.

Friends: Soul to Sole

Position (Figure 24.55)

Baby and therapist: Any comfortable position and any adaptation of hand placement.

To minimize guarding or defensive responses to this handhold, you may initiate treatment with the Air Hug Hold (see The Ahh), connect with the dorsal aspect of the baby's foot, or gradually transition from firm to light pressure contact.

Therapist: Conscious softening through the palm and digits may ease the baby's connection and deepening into stillness.

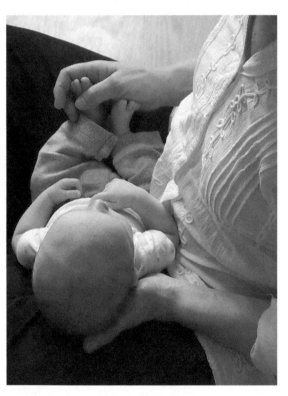

Handholds useful for combining with Friends: Soul to Sole include: MASS, the Hula Hoop (use the ventral aspect of arm), and Floating Air Balloons.

Therapeutic Indications

Hospitalizations or medical care (same as above), with legs secured to diminish unsafe movements during caregiving experiences, including heel sticks and/or IV placement.

States of hyperarousal, disorganization, fight-flight, shutdown, or shock withdrawal.

Initiation of treatment with medically acute, fragile infant.

Structural Changes and Therapeutic Processes

Settling, and softening of facial expression.

Deepening/descending.

Vertical decompression.

Deep restful state.

Figure 24.55. Friends: Soul to Sole.

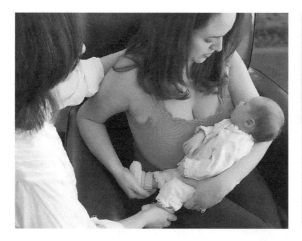

Figure 24.56. Friends: Soul to Sole, mommy and baby.

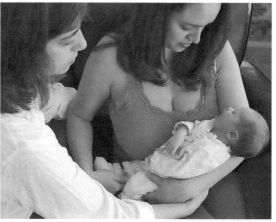

Figure 24.57. Friends: Soul to Sole, mommy and baby, adaptation for sacral hold with baby.

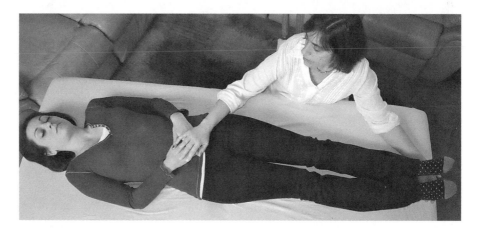

Figure 24.58. Friends: Holding Hands and Soul to Sole, adult handhold adaptation.

Blending Handholds:
Friends Holding Love—Mommy and Baby

The handholds may be easily combined to meet the baby's needs. As an example, blending Friends with Holding Love might unfold in the following sequence: First, a connection is formed by the mommy holding one of the baby's hands, and you holding the baby's other hand (Figure 24.59). Then you may offer a sense of security or grounding with Soul to Sole (Figure 24.60). The mommy continues to hold the baby's hand, while creating a soft contact overlying the baby's heart, coupling Holding Love with Friends. You join this heartwarming connection by resting the baby's hand (still held in your hand) over the mother's (Figure 24.61). You then support a heart-to-heart connection by gently holding along the back of the mother's heart, harmonizing with the heart union of mommy and baby and embracing their full circle of love (Figure 24.62).

Combining handholds may be less elaborate, as you create congruency by linking therapeutic processes in simplified handholds. For instance, matching Floating Air Balloons with Friends: Soul to Sole may offer the baby supportive grounding through the soles of the feet, in the context of treating difficult oral intubations or prolonged intubation (Figure 24.63).

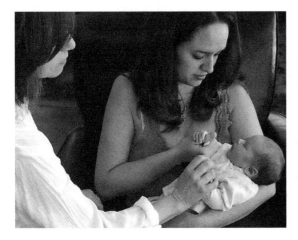

Figure 24.59. Start with Holding Hands.

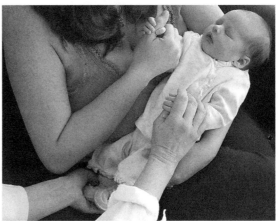

Figure 24.60. Add Soul to Sole.

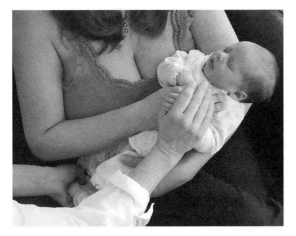

Figure 24.61. Mommy and baby hug baby's heart; therapist and baby hug baby's heart.

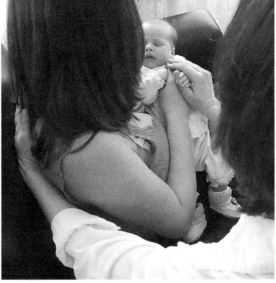

Figure 24.62. Therapist holds the heart union of mommy and baby.

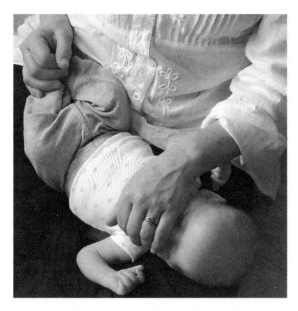

Figure 24.63. Blending handholds:
Floating Air Balloons and Soul to Sole.

Mama Bear's Care:
The Experience of Love as Protection

Soothing Surroundings

Position (Figure 24.64)

Baby: Facing you and supported along your belly in sidelying; baby may be rolled toward you to a slightly prone position for increased comfort.

Therapist's arms: Holding baby along the length of the body, with your forearms in a cross-cradle position forming a supportive blanket. Baby's face and head may be covered by your arm or hand, creating a sense of protection from the intensity of bright lights or loud sounds.

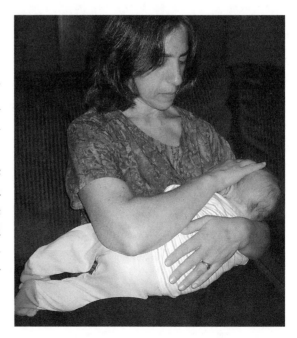

Figure 24.64. Soothing surroundings.

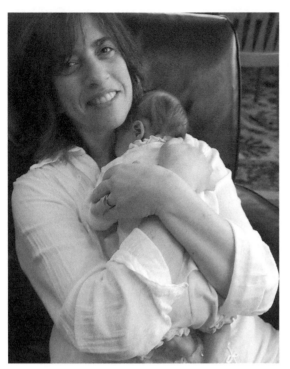

Figure 24.65. Protection from pain.

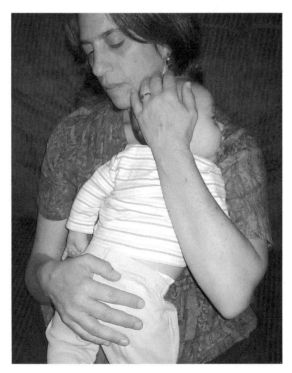

Figure 24.66. Bathing in Mama Bear's Love.

Protection from Pain

Position (Figure 24.65)

Baby: Supported in an upright position, ideally on your left side for a heart-to-heart connection.

Therapist: Semireclined, allowing baby's weight to be distributed for added comfort; therapist crosses arms over baby, creating a posture of shielding and safety.

Bathing in Mama Bear's Love

Position (Figure 24.66)

Baby: Supported in an upright position, ideally on your left side for a heart-to-heart connection.

Therapist: Semireclined, allowing baby's weight to be distributed for added comfort. Use one hand to support the baby's lower body, while the other arm connects along the baby's upper body and gently cups the baby's head.

You are connecting with the softness in the heart, allowing the baby to lie in the fullness of love.

Therapeutic Indications for Mama Bear's Care

Difficult delivery or C-section.

Experience in NICU and/or hospitalization.

Sensory system hyperarousal or withdrawal states.

Adoption and/or limited contact with family or experiences of being nurtured.

Surgery.

Structural Changes and Therapeutic Processes

Softening and molding into therapist.

Deepening/descending.

Sense of broad unified pulsing of baby and therapist.

Expansive stillness.

Profound peace.

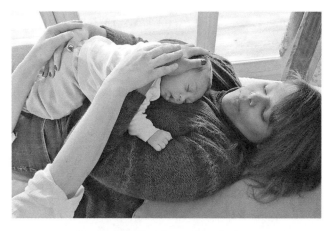

Figure 24.67. Mama Bear's Care: Bathing in Mama Bear's Love, mommy and baby.

Adult Handhold Adaptations

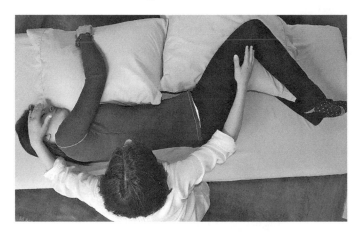

Figure 24.68. Soothing surroundings.

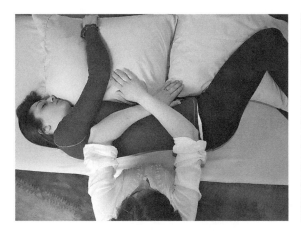

Figure 24.69. Protection from pain.

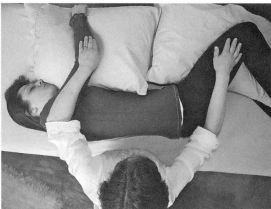

Figure 24.70. Bathing in Mama Bear's Love.

The Ahh (Air Hug Hold)

The Open Door: Single-Hand Air Hug Hold

I named this the Ahh (Air Hug Hold) to signify that the therapist is not making contact with the skin of the baby but rather is hugging the air around the skin of the infant.

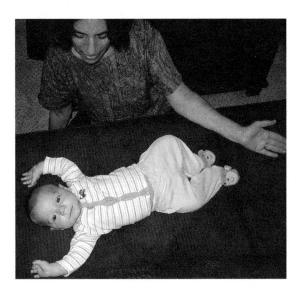

Figure 24.71. The Ahh (Air Hug Hold):
The Open Door: Single-Hand Air Hug Hold.

Position

Baby: Any position. Beneficial to determine if moving baby to alternative position will ultimately magnify stress level, or improve comfort level.

In general, therapist uses maximal telescoping out to the horizon and back to make more space for the baby.

Therapist usually diverts eye gaze.

You may find it beneficial to use nondominant hand to further diminish sense of physical proximity.

Position your hand facing upward 6–9 inches from baby's feet; fingertips are pointing away from baby and hand is generally parallel to the baby's midline and angled slightly upward (Figure 24.71).

Therapeutic Indications

Hyperresponsivity or shutdown in response to close proximity and/or touch.

Shutdown or deep freeze.

Shock posture.

Intermittent periods of disorganized, abrupt movements impeding self-quieting actions.

Progravity postures inhibiting flexed and/or comfortable positions.

Physiological difficulties (increased heart rate and/or respiratory rate, decreased oxygen saturation).

Therapeutic Processes and Structural Changes

Transition from shutdown state to sleep or drowsy state.

Flexed postures maintained more easily with blanket rolls.

Shift in physiology toward regulated cardiac and respiratory functions.

Increased periods of sleep following treatment.

Improved physiologic, motor, and state responses to caregiving.

Improved physiological responses to the opening of isolette doors.

Sense shifts in fluid body from disorganized to organized.

Baby's Bookends: Two-Handed Air Hug Hold

Position

Baby: Any position. Beneficial to determine if moving baby to alternative position will ultimately magnify stress level, or improve comfort level.

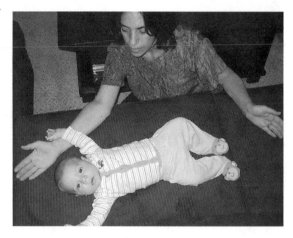

Therapist: Two hands facing upward 4–6 inches from baby's feet and head; fingertips are pointing away from baby and hands generally parallel to the baby's midline and angled slightly upward (Figure 24.72).

Therapeutic Indications

As above, with decreased intensity of physiological characteristics, postural functions, and motor actions.

Figure 24.72. The Ahh (Air Hug Hold): Baby's Bookends: Two-Handed Air Hug Hold.

Therapeutic Processes and Structural Changes

As above.

Frequent experience of partial or shortened time period for vertical or lateral decompression.

Weak, and often rhythmic sucking on endotracheal tube, omogastric tube, or empty oral cavity without oral stimulus.

Baby's Blanket over a Gentle Breeze
Alternative: Two-Handed Air Hug Hold

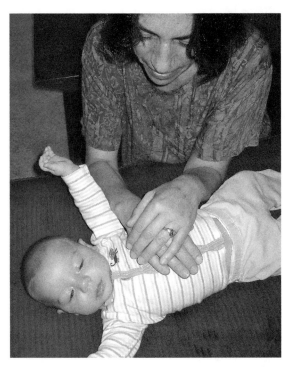

Figure 24.73. The Ahh (Air Hug Hold): Baby's Blanket over a Gentle Breeze.

Position

Baby: Any position. Beneficial to determine if moving baby to alternative position will ultimately magnify stress level, or improve comfort level.

Therapist: Cups hands facing down 1–2 inches above baby's chest, or chest and abdomen; palms are soft, and fingers are gently spread apart to form a lattice over baby. Elbows are resting on surface if possible (Figure 24.73).

Therapeutic Indications

As above, except less hyperresponsivity or shutdown in response to close proximity and/or touch.

Frantic movements; frequent, abrupt motor actions.

Nurse suspects painful experiences disrupt sleep.

Therapeutic Processes and Structural Changes

As above, in The Open Door and Baby's Bookends, with exception that the state of the baby's system usually shifts from hyperarousal levels to sleep.

Vertical and lateral decompression are expressed with a greater length of time and/or increased intensity.

Settling of abrupt or frantic motor actions with gradual transition to quiet body postures.

Weak and often rhythmic sucking on endotracheal tube, omogastric tube, or empty oral cavity without oral stimulus.

Brief motor actions as expressions of self-regulation, such as partial movements of hand to face, or hand to mouth.

Adult Handhold Adaptation

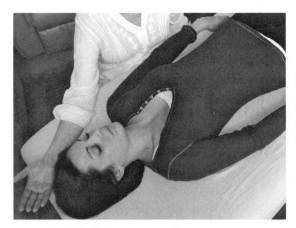

Figure 24.74. Open Door.

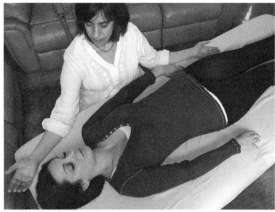

Figure 24.75. Bookends.

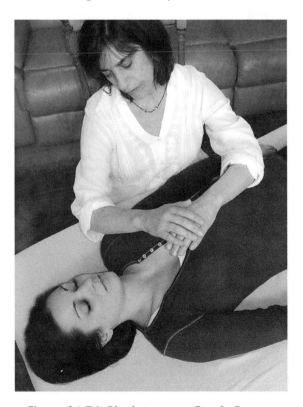

Figure 24.76. Blanket over a Gentle Breeze.

The MASS (Magnified Anterior Sacral Softening)

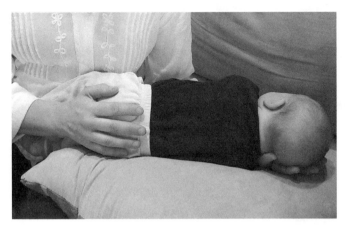

Figure 24.77. The MASS.

Position

Baby: Supported on therapist's lap in any comfortable position.

Therapist's right or left hand (dominant hand may be favorable): Contour palm and digits to support a uniform contact with baby's sacrum (Figure 24.77).

Magnified Hand: A "magnified hand" describes the therapist's shift in perception of certain qualities within their hand(s) while treating an infant. The attention is magnified but not the actual pressure being used by the therapist in the hands.

Therapist's hand takes on a light and airy consistency.

Hand is sensed as expansive like a gentle cradle that is larger than life.

Hand is perceived as shifted away from baby (1–2 inches).

Union is experienced along anterior sacrum, and connection extends anteriorly through pelvis and abdomen.

Therapeutic Indications

Increased muscle tone with postural and/or mobility discomforts.

Irritability or hyper-responsive sensory system.

Fatigue and/or discomfort through abdomen following medical tests.

Inguinal or umbilical hernia.

Ascites/gastroschisis/omphalocele.

Following necrotizing enterocolitis (NEC).

Following colostomy.

Therapeutic Processes and Structural Changes

Intraosseous expansion through sacrum.

Decompression through pelvis.

Softening through taut or dense visceral structures.

Increased life force through abdominal cavity.

Facial expressions indicating easing of discomfort.

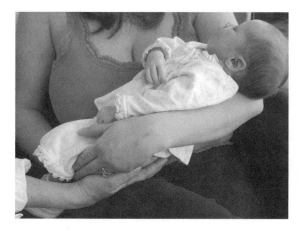

Figure 24.78. The MASS, mommy and baby.

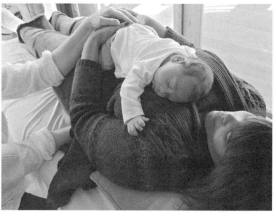

Figure 24.79. The MASS, mommy and baby.

Adult Handhold Adaptations

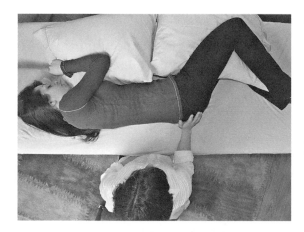

Figure 24.80. Single-hand.

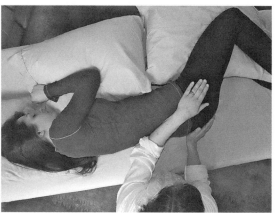

Figure 24.81. Two-handed adaptation

The Hula Hoop: Embracing the Circle of Love

This handhold is dedicated to my daughter Olivia for bringing me joy through her epic sense of humor, and guiding me to know the depth and breadth of love.

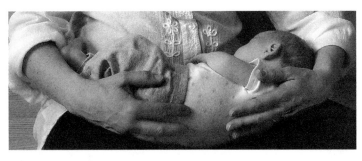

Figure 24.82. The Hula Hoop: Embracing the Circle of Love.

Position (Figure 24.82)

Baby: Supported in sidelying on your lap, or in blanket rolls forming a nest. Baby is positioned facing you.

Therapist: Arms extend forward forming an open circle. You soften the ventral aspect of the hands and forearms, conforming and supporting the baby posteriorly.

Therapeutic Indications

Experience in NICU and/or hospitalization.

Sensory system hyperarousal or withdrawal states.

Adoption and/or limited contact with family or experiences of being nurtured.

Therapeutic Processes and Structural Changes

Generalized softening, with broad unified pulsing.

Slowing of breath and smooth respiration.

Deep stillness followed by peaceful state.

Little Hula Hoops
Embracing the Circle of Love with Babies in Isolettes

The therapist may support parents' comfort in holding their baby during early NICU experience. Isolette is lowered, allowing parents to sit and extend their arms through the isolette portholes. While settling and slowing their breathing, parents may encircle the baby by placing arms on the blanket roll nest. If beneficial, you may support the baby and parent, while the parent shifts forearms and hands forming a circle with the baby (Figures 24.83 through 24.86).

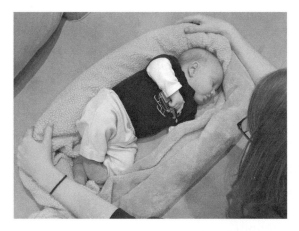

Figure 24.83. Mommy encircles baby by placing arms around blanket nest.

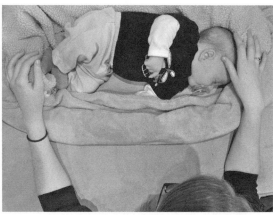

Figure 24.84. Mommy softens the embrace with slow movements and soothing touch.

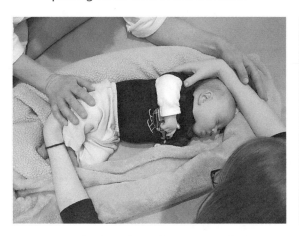

Figure 24.85. Therapist supports baby and mommy through Primary Respiration or stillness.

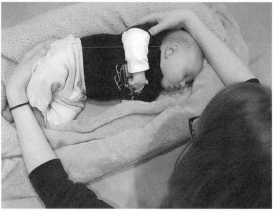

Figure 24.86. Mommy embraces baby and creates a sense of safety in their circle of love.

Preparation and Position

Discuss a plan with the nurse, especially for guidance in managing the baby's temperature.

Create ease for the mom or dad by lowering the isolette, and placing pillows along the back and sides of each parent's chair.

Reposition the baby in sidelying, ensuring comfort in a supportive blanket roll nest.

Therapeutic Benefits

Meets the longing for connection in the attachment process.

Nurtures the baby's experience of touch as loving.

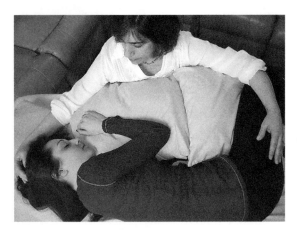

Figure 24.87. The Hula Hoop, adult handhold adaptation.

Supports the parent's confidence and sense of contribution in caring for the baby.

Fosters the baby's physiological stability and sensory system regulation.

Creates ease for the parents in supporting their baby's development.

Therapeutic Processes and Structural Changes

Baby's disorganized or excess movements diminish.

Slowing of baby's heart rate or respiration, with increased oxygen saturation for improved physiological stability.

Profound sense of love and unity.

Useful for babies unable to participate in kangaroo care, or before or after kangaroo care. Kangaroo care fosters a loving connection between the parent and baby through skin-to-skin contact. The baby is dressed only in a diaper, and positioned upright on the parent's bare chest, resembling the kangaroos' method of caring for their young. The organic nature of this experience is evident, as the mother's chest temperature accommodates to her baby's needs, cooling if her baby is too warm, or rising to create warmth as needed. The benefits are extensive, with the baby demonstrating improved breathing, stable heart rate, and more rapid brain development. Discharge from the hospital is earlier, as the baby regulates stress hormones, improves sleep, and increases weight gain. Benefits for the mother include an increase in milk supply, regulation of stress hormones, improved confidence, and improved coping methods.

Conclusion

Encircling the baby and his or her family with acceptance and understanding is central to the therapeutic and healing process in the NICU. The images of the NICU handholds may be assimilated by you, and brought into consciousness as a light mist expanded throughout a wide perceptual field. While treating the NICU baby, joint awareness emerges seamlessly as you magnify connection, and the baby orients toward therapeutic options. Clarity is illuminated as the baby expresses unity throughout his or her physiological and sensory systems, welcoming the health found in the strength of wholeness.

CHAPTER 25

Biodynamic Treatment Methods Fostering Digestion in Babies

by Phyllis Aries, MA, BCST, OTR

The nature and complexity of digestion, an essential component of baby's health, are reflected in expression of vitality and capacity for tranquility. The digestion handholds harmonize with biodynamic processes for a gentle unfolding of sound integration. The information in this chapter is presented similarly to the format of the NICU handholds chapter, with photographs and text illustrating and describing a range of handholds that enhance digestion.

Most of the digestion handhold descriptions incorporate a complementary treatment adaptation, illustrated here in photographs of mommy and baby or daddy and baby. All handhold descriptions also include photographs illustrating adaptation(s) for working with adults.

As with the NICU handholds in the previous chapter, variations are outlined here for two of the digestion handholds (the Poncho and the LACE). For example, the Poncho is adapted to include Poncho with a Scarf, Poncho over a Gentle Breeze, and Wearing a Poncho on the Digestive Hammock.

All of these skills are based on your perception of Primary Respiration or stillness in yourself first and then the baby.

The Digestive Hammock

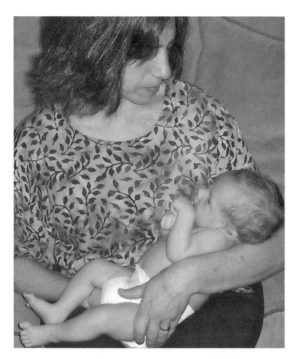

Figure 25.1. The Digestive Hammock.

Position (Figure 25.1)

Baby: Sitting semireclined on therapist's lap.

Therapist's left arm: Cradling baby against therapist's body and inner aspect of left arm.

Therapist's left hand: Supports left side of baby's pelvis, with therapist's thumb over descending colon, and therapist's palm and digits along side of descending colon.

Therapist's right hand: Under sacrum.

Therapeutic Indications

Constipation.

Runny stools.

Low motility or limp digestive tract.

Swollen and/or inflamed descending colon.

Irritability and/or digestive difficulties.

Therapeutic Processes and Structural Changes

Heat release through descending colon and sacrum.

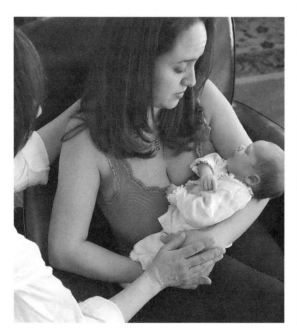

Figure 25.2. The Digestive Hammock, mommy and baby.

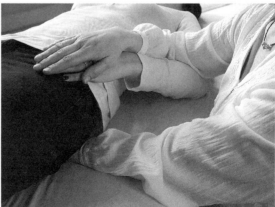

Figure 25.3. The Digestive Hammock, adult handhold adaptation.

Increased vitality through digestive tract.

Decompression through pelvis.

Gas and/or bowel movement.

Figure 25.2 shows an adaptation, with the therapist's hands supporting the mother who is cradling her baby.

Figure 25.3 shows an adaptation working with an adult. Your right hand is over the client's hand which is placed over the area of the sigmoid colon. The left hand is making nonspecific contact with the client's sacrum.

The Poncho

Position (Figure 25.4)

Baby: Sitting on therapist's lap, facing sideways.

Therapist's left hand: Supporting baby's occiput, neck, and shoulders for upright positioning.

Therapist's right hand: Thumb is along the front of baby's right shoulder, and fingers extend to baby's left shoulder. Palm and wrist are along volar aspect of pharynx and chest.

Therapeutic Indications

Reflux.

Swollen or inflamed esophagus.

Emesis (vomiting).

Irritability.

Therapeutic Processes and Structural Changes

Heat release through esophagus.

Disorganization resolving into expansion.

Breathing shifts from rapid, intermittent respirations to slow, smooth respirations.

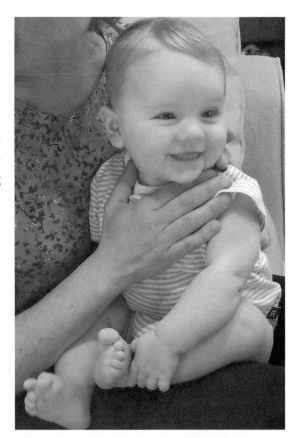

Figure 25.4. The Poncho.

Figure 25.5 shows an adaptation, with the therapist's hands supporting the mother who is cradling her baby.

Figure 25.6 shows an adaptation working with an adult. Your right hand is over the client's sternum. The left hand is making nonspecific contact with the client's mid-thoracic spine.

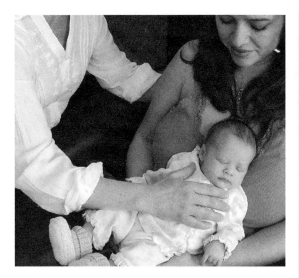

Figure 25.5. The Poncho, mommy and baby.

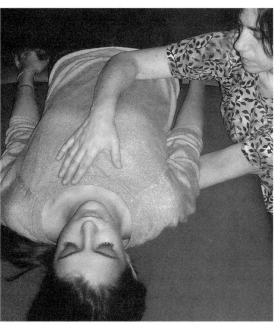

Figure 25.6. The Poncho, adult handhold adaptation.

Poncho with a Scarf

Adaptation (Figures 25.7 and 25.8)

Therapist's right hand: Baby may be sucking on pacifier or your gloved right index finger. Right thumb is along baby's right side of pharynx. Right index and middle are on left side of pharynx. Palm and wrist are along volar aspect of pharynx and chest.

Therapeutic Indications

Swollen or inflamed pharynx or esophagus. Oral-motor incoordination.

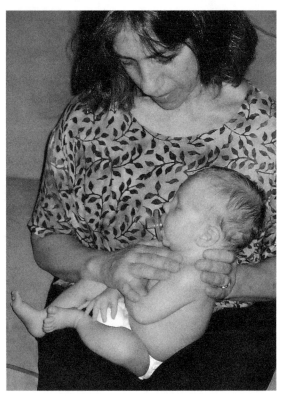

Figure 25.7. Poncho with a Scarf.

Therapeutic Processes and Structural Changes

Heat release through pharynx or esophagus.

Hyoid expands laterally and anteriorly.

Oral cavity decompression.

Oral-motor coordination.

Figure 25.9 is an adaptation for adult clients. The left hand cups the nape of the neck. The right hand makes gentle contact with the trachea with just the thumb and index finger.

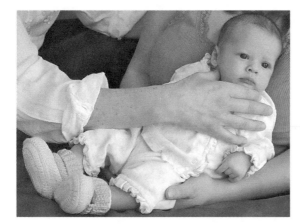

Figure 25.8. Poncho with a Scarf, mommy and baby.

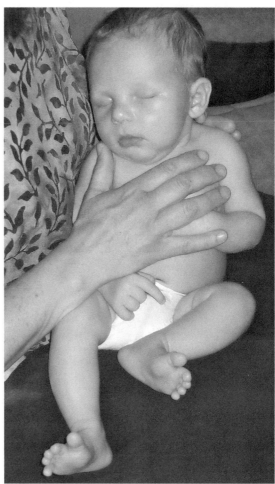

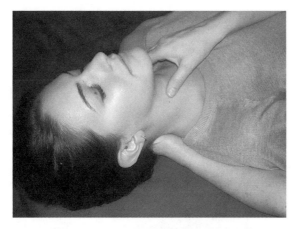

Figure 25.9. Poncho with a Scarf, adult handhold adaptation.

Figure 25.10. Poncho over a Gentle Breeze.

Poncho over a Gentle Breeze

Adaptation (Figure 25.10)

Telescope away a small distance with an image of a gentle breeze lifting the poncho.

Therapeutic Indications

Respiratory difficulties.

Presence of fear and/or defensive tissues.

Therapeutic Processes and Structural Changes

Deepening/descending.

Disorganization resolving into comfort, with rhythmic respiration.

Sense of feeling settled.

Figure 25.11 shows the therapist supporting both mom and baby. The right hand is held about one inch off of the baby's upper thoracic area. The left hand supports the mother's lower back.

Figure 25.12 shows an adaptation for the adult client. The right hand of the therapist is over the upper sternum of the client. The left hand gently supports the middle of the client's neck.

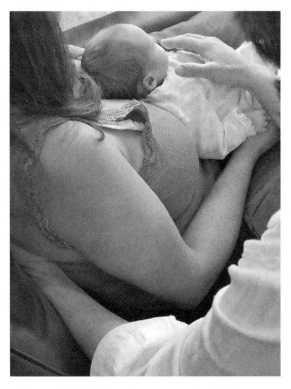

Figure 25.11. Poncho over a Gentle Breeze, mommy and baby.

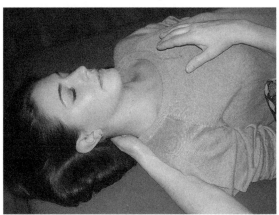

Figure 25.12. Poncho over a Gentle Breeze, adult handhold adaptation.

Wearing a Poncho on the Digestive Hammock

Position (Figure 25.13)

Baby: Sitting on therapist's lap, supported by therapist's left arm.

Therapist's left hand (Hammock): Left arm supports baby's body in sitting, while left thumb is over descending colon and fingers wrap around left side of baby's pelvis.

Therapist's right hand (Poncho): Thumb is along the front of baby's right shoulder, and fingers extend to baby's left shoulder. Palm and wrist are along volar aspect of pharynx and chest.

Option for therapist's right hand (Poncho with a Scarf): Baby is sucking on pacifier or gloved index finger. Your right thumb is along baby's right side of pharynx. Right index or middle finger is on left side of pharynx, as seen in Figure 25.7.

Therapist's right palm over esophagus, and forearm over baby's abdomen.

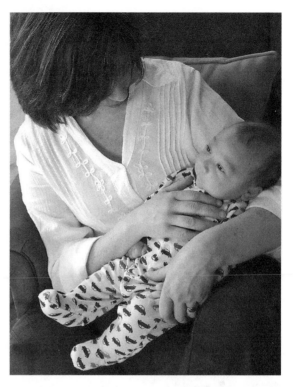

Figure 25.13. Wearing a Poncho on the Digestive Hammock.

Therapeutic Indications

Reflux with inflammation through pharynx and/or esophagus.

Constipation.

Irritability during or following eating.

Tendency for bearing down or flexion movements.

Tightness through axial flexor musculature.

Therapeutic Processes and Structural Changes

Decompression through pelvis.

Heat release through descending colon and/or pharynx.

Slowing of respiration.

Bowel movement.

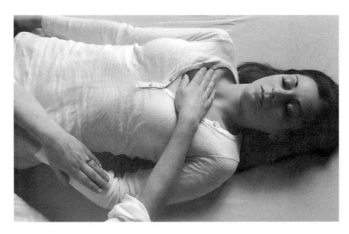

Figure 25.14. Wearing a Poncho on the Digestive Hammock, adult handhold adaptation.

Figure 25.14 shows an adaptation with an adult client. Your right hand spans the client's manubrium and proximal ends of the clavicles, while overlying the esophagus. The client's left hand rests over their descending colon. Your left forearm supports the client's hand, and your left hand extends onto the client's forearm.

The Digestive Seam Suck

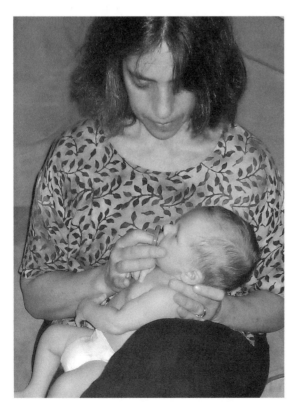

Figure 25.15. The Digestive Seam Suck.

Position (Figure 25.15)

Baby: Sitting on therapist's lap or lying in bassinette.

Therapist's left hand: Support baby's neck and occiput.

Therapist's right hand: Right thumb on right cheek seams and right long finger on left cheek seams.

Therapeutic Indications

Oral-motor incoordination.

Low motility or limp digestive tract.

Digestive tract malformation.

Following NEC (necrotizing enterocolitis).

Irritability and/or digestive difficulties.

Therapeutic Processes and Structural Changes

Decompression through pharynx and oral cavity.

Rhythmic sucking pattern.

Intra-oral suction pressure.

Suck-swallow coordination.

Figure 25.16 shows an adaptation with an adult client. Your right hand supports the base of the neck. The left hand gently contacts the cheek seams of the client.

The Digestive Cradle

Position (Figure 25.17)

Baby: Prone on therapist's lap or held in side-lying, facing away from therapist.

Therapist's left arm: Upper arm and forearm support baby's head. Wrist, palm, and digits gently span across inferior aspect of oral cavity, pharynx, esophagus, and stomach.

Therapist's right hand: Forearm extends between baby's lower extremities, and gently supports baby's lower body. Wrist and hand form a soft connection with baby's abdomen.

Option: Therapist is sitting with left leg bent over the top of the right leg in such a way that the therapist's knees are almost on top of one another (the so-called tailor-sit). Baby held prone, with the head to the left side of therapist's lap. Baby's head rotated to the right, and head resting over therapist's left forearm with the top of the head lower than the chin.

Therapist's left hand: Placed under oral cavity or pharynx and possibly extending down along portion of esophagus.

Therapist's right hand: Forearm along right side of baby's pelvis, with palm or digits along abdomen. Thumb may extend up along esophagus.

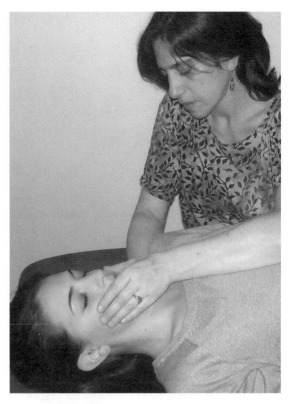

Figure 25.16. The Digestive Seam Suck, adult handhold adaptation.

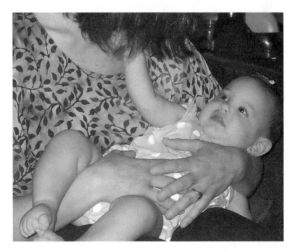

Figure 25.17. The Digestive Cradle.

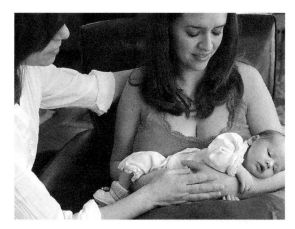

Figure 25.18. The Digestive Cradle, mommy and baby.

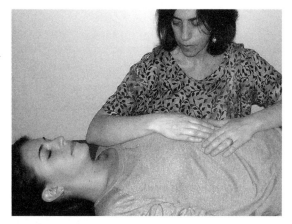

Figure 25.19. Arm position, distant view.

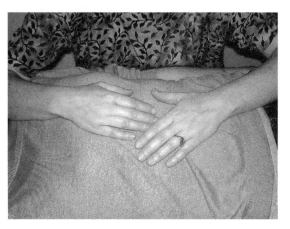

Figure 25.20. Hand position, close view.

Create less pressure on baby's abdomen by having right hand along open space in lap.

Therapeutic Indications

Low motility and/or limp digestive tract.

Reflux.

Swollen or inflamed pharynx or esophagus.

Irritability and/or digestive difficulties.

Gas.

Therapeutic Processes and Structural Changes

Heat release through digestive tract.

Bowel movement.

Lengthening through axial musculature.

Organization of suck-swallow improved.

Figure 25.18 shows a variation in which the right hand of the therapist is over the mother's hand around the baby's abdomen. The left hand of the therapist supports the mother's heart from around the fifth thoracic vertebra.

Figures 25.19 and 25.20 show an adaptation with an adult client. Your right hand rests gently over the lower sternum and xiphoid process of the client. The left hand is over the epigastric area of the client and has a little contact with the opposite hand. Make sure your arms are supported. It is important to negotiate the contact shown here since your arms are resting on the client's torso.

The PASS (Pharyngeal Anterior Sacral Softening)

Position (Figure 25.21)

Baby: Sidelying or prone on therapist's lap.

Therapist's left hand: Cradling and supporting underneath oral cavity or mandible or pharynx.

Therapist's right hand: Thumb along left side of sacrum. Digits span toward right side of sacrum.

Loosen and lighten hold along sacrum.

Use telescoping and hold as a continuum between pharynx and sacrum.

Sense the anterior aspect of the sacrum and entire abdominal area, while telescoping to maintain an open expansive connection.

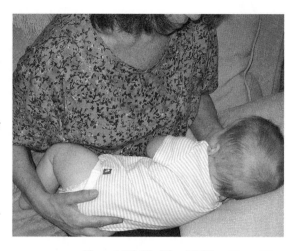

Figure 25.21. The PASS (Pharyngeal Anterior Sacral Softening).

Therapeutic Indications

Low motility or limp digestive tract.

Diminished life force through abdomen.

Swollen or inflamed stomach, intestines, colon, pharynx, or esophagus.

Constipation (hard, dry, painful, or infrequent bowel movements).

Therapeutic Processes and Structural Changes

Decompression through pelvis and sacrum.

Heat release through continuum of pharynx to sacrum.

Decompression through oral and/or abdominal cavity.

Increased motility and life force through abdomen.

Figure 25.22 shows a variation with your right hand over the sacrum of the baby and the

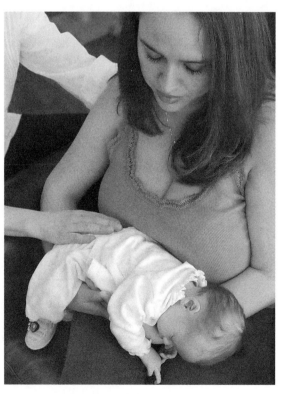

Figure 25.22. The PASS, mommy and baby.

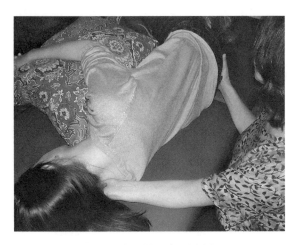

Figure 25.23. The PASS,
adult handhold adaptation.

left hand supporting the heart of the mother around her mid-dorsal spine.

Figure 25.23 shows an adaptation with an adult client. Your right hand contacts the client's sacrum and the left hand supports the client's neck and lower part of the mandible.

The P-A Jump Rope (Pharyngeal-Anal Jump Rope)

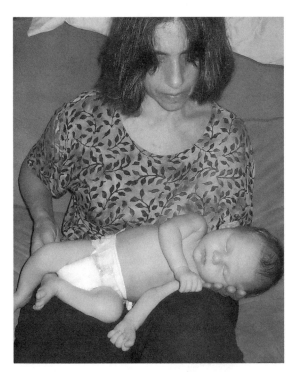

Figure 25.24. The P-A Jump Rope
(Pharyngeal-Anal Jump Rope).

Position (Figure 25.24)

Baby: Lying on therapist's lap in a reclined prone or sidelying position, facing away from therapist. If baby is prone, therapist may use a tailor sit position, with the left leg up. Pressure on baby's belly is relieved by positioning the belly in opening created by tailor sit.

Therapist's left hand: Hand is placed on top of your left knee and under baby's head, supporting under baby's maxilla, oral cavity, mandible, and pharynx. If possible, drape baby's head over your knee so the chin is slightly higher than the top of the head.

Therapist's right hand: Index finger pad is positioned lightly on anus (without removing diaper, clothing, or blanket).

Therapeutic Indications

Constipation, runny stools, gas.

Inflamed descending colon.

Low motility.

Limited activity or life force in intestines, colon, and/or stomach.

Therapeutic Processes and Structural Changes

The metaphor of a jump rope is used here as an image of the baby's undeveloped digestive tract from mouth to anus. The image of a jump rope allows for greater flexibility in the abdominal cavity of the baby and makes it easier to sense Primary Respiration since the jump rope is sensed as moving very slowly. This stimulates digestion, absorption, and elimination in the baby.

Unity of digestive tract as jump rope.

Wavelike or pulsing motions of jump rope.

Quieting of jump rope motions.

Decompression through jump rope.

Heat release through pharynx and/or anus.

Lengthening through body vertically.

Decreased inflammation of descending colon.

Figure 25.25 is a variation with an adult. The left hand is similar to Figure 25.23 but the right hand is several inches away from the lower sacrum and coccyx.

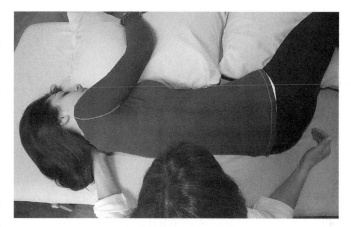

Figure 25.25. The P-A Jump Rope, adult handhold adaptation.

The OASIS (Oral Autonomic Sucking Inversion Softening)

Position (Figure 25.26)

Baby: Supine on therapist's lap.

Therapist's left hand: Supports baby behind the head, neck, and shoulders.

Therapist's right hand: Gloved index is in baby's mouth (option of finger against pacifier). Your thumb is against the baby's right side of pharynx, and long finger is on left side of pharynx. Palm and forearm are along the anterior aspect of the baby's body.

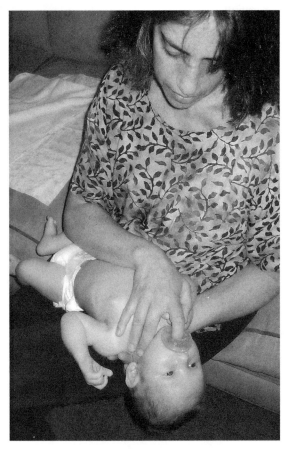

Figure 25.26. The OASIS (Oral Autonomic Sucking Inversion Softening).

Therapeutic Indications

Need for autonomic regulation.

Pharyngeal inflammation.

Pharyngeal and hyoid compression.

Disorganized or dysfunctional sucking pattern.

Axial flexor tightness.

Therapeutic Processes and Structural Changes

Decompression through pharynx.

Hyoid gliding anteriorly and expanding laterally.

Heart rate and respiratory regulation.

Lengthening through anterior body.

Rhythmic sucking pattern.

Tongue shaping and intra-oral suction pressure.

Comfort with self and in the world.

Figure 25.27 shows a variation with mom and baby. Again, you support the mom around her

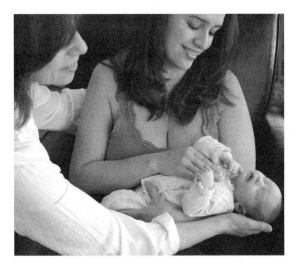

Figure 25.27. The OASIS, mommy and baby.

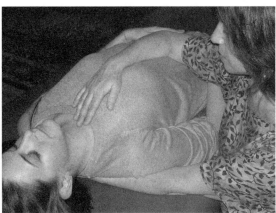

Figure 25.28. The OASIS, adult handhold adaptation.

heart with your left hand over the mid-thoracic spine. The right hand supports the occiput of the baby.

Figure 25.28 shows an adaptation with an adult. Your right hand is over the sternum and manubrium of the client. The left hand supports the base of the neck and upper thoracic spine. The spinous processes of the client's vertebra are in the palm of your hand.

The PALACE (Pharyngeal Anterior Lateral Abdominal Creation Energy)

Position (Figure 25.29)

Baby: On therapist's lap in sidelying (slightly supine), facing away from therapist.

Therapist's left hand: Supporting baby's head under mandible and pharynx.

Therapist's right hand: Thumb along ascending colon, and ring/little fingers along descending colon. Palm over abdomen.

Option: Use magnified hand as described above to expand throughout pelvis.

Therapeutic Indications

Limited motility.

Limp digestive tract.

Pharyngeal inflammation.

Abdominal inflammation.

Following NEC (necrotizing enterocolitis)

Therapeutic Processes and Structural Changes

Heat release through pharynx and abdomen.

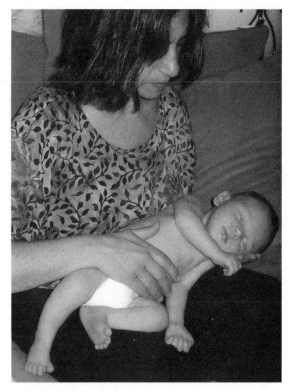

Figure 25.29. The PALACE (Pharyngeal Anterior Lateral Abdominal Creation Energy).

Increased life force through abdominal cavity. (Life force is expressed as an underlying potential for action, sensed as vitality, energy, or subtle aspects of movement.)

Increased motility.

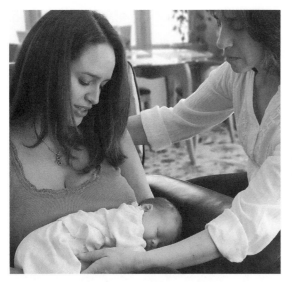

Figure 25.30. The PALACE, anterior view.

Figures 25.30 and 25.31 show a variation with mom holding her baby. Your right hand supports the heart of the mom in back. The left hand is around the infant's abdomen. It can also be over the mother's hand if it is already over the baby's abdomen.

Figure 25.32 is an adaptation with an adult. Your right hand is adjacent to the superior ridge of the pubic symphysis. The left hand is over the anterior neck and throat area. This must be done with a great deal of delicacy.

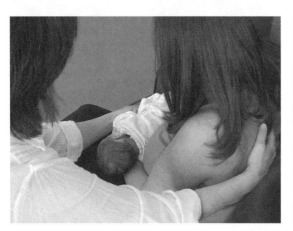

Figure 25.31. The PALACE, posterior view.

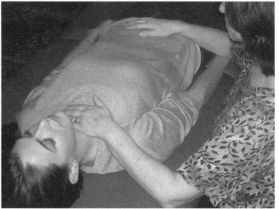

Figure 25.32. The PALACE,
adult handhold adaptation.

Sitting on Mother Earth's Lap

Position (Figure 25.33)

Baby: Sitting upright on therapist's lap (facing sideways may be easiest). If possible, allow baby's legs to be positioned with an obtuse hip angle (hip angle is open so baby's thighs are not compressing abdominal structures).

Therapist's right hand: With baby facing toward your right, hand acts as front of Poncho. Thumb is along the front of baby's right shoulder, and fingers extend to baby's left shoulder. Palm and wrist are along anterior aspect of pharynx and chest. Forearm extends down anterior aspect of abdomen.

Therapist's left hand: Supporting baby's head, neck, and shoulders posteriorly.

Use your lap as a treatment "hand," open and receiving, while offering loving and grounded support.

Therapeutic Indications

Reflux, irritability.

Hyper-responsive or disorganized sensory system.

Excessive sympathetic nervous system activation.

Facial expression or crying as indications of pain.

Bonding with family compromised.

Therapeutic Processes and Structural Changes

Heat release through sacrum.

Broad slow pulsing in unison with therapist.

Deepening/descending.

Physiological regulation.

Deep restful state.

Softening of facial expression.

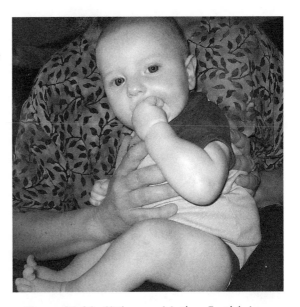

Figure 25.33. Sitting on Mother Earth's Lap.

Figure 25.34 shows an adaptation for the adult client. The client is in left sidelying postion. Your left hand supports the occiput and the right hand and arm cradle the back of the right leg and buttocks of the client. Please remember to use bolsters and pillows to support your arms when necessary.

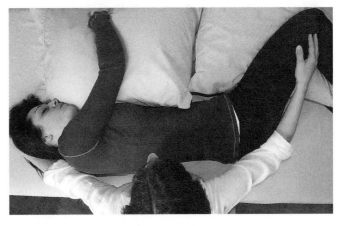

Figure 25.34. Sitting on Mother Earth's Lap, adult handhold adaptation.

The Candy Cane

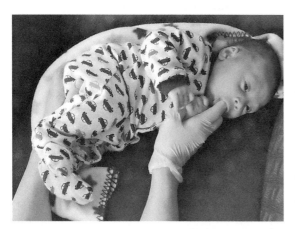

Figure 25.35. Unified wholeness in the shape of a candy cane, intra-oral treatment with gloved index finger.

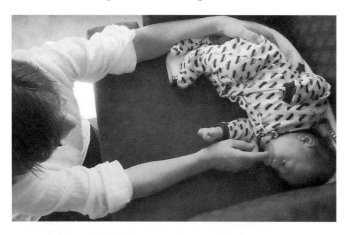

Figure 25.36. Intra-oral treatment through contact with pacifier.

Position

Baby: On therapist's lap or comfortable surface, facing therapist in sidelying, or supported in a semireclined sitting position.

Therapist's right hand: Place gloved index finger with pad along tongue surface for intra-oral position (Figure 25.35). Alternatively, connect index finger pad with pacifier (Figure 25.36).

Therapist's left hand: Cradle sacrum in palm.

You may create a sense of unified wholeness, imaging the shape of a candy cane between your hands, and using telescoping methods (cycle of attunement).

Therapeutic Indications

Oral-motor incoordination.

Sensory system hyperarousal states.

Irritability in relation to digestive processes.

Pharyngeal or esophageal inflammation.

Low motility or limp digestive tract.

Therapeutic Processes and Structural Changes

Tongue shaping and formation of tongue's central groove.

Rhythmic tongue and jaw motions.

Increased intra-oral suction pressures.

Postural softening with behavioral organization.

Heat release through pharynx or esophagus.

Increased motility and vitality through digestive tract.

Sensation of unified wholeness from oral cavity to abdomen.

Deepening/descending.

Broad, expansive vertical or lateral decompression.

Figure 25.37 shows a variation with an adult. Your left hand is under the sacrum. Your right hand is using two fingers to approximate the client's mouth, remaining off of the skin's surface.

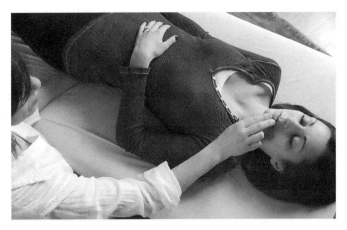

Figure 25.37. The Candy Cane, adult handhold application

Nonna's Touch: Linking Love with Nutrition

Nonna means grandmother in Italian, and this handhold was named by NICU nurse Fran, with fondness for her grandmother's loving persuasions to eat more food.

Position (Figure 25.38)

Baby: Supported on therapist's lap in a right-sided sidelying, or reclined sitting position.

Therapist's left arm: Supports and cradles the baby through the length of the body.

Therapist's right hand: Overlying the baby's heart, diaphragm, and stomach.

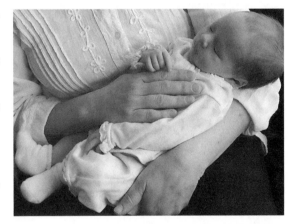

Therapeutic Indications

Respiratory irregularities during or after feeding experiences.

Sensory system hyperarousal with the presentation of scents, sights, or position changes typical in feeding preparations.

Figure 25.38 Nonna's Touch.

Irritability with feeding or digestive processes.

Delays in attachment processes or self-soothing skills.

Connections through the heart, diaphragm, or stomach characterized as strain patterns or irregular textures.

Therapeutic Processes and Structural Changes

Deepening/descending.

Heat release and softening through structures.

Period of resolving into settling and expansion.

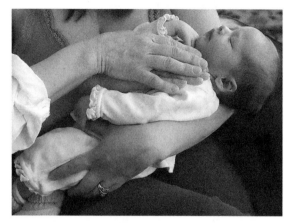

Profound stillness.

Figures 25.39 and 25.40 show a variation with mom cradling her baby. As illustrated in both figures, you place the palm of your right hand directly over the mother's right hand. Your left hand supports the mother's heart in back.

Figure 25.41 is an adaptation with an adult client. Your arms are shaped to encircle the heart, diaphragm, and stomach. Your left hand rests superior to the heart (left breast), and your forearm and arm encompass diaphragm and stomach. Your right hand approximates heart, diaphragm or stomach, depending on treatment needs. With a female client, this adaptation is for a female therapist.

Figure 25.39. Nonna's Touch, anterior view.

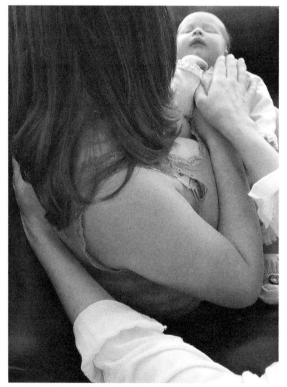

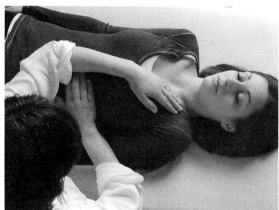

Figure 25.40. Nonna's Touch, lateral and posterior view.

Figure 25.41 Nonna's Touch, adult handhold adaptation.

ACE (Abdominal Creation Energy): Holding Sacrum and Anterior Abdomen

Position (Figure 25.42)

Baby: Supported on therapist's lap or comfortable surface in sidelying or supine.

Therapist's dominant hand: Use palm and full length of digits to gently cup sacrum.

Therapist's nondominant hand: Soften hand and approach the baby's abdomen slowly. It may be beneficial to use distant telescoping, conveying respect and acceptance for any guarding through this area. The palm and digits are rounded, distributing pressure gently and evenly over the baby's abdomen.

Therapeutic Indications

Irritability during or following feeding.

Milk or formula in mouth, or sucking and swallowing movements following feeding.

Sensation of inflamed, limp digestive tract (especially through small intestine and ascending/transverse colon).

Apparent slow motility, with discomfort between feedings, expressed as diffuse squirming or frequent periods of flexion through thoracic-lumbar-sacral spine.

Diagnosis or symptoms of reflux.

Therapeutic Processes and Structural Changes

Quieting of motor actions.

Deepening followed by reorganization process.

Broad pulsing and expansive decompression.

Increased life force through abdominal cavity.

Increased motility.

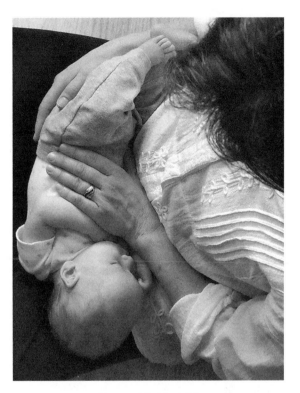

Figure 25.42. ACE
(Abdominal Creation Energy).

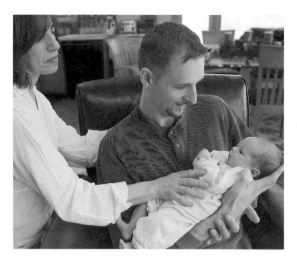

Figure 25.43. ACE, daddy and baby.

Figure 25.43 shows a variation with a father cradling his baby. Your left hand is supporting the heart of the father in back. Your right hand is over the baby's abdomen.

Figures 25.44 and 25.45 show an adaptation with an adult client. Your left hand is over the umbilicus of the client, while the right hand is making a nonspecific contact with the client's sacrum.

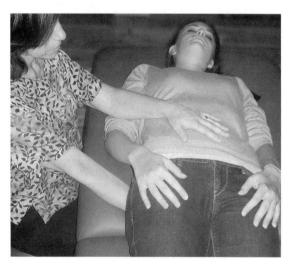

Figure 25.44. Wide, gentle hand position on abdomen.

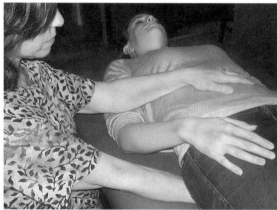

Figure 25.45. Posterior sacrum, softening and settling through palms.

LACE (Localized Abdominal Creation Energy)

LACE Option: Holding Sacrum and Descending Colon

Position (Figures 25.46, 25.47, and 25.48)

Baby: Optimal positioning includes access to full length of descending colon. If possible, avoid supported sitting as colon may be shifted into shortened position. Baby may be in bassinette or supported on therapist's lap, with supine or right-sidelying as the easiest treating positions.

Therapist's left hand: Use palm and full length of digits to gently cup sacrum.

Therapist's right hand: Use distributed pressure of finger shafts or palm to connect with descending colon. Shifting to digit pads as treatment progresses may be beneficial for managing gas bubbles or highly compressed or inflamed areas. In some circumstances, as shown in Figure 25.47, the therapist places a gloved finger, usually the index finger, into the mouth of the baby. The baby will usually suck on the finger, which creates a gentle lifting of

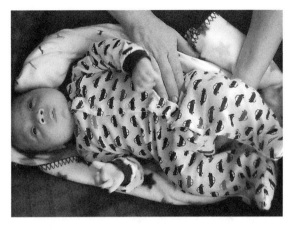

Figure 25.46. LACE, holding sacrum and descending colon.

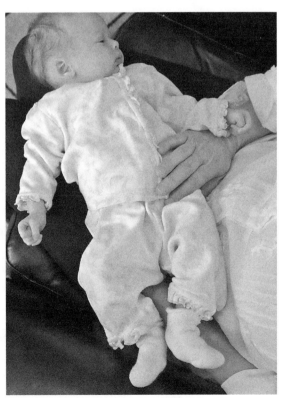

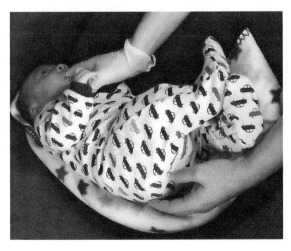

Figure 25.47. LACE, holding sacrum and anus.

Figure 25.48. LACE, holding sacrum and descending colon.

the colon and is beneficial in connecting the whole digestive tract of the infant to the function of the colon.

Therapeutic Indications

Constipation.

Gas or digestive discomfort.

Runny stools and/or diaper rash.

Bowel movements often occur with bearing down, and color changes to red, with increased intra-cranial pressure.

Irritability, breath holding, or bradycardia (low heart rate) before or during bowel movements.

Therapeutic Processes and Structural Changes

Quieting of body movements.

Deepening/descending.

Intense heat release through descending colon.

Vibratory or rhythmic component often precedes a reorganization.

Deep stillness and broad decompression with settling and softening of structures.

Period of diffuse squirming movements, with expelling of gas, or bowel movement during or after treatment.

LACE Option: Holding Sacrum and Anus

Position

Baby: Supported on therapist's lap or bassinette in supine, sidelying, or prone.

Therapist's left hand in single-hand placement (Figures 25.47 and 25.49): The pad of the thumb or another digit may be used to softly approximate the anus, while the other digits or palm extend along the sacrum.

Two-handed position (Figure 25.50): Use the index or long finger pad of the right hand to softly approximate the anus. Settle into a gentle receiving manner. Use palm or full length of digits of the left hand to gently cup sacrum.

Therapeutic Indications

Same as above.

May be preferred for gas, diaper rash, or runny stools.

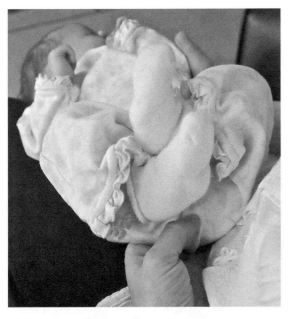

Figure 25.49. LACE, holding sacrum
and anus, single-hand.

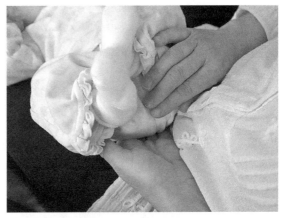

Figure 25.50. LACE, holding sacrum
and anus, two-handed.

Therapeutic Processes and Structural Changes

Same as above, with the addition of slow streaming or intense heat release from anus.

LACE Option: Holding Descending Colon and Anus

Position (Figure 25.51)

Baby: Supported on therapist's lap or bassinette in supine, sidelying, or prone.

Therapeutic Indications

Same as above.

May be preferred to treat prolonged periods of constipation.

Therapeutic Processes and Structural Changes

Same as above.

Figure 25.52 is a variation with mom cradling her baby. Your right hand is

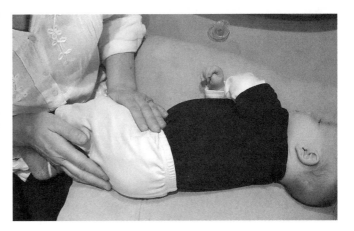

Figure 25.51. LACE, holding descending
colon and anus.

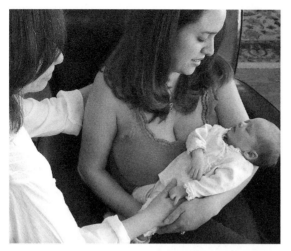

Figure 25.52. Descending colon and sacrum, mommy and baby.

over the lower abdomen and sigmoid colon of the baby. Your left hand supports the heart of the mother in back.

Figures 25.53 and 25.54 show a variation with an adult client. Your right hand makes a non-specific contact with the client's sacrum. The left hand is over the anterior superior iliac spine of the client. The fingers of the left hand are over the sigmoid colon of the client.

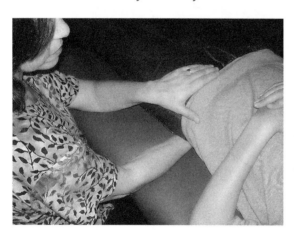

Figure 25.53. Adult handhold, with palm and shafts of digits for distributed pressure.

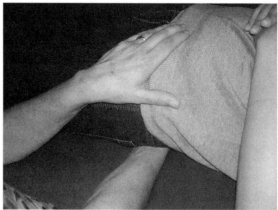

Figure 25.54. Digit pads for managing gas bubbles.

The HH (Hiccup Helper)

Position (Figure 25.55)

Baby: Supported to permit both of therapist's hands to be free and have easy access to diaphragm.

Therapist: Thumb or finger pads (usually thumb, index, and long fingers) of both hands along borders of diaphragm.

Location of digit pads are adjusted in relation to areas of diaphragm sensed as uncomfortable. Initially placing shaft of digits along diaphragm may allow easier perception of tight or painful areas. Position digit pads on opposite sides of diaphragm to permit an open treatment space.

Therapeutic Indications

Imbalances and/or tightness through diaphragm.
Hiccups.

Therapeutic Processes and Structural Changes

Pulsing, often rapid and then shifting to a broad slow beat.

Heat release along finger pads.

Disorganization resolving into expansion.

Softening through diaphragm.

Hiccups cease.

Figure 25.56 shows an adaptation with an adult client. Your left hand spans across the client's abdomen and makes contact with the costal arch of the client. Your right hand is over the lower rib cage of the client's left side.

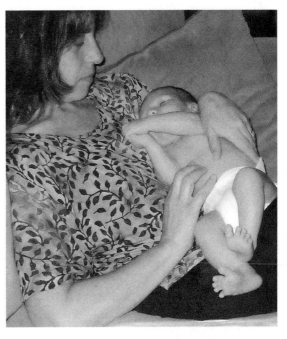

Figure 25.55. The HH (Hiccup Helper).

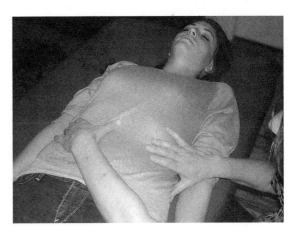

Figure 25.56. The HH,
adult handhold adaptation.

The Water Slide: Treating the Salivary Glands

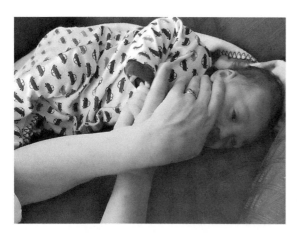

Figure 25.57. The Water Slide.

Position (Figure 25.57)

Baby: Supported on therapist's lap or a comfortable surface in the sidelying position. If needed, use blanket rolls to fully support baby in sidelying. Position the baby to face you.

With the baby in left sidelying, use your left hand on the baby's face, with right hand positioned along the anterior pharynx or esophagus.

With the baby in right sidelying, use your right hand on the baby's face, with left hand positioned along the anterior pharynx or esophagus.

Therapist: Place the thumb or palm in front of the baby's mouth. The thumb or palm may aid the baby in stabilizing the pacifier in his or her mouth. If preferred, use your gloved index finger in the baby's mouth.

Therapist: Gently drape the hand over the lateral aspect of the baby's face, spanning the sublingual, submandibular, and parotid glands. Your palm cups the lateral aspect of the baby's mouth and mandible, while your digits extend toward the baby's ear. If drooling appears to affect the baby's skin, adjust the contact for comfort. Using distant telescoping may be beneficial for connecting with the layers of skin and fascia overlying the glands.

Therapeutic Indications

Difficulty managing saliva, with increased drooling.

Skin irritation in relation to saliva.

Diagnosis of reflux.

Tendency for increased saliva production or emesis.

Sensation of inflammation or compression through facial structures and/or salivary glands.

Therapeutic Processes and Structural Changes

Deepening, with softening through facial structures.

Broad unified pulsing.

Periods of disorganization resolving into reorganization.

Stillness and expansive decompression.

Figures 25.58 and 25.59 show a variation with an adult client. Your right hand is contacting the right mandible and maxilla of the client. Your left hand supports the client's neck. After several minutes, repeat on the other side of the client's face.

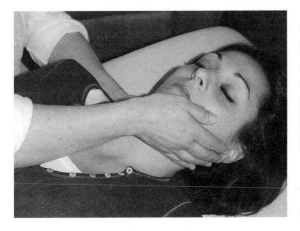

Figure 25.58. Connecting with skin and fascia overlying salivary glands.

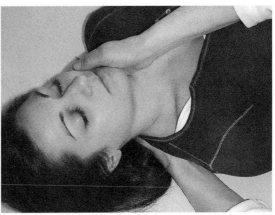

Figure 25.59. Supporting through shoulders posteriorly.

The COOO (Cervical Oral Occipital Opening)

Position (Figure 25.60)

Baby: Held on therapist's lap in supine or semi-sidelying.

Therapist's nondominant arm: Hand supports baby's occiput, cervical spine, and shoulders. Forearm and elbow are supportive, connecting with the baby's upper and lower body along the posterior aspect.

Therapist's dominant arm: Index finger is positioned on the pacifier, or gloved index finger is placed intra-orally along the central groove of the baby's tongue. Forearm and elbow connect with the baby anteriorly.

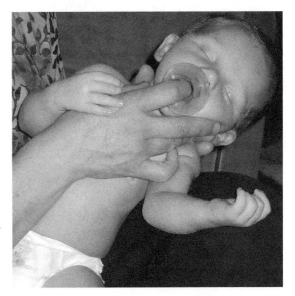

Figure 25.60. The COOO (Cervical Oral Occipital Opening).

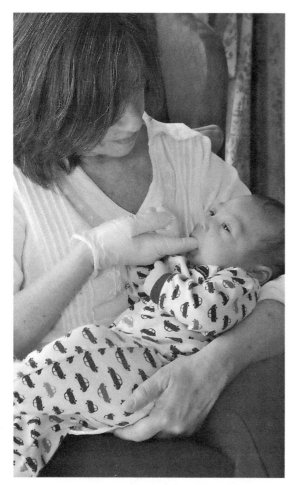

Figure 25.61. The COOO,
alternative handhold.

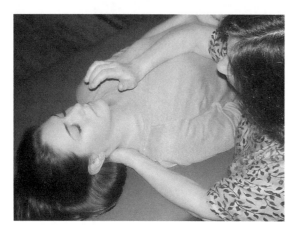

Figure 25.62. The COOO,
adult handhold adaptation.

Alternative handhold (Figure 25.61):

Therapist's nondominant arm: Cradles baby with the use of the lateral and anterior aspects of the elbow area as the treating hand. Allow a softening through the arm and forearm to create an open and expansive sense, while supporting the baby with a slow tempo and telescoping.

Therapist's dominant hand: Gloved index finger is positioned with the pad contacting the baby's palate.

Therapeutic Indications

Oral-motor incoordination.

Pharyngeal or esophageal inflammation.

Sensory system hyperarousal states.

Irritability with feeding or digestive processes or generalized irritability.

Possible strain and/or compression through the craniocervical junction or jugular foramen.

Possible activation of the hypothalamic-pituitary-adrenal axis (use palm facing upward position for intra-oral digit to connect finger pad to palate).

Therapeutic Processes and Structural Changes

Gradual shift from sensory system hyperarousal to states of behavioral organization and regulation.

Deepening/descending.

Broad pulsing.

Heat release through pharynx or esophagus.

Expansive decompression or deep stillness.

Softening and shifting of strain or structures, with improved tongue shaping, timing of tongue and jaw movements, and organization of sucking pattern.

Figure 25.62 is an adaptation with an adult. The heal of your right hand is over the manubrium of the client. The left hand supports the lower neck of the client.

The Party Invitation: Welcoming the Vagus Nerve

Position

Baby: Supported in sidelying on your lap or a comfortable surface.

Therapist: With the baby in right sidelying, your right hand supports the baby's pelvis, centering the sacrum in the palm, and providing a sense of gentle grounding (Figure 25.63). The left hand cradles the side of the baby's head, positioning the jugular foramen in the center of your palm. This hand offers the soft comfort of a fluffy featherbed, with a gentle feeling of acceptance (Figure 25.64).

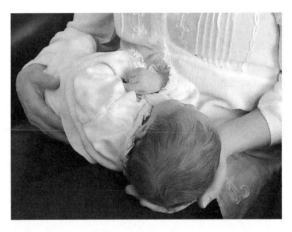

Figure 25.63. Dominant hand cups sacrum.

With the baby in left sidelying, your left hand supports the baby's pelvis, and the right hand cradles the side of the baby's head, as above.

As the treatment progresses, you may sense a localized area of density or compression. Remaining in this open-palm position or adjusting the hand that cradles the baby's head is your choice. Frequently, distant telescoping while remaining in the open-palm position supports the baby for deep stillness and decompression.

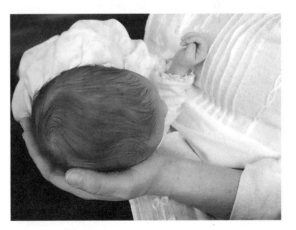

Figure 25.64. Nondominant hand creates featherbed cradle for baby's head.

Therapeutic Indications

Difficult delivery or C-section.

Sensory system hyperarousal states.

Irritability during or between feedings.

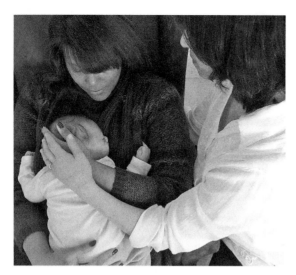

Figure 25.65. Embracing mommy and baby's gentle connection, while a fluffy pillow is offered to support baby's temporal and occipital areas.

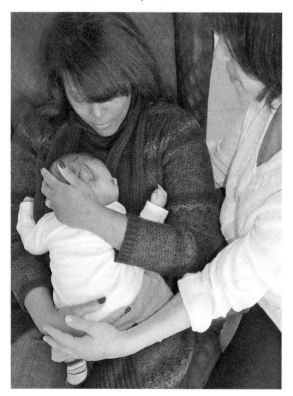

Figure 25.66. Sacral hold creates a cradle of warmth as mommy softly holds her baby's head.

Diagnosis of reflux.

Pharyngeal and/or esophageal inflammation.

Tendency for belly posture (flexed lower spine).

Therapeutic Processes and Structural Changes

Deepening/descending.

Heat release through sacrum.

Softening and lengthening through spine and/or abdominal viscera.

Profound stillness.

Decompression and/or expansion through cranium.

Figures 25.65 and 25.66 show two variations with a mom holding her baby. It is always appropriate for the therapist to place a hand over the mother's hand, with permission. Your left hand alternatively supports the hand around the baby's occiput, as in Figure 25.65, or over the sacrum, as in Figure 25.66.

Figure 25.67 shows a variation with the mom supine and her baby lying over her heart. Your right hand is under the mother's heart and the left hand is over the side of the baby's face. Again, it will be necessary to support your arms to maintain this position for very long.

Figure 25.68 shows an adaptation for an adult client. Your left hand is over the side of the client's ear. This is very light contact. The right hand is cupping the client's sacrum.

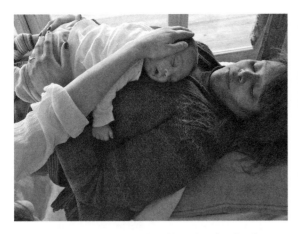

Figure 25.67. Table offers featherbed of support.

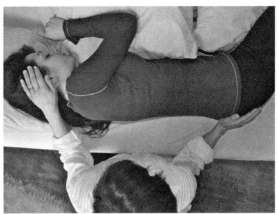

Figure 25.68. The Party Invitation, adult handhold adaptation.

The Sandwich

Position (Figure 25.69)

Baby: Supported in bassinette or comfortable surface in sidelying position.

Therapist's nondominant arm: Supports the baby posteriorly, with digit pads contacting the occiput, cervical spine, or shoulders according to the baby's comfort. Your hand, forearm, and elbow extend inferiorly along the center of the baby's body.

Therapist's dominant arm: Supports the baby anteriorly, as digit pads connect with the pharynx or esophagus according to baby's comfort. Your hand, forearm, and elbow extend inferiorly, aligned with the digestive structures as possible.

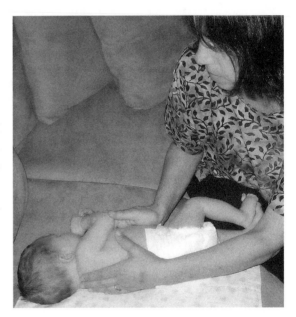

Figure 25.69. The Sandwich.

Therapeutic Indications

Oral-motor incoordination, with limited tongue shaping, and shifting of tongue superiorly and/or anteriorly in oral cavity.

Inflammation through pharynx and esophagus.

Low motility and/or limp or inflamed digestive tract.

Irritability during or following feedings.

Residuals and/or emesis. Residuals are the amount of liquid remaining in the stomach prior to the next feeding, measured as a function of gastric emptying. To determine the quantity of residuals, a syringe is used to extract liquid from the baby's stomach through the nasogastric or omogastric tube (i.e., feeding tubes inserted through the baby's nose or mouth). Emesis is the term commonly used to signify vomiting.

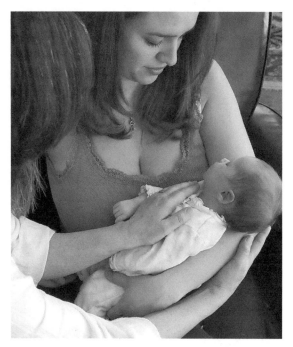

Figure 25.70. The Sandwich, mommy and baby.

Therapeutic Processes and Structural Changes

Heat release through pharynx and esophagus.

Tendency for sudden short bursts of movement through extremities with deepening and descending.

Periods of disorganization followed by reorganization with a broad expansive decompression or profound stillness.

Sensation of a posterior and inferior shift through the digestive tract, followed by a gentle settling.

Figure 25.70 shows a variation with mom holding her baby. Your right arm supports the mother's arm beneath the baby. In this case it is the left arm of the mother holding her baby. When mom shifts her baby to her other arm,

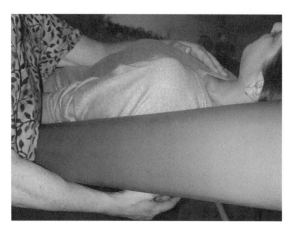

Figure 25.71. Posterior hand placement under table.

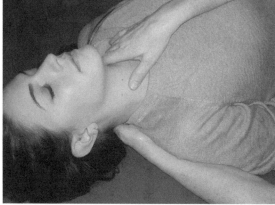

Figure 25.72. Broaden and lengthen forearm contact anteriorly.

the therapist also switches hands. Your left hand in this case is placed over the upper chest area and shoulder of the baby.

Figures 25.71 and 25.72 show an adaptation for an adult client. As illustrated in Figure 25.71, you place your right hand under the table approximately where the lower neck of the client is located above it. The left hand is over the manubrium of the client. Figure 25.72 is a little more intimate. Your right hand is above the manubrium over the area of the thyroid in the anterior neck of the client. The left hand is directly below the right hand under the client's lower cervical spine.

Conclusion

As the baby grows to understand the peaceful nature of biodynamic processes, a gentle expression of trust emerges. The baby opens to greater exploration, presenting discomforts to the therapist for shared awareness. While immersed in an endeavor to discern the baby's unique qualities and needs, the therapist may inadvertently interrupt the flow of trust, even with heartfelt intent to soothe and nurture the baby. Expanding the treatment space creates a sphere of acceptance, as the therapist mirrors safety through a reflection of deep trust in the earth's support. The baby senses that expectations have been suspended, and bathes in the texture of acceptance, welcoming union within the therapeutic process.

CHAPTER 26

Sing Them to Heaven

by Laurie Park, LCAT, MT-BC

Where words fail, music speaks.

Hans Christian Andersen

Saint Augustine said, "Those who sing pray twice." In the neonatal intensive care unit (NICU), people often find themselves praying, pleading, hoping, and sometimes begging a "higher power" to spare the life of their little one. The NICU can be an incredibly overwhelming environment for all who enter. This includes, but is not limited to, the baby who was born much too soon, the traumatized parents, the medical staff who are ready for anything at the slightest alarm, and the extended families, who feel completely helpless as they suffer from a distance. What you expect would be the happiest time of your life suddenly turns into a horrific case of your worst nightmares. Anyone who enters can certainly feel the intense energy that consumes the room. In the meantime, medical personnel are putting forth every effort to protect infants from any danger that may befall them.

Sometimes, for a variety of reasons, mothers can give birth at unexpected times, which often can be dangerous for the babies. When a child is born in imminent danger, he or she is whisked away from the parents and quickly assessed so care can be determined. It is all about survival at this point. The "team" consists of parents, doctors, nurses, therapists, social workers, and others. The goal is survival—to sustain life. Unfortunately, this is not always the outcome. Some babies will live for moments, some days, some even months. Some will not survive.

We know that, if we could create a less stressful atmosphere for these fragile infants, they would certainly benefit and ultimately have better outcomes. It is vital to take into consideration the cultural, religious, and social needs of each family unit. As the music therapist in the NICU, it is part of my responsibility to change the feeling of the environment and to address some of these needs.

Loewy, Hallan, Friedman, and Martinez (2005) emphasize the importance of utilizing songs-of-kin and supporting the mother's and father's vocal interaction with their baby in the NICU during music therapy sessions. In reviewing cases for this essay, I took note of the following patients and their special song that defined their "story."

"You Are My Sunshine"

One mother happened to be from a particularly musical family. We would often sing in harmony to her child. When family members would visit, they would join us and we would all sing around the crib. The song selection would vary from day to day: "The Itsy Bitsy Spider," "Jesus Loves Me," "Twinkle, Twinkle Little Star," and so on. The one song the family always included was "You Are My Sunshine." The mother told me: "Music is life. Music is all we can do for him. Music is the sun. He has never seen the sun so this is sunshine to him." And so we would sing:

> You are my sunshine
> My only sunshine.
> You make me happy
> When skies are gray.
> You'll never know dear
> How much I love you.
> Please don't take my sunshine away.

This became the mom's mantra during the course of her son's hospital stay. Months passed, until the baby eventually died. The mother asked if I would join her in singing at his funeral. To witness this mother singing to her child one last time as she laid him to rest was an incredibly powerful experience. She wore a white dress and explained that it was her Mother's Day dress and that being his mother was the greatest gift she had ever received. She too was a gift to him. The way he would look into his mother's eyes as she sang was priceless. A couple of years after he passed away, I received a call from this mother to ask if we could record some of the songs we sang to her son as a special gift for father's day. She said the songs remain in her heart with the memories of her son and she wanted to share them with his daddy.

"Amazing Grace"

I do not always have the benefit of knowing the families before I am called in to work with them, which often is at the end of their child's life. This requires a quick, sensitive assessment of the situation and a decision about what I might be able to offer. I happened to be in one of the NICU rooms meeting with a parent at the time of the untimely death of another baby in the room. The mothers in the room quickly responded to this despondent mother's grief. They coddled and comforted her to the best of their ability, offering what support they could, and then drifted back to their own baby's isolettes to keep a watchful eye on their baby's every breath. I then offered to sing a song and asked if she had anything in mind. She immediately responded, "Do you know 'Amazing Grace?'" The chaplain had recently baptized the baby and sang this song to the family. As I sang, the mother held her baby in her arms, rocking her deceased infant.

In the confined environment of the room, this particular death affected many people in the NICU at this time. The baby had been doing quite well then quickly took a turn for the worse and died rather suddenly. The other mothers in the room were heartbroken for their friend. They had formed a bond over the course of the weeks and months in the NICU, and now agreed to watch over each other's babies, fearing the same could happen to their child. Due to the severity of medical conditions in the unit, this group of women had unfortunately witnessed many ups and downs during this time, watching in fear, by virtue of having a connection that no one else can understand. The amazing grace of these women gave them the strength they needed to support one other and swaddle each other's babies with a blanket of love and protection.

"Miracle"

One morning that started out ordinarily ended as one of the most profound days of my career. I was paged to the NICU at a family's request, for a patient I had seen for many months. Today was the day when this family would withdraw support and say goodbye to their child. Their baby had been suffering for many months from a variety of medical complications. The medical team had determined that there was nothing else they could do. The neonatologist turned to me and said, "We have done everything we can do, now it's up to you." I had never actually been with a patient who was actively dying, so I wasn't quite sure what to expect. The nurse pulled the thin curtain to guide me into the space where the family was holding the baby.

The mother had removed her shirt so she could hold her bare infant, skin to skin, heart to heart. Tears streamed down both parents' cheeks as they embraced.

I had worked with this family for some time and was familiar with the songs that were most special to them. They especially loved Celine Dion's *Miracle* album. I sang one song after the other, sometimes singing, sometimes humming, and sometimes offering periods of silence. This process went on for well over an hour and I too shed some tears as I experienced an intimate, sacred moment with this family. The nurses had silenced the monitors so we would not be distracted by the sound of the slowing rate of his vitals. I continued to play as we watched the tubes fill with blood. The nurse nodded to let me know that he had died. I stopped playing and the mother grabbed my arm and said, "Don't stop playing! You have to sing him to heaven!" I quickly returned to the comfort of the melody and played for several more minutes, not knowing what to expect. How long would it take for him to get there? She then looked at me and said, "Okay, he's there," and smiled.

I was forever changed by this powerful experience and thought to myself that if I never worked another day, this was the day I was meant to be a music therapist. The music provided such comfort at what was the most difficult day of their lives. The day they chose to give their child the gift of peace even though it meant that they would no longer be able to hold him in their embrace.

About a year and a half later I was called by labor and delivery to sing to their newborn daughter in the well-baby nursery. I was once again humbled that the family would include me in such an intimate time of their lives. We again exchanged a similar smile, this time to celebrate a "miracle."

"Miracle"

You're my life's one Miracle,
Everything I've done that's good
And you break my heart with tenderness,
And I confess it's true
I never knew a love like this till you....
You're the reason I was born
Now I finally know for sure
And I'm overwhelmed with happiness
So blessed to hold you close
The one that I love most
With all the future has so much for you in store
Who could ever love you more?
The nearest thing to heaven,
You're my angel from above
Only God creates such perfect love.

When you smile at me, I cry
And to save your life I'll die
With a romance that is pure heart,
You are my dearest part
Whatever it requires,
I live for your desires
Forget my own, needs will come before
Who could ever love you more?
Well there is nothing you could ever do,
To make me stop, loving you
And every breath I take,
Is always for your sake
You sleep inside my dreams and know for sure
Who could ever love you more?

"Handprint on My Heart"

A ritual that is performed at our facility offers the opportunity to create a handprint canvas (Figures 26.1 and 26.2). This process can occur prior to the child's death or after, depending on the circumstances. It can be a very cathartic experience for the family—the act of painting the child's palm, laying their hand on the canvas and gently pressing their imprint onto the page, then cleansing the ink from their hands and feet. It is often the last "activity" that is experienced together. Parents have often expressed gratitude for this gift from their child. The canvas may include the patient's hand or footprints, as well as those of the parents and siblings if they so choose. The nurse usually plays a key role in facilitating this ritual, applying expertise to positioning the infant so that his or her IV and a multitude of other tubing does not interfere with the act of making the imprints. All present serve an important role in creating this legacy. During a recent experience we included music while we were preparing to do handprints of an infant that had been declared a DNR. The mother held her baby and we sang:

Hold on to me
And I'll hold on to you.
Hold on to me,
I am loving you.
Hold on to me
And I'll hold on to you.
Holding on to each other

The doctor passing by commented that he had never seen this mother at such peace.

My twenty years as a clinician in a variety of settings has led me to the place I am now. I did not originally envision my work having such an emphasis on end of life, but this path has been the most rewarding. I am humbled in the

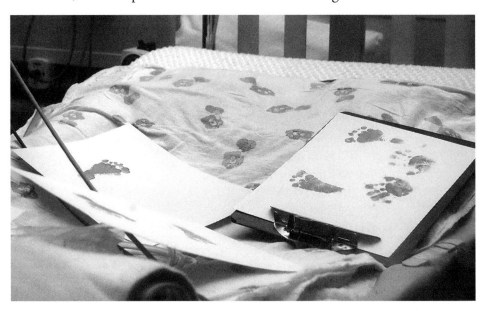

Figure 26.1. On the morning of her baby's death I was met by this grieving mother in the Children's Hospital lobby. As I tried to console her, all she could say was "Thank you so much for the gift of my child's handprints."

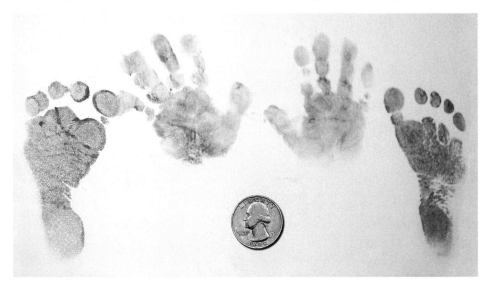

Figure 26.2. "You'll be with me like a handprint on my heart," from the song "For Good," in the Tony award-winning musical *Wicked*.

presence of the patients and families I work with. Their courage and strength enrich my faith in the human spirit and I thank them for allowing me into their lives, leaving a handprint on my heart forever.

SECTION IV

. . .

Healing Principles

CHAPTER 27

Accessing a Spiritual Resource

by Michael Kern, DO, BCST, ND

The exercise described here is one that I sometimes teach in seminars once a certain degree of settling and stillness has entered the group. I refer to this exercise as "accessing a spiritual resource" and it involves using visualization to develop a relationship with the deepest, most complete, truest sense of ourselves. We can then use the form of this visualization to open ourselves to healing and guidance from the realm of the transpersonal, beyond our usual limited sense of self. This exercise is an adaptation of Vajrayana Buddhist practices and it involves four stages:

- Grounding and orientation
- Visualization
- Communion
- Dissolution and embodiment

Grounding and Orientation

Sit upright on a chair or on the floor, with your back comfortably supported as necessary. Establish some orientation and grounding by feeling your feet touching the floor and your bottom on the cushion or chair. Then bring attention to your vertebral column to explore the sense of your midline. Don't be concerned about which aspect of the midline you sense or the depth of function that you notice, but just be with whatever shows. Are there any areas of pain or discomfort, or of ease and lightness? Can you simply notice how this is, without trying to change or fix anything? How are you right now in relation to your midline? Do you feel a bit off to one side, or perhaps even twisted? As you acknowledge how things are, can you start to settle with this?

Visualization

When ready, see if you can find an image, a symbol, or a being that represents for you your deepest nature, your truest and most complete sense of yourself. This symbol or being should signify your deepest and fullest potential, untainted by unresolved experiences. For example, you may choose a light, a cross, a star, or a crystal, or an image of Jesus, Buddha, Mary, Tara, Krishna, or Moses, and so on. Take your time to choose a symbol or being that has special meaning and significance for you. Then start to visualize it in the space in front of you or above your head. As you do this visualization you may start to sense the presence of your symbol or being, as if it's right there in the room with you.

Communion

Can you allow a dialogue to commence between you and the symbol or being in front of you or above your head? What would this symbol or being transmit or say to you right now? Can you open yourself to receive it? Is there anything that you'd like to ask or say to this symbol or being? Can you sit quietly for some minutes to allow this dialogue and communion? Stay there until you've received as much as you can of the message transmitted to you.

Dissolution and Embodiment

Visualize your symbol or being moving toward you and literally dissolving into your body so that it becomes part of you. In this way you can embody the qualities carried by your symbol or being; it becomes a part of you and you've become part of it. Then slowly re-orient your attention back to the room where you are sitting. What have you received? What can you take away with you to encompass in your daily life?

CHAPTER 28

Showing Patience

from Engaging in Bodhisattva Behavior,
by Shantideva, translated from the Tibetan,
as clarified by the Sanskrit,
by Alexander Berzin, 2004

To say that the text is meant for use in meditation means that the whole or selected parts are to be read or recited from memory each day, aloud or silently, and reflected upon. This implies that the verses all connect with each other to form a flowing presentation of the various topics. The text does not consist of disjointed verses. Preservation of the flow of presentation or argument, then, is one of the main criteria I have used for establishing the context in which each verse needs to fit. I have therefore tried, as much as possible, to preserve the flow by adding conjunctions and so on, in parentheses, to help make the connections clearer.

One and a half verses from Sanskrit are missing from the Tibetan, and I have added them in parentheses. When words and phrases in the Sanskrit version have been omitted in the Tibetan translation, and they fit in well with the context, I have also added them in parentheses.

The greatest apparent source of discrepancies, however, is the difficulty of rendering the complexities of Sanskrit grammar into Tibetan. The two languages are extremely different in structure. Sanskrit is one of the most highly inflected Indo-European languages, while Tibetan belongs to the Sinitic family of languages and is far less inflected. Moreover, it is inflected according to different parameters. When the Tibetan is obviously trying to render the Sanskrit construction, and the verb or noun forms are ambiguous in Tibetan due to the limitations of Tibetan grammar, I have followed the Sanskrit grammar.

Occasionally, the order of the phrases in the verses do not correspond with each other, and change the emphasis in the verse. When the Sanskrit ordering gives an emphasis that fits better into the context of the flow of the verses, or is more poetic, I have followed the Sanskrit. When it has not made much difference, I have followed the Tibetan.

(1) Whatever generosity,
Offerings to the Blissfully Gone (Buddhas) and the like,
And positive deeds I've amassed over thousands of eons—
One (moment of) hatred will devastate them all.

(2) As no negative force resembles anger,
And no trial resembles patience,
I shall therefore meditate on patience,
With effort and in various ways.

(3) When the thorn of anger lodges in my heart,
My mind doesn't feel any peace,
Doesn't gain any joy or pleasure,
Doesn't fall asleep, and becomes unstable.

(4) Even those on whom he lavishes wealth and honor
And those who've become dependent on him
Get provoked to the point of murdering
A lord who's possessed with anger.

(5) Friends and relations get disgusted with him,
And though he might attract (others) with gifts,
   he isn't regarded with trust and respect.
In brief, there's no way at all in which
A raging person is in a happy situation.

(6) Hence the enemy, rage,
Creates sufferings such as those and the like,
While whoever clamps down and destroys his rage
Will be happy in this (life) and others.

(7) Finding its fuel in the foul state of mind
That arises from its bringing about things I don't want
And it's preventing what I wish,
Anger, once enflamed, destroys me.

(8) Therefore, I shall totally eradicate
   The fuel of that enemy,
   For this enemy hasn't a mission
   Other than injuring me.

(9) No matter what happens,
   I shall never let it disturb my good mood.
   For if I've fallen into a foul mood, what I want
     will not come about,
   And my constructive behavior will fall apart.

(10) If it can be remedied,
   Why get into a foul mood over something?
   And if it can't be remedied,
   What help is it to get into a foul mood over it?

(11) For myself and my friends,
   Suffering, contempt, verbal abuse,
   And disgrace aren't things that I'd wish for;
   But for my enemies, it's the reverse.

(12) The causes for happiness rarely occur,
   While the causes for sufferings are overly abundant.
   But, without any suffering, there wouldn't be the determination
     to be free;
   Therefore, mind, you must think to be firm.

(13) If devotees of Durga[1] and people of Karnata[2]
   Pointlessly endure the torments of burning
   And cutting themselves, and the like,
   Then why am I such a coward for the sake of liberation?

(14) There isn't anything that doesn't become easier
   Once you've become accustomed to it;
   And so, by growing accustomed to minor pains,
   Greater pains will definitely become bearable.

(15) Don't you see (this) with problems, (borne)
    without a (great) purpose,
From snakes and mosquitoes,
Discomforts such as hunger and thirst,
As well as rashes and the like?

(16) (So,) I shall not be soft
Regarding such things as heat and cold, rain and wind,
Also sickness, captivity, beatings, and the like;
For if I've acted like that, the injury is worse.

(17) There are some who, seeing their own blood,
Develop exceptional courage and resolve;
And there are some who, seeing the blood of others,
Collapse and faint.

(18) That comes from their states of mind being
Either of a resolute or a cowardly type.
Therefore, I must be dismissive of pains
And must not be thrown off by suffering.

(19) Even when he's in agony, someone skilled
Will never let the composure of his mind be stirred;
And in a war that's waged against disturbing emotions,
Bruises abound, when fighting the battle.

(20) Those who, having been dismissive of suffering,
Destroy the enemies, anger and so on,
They are the heroes who have gained the victory;
The rest (merely) slay corpses.

(21) Furthermore, there are advantages to suffering:
With agony, arrogance disappears;
Compassion grows for those in recurring samsara;
Negative conduct is shunned; and joy is taken as being constructive.

(22) As I don't get enraged
With great sources of suffering, for instance with bile,
Then why get enraged with those having limited minds?
All of them, as well, are provoked by conditions.

(23) For example, without being wished for,
   Their sicknesses arise;
   And likewise, without being wished for,
   (Their) disturbing emotions also strongly arise.

(24) Without thinking, "I shall get enraged,"
   People just become enraged;
   And without thinking, "I shall arise,"
   Likewise, rage arises.

(25) All mistakes that there are
   And the various sorts of negative behavior—
   All arise from the force of conditions:
   There aren't any under their own power.

(26) A collection of conditions
   Doesn't have the intention, "I shall create";
   And what it's created didn't have the intention,
   "I'm to be created."

(27) The darling (the Samkhyas[3]) call "primal matter"
   And what they imagine to be "the self"—
   They don't think with some purpose, "I shall come into being
      (to cause some harm),"
   And then come about.

(28) (In fact,) as they haven't arisen, they do not exist,
   So what would have then had the wish to arise?
   And, since (a static sentient self) would be something that was
      permanently occupied with an object,
   It would never come to cease (being so).

(29) But if the self were static (and nonsentient, like Nyaya[4] asserts),
   It would obviously be without actions, like the sky;
   So even if it met with other conditions,
   What activity could something unchangeable have?

(30) If even at the time of the action, it (remains) as before,
   What could have been done by it from the action?
   And if there were something called "This is its action,"
   Which is the one that made them connected?

(31) Thus, everything's under the power of others,
    And the powers they're under aren't under their (own) power.
    Having understood this, I shall not become angry
    With any phenomenon—they're like magic emanations.

(32) And if I said, then, "Warding off (anger) would indeed be unfitting,
    For who (or what) can ward off what?"
    I'd assert that it's not unfitting,
    Since, by depending on that, the continuity of suffering
        can be cut.

(33) Thus, when seeing an enemy or even a friend
    Acting improperly, I'll remain relaxed,
    Having reflected that it's arising
    From some such condition as this.

(34) If all embodied beings had things
    Turn out as they liked,
    Then, since no one wishes ever to suffer,
    It would never come about that anyone suffered.

(35) People hurt themselves
    With such things as thorns, because of not caring,
    And, in a fury, because of desiring to obtain women
        and the like,
    With such acts as refusing food,

(36) There are some who destroy themselves
    By hanging themselves, jumping off cliffs,
    Eating poison and unhealthy foods,
    And through negative acts (bringing worse rebirth states).

(37) When people kill even their beloved selves
    From coming under the power of disturbing emotions,
    How can it be that they wouldn't cause injury
    To the bodies of others?

(38) When I can't even develop compassion, once in a while,
    For those like that, who, with disturbing emotions arisen,
    Would proceed to such things as killing themselves,
    At least I won't get enraged (with them).

(39) (Even) if acting violently toward others
  Were the functional nature of infantile people,
  Still, it'd be as unfitting to get enraged with them
  As it would be for begrudging fire for its functional nature
    of burning.

(40) And even if this fault were fleeting instead,
  And limited beings were lovely by nature,
  Well, still it would be as unfitting to get enraged
  As it would be for begrudging the sky for the (pungent) smoke
    that was rising (in it).

(41) Having set aside the actual (cause of my pain),
    a staff or the like,
  If I become enraged with the person who wielded it,
  Well he, in fact, was incited by anger, so he's secondary (too).
  It would be more fitting to get enraged with his anger.

(42) Previously, I must have inflicted
  Such pain on limited beings,
  Therefore, it's fitting that harm comes to me,
  Who've been a cause of violence toward limited ones.

(43) Both his weapon and my body
  Are the causes of my suffering.
  Since he drew out a weapon and I a body,
  Toward which should I get enraged?

(44) Blinded by craving, I've grabbed hold of a painful boil
  That's shaped like a human and can't bear to be touched,
  And so when it's bruised,
  Toward what should I get enraged?

(45) Childish me, I don't wish to suffer
  And yet I'm obsessed with the cause of my suffering.
  Since it's my own fault that I get hurt,
  Why have a grudge toward anyone (else)?

(46) It's like, for example, the guards of the joyless realms
And the forest of razor-sharp leaves:
This (suffering too) is produced by my impulsive karmic behavior;
So toward what should I be enraged?

(47) Incited by my own karmic behavior,
Those who hurt me come my way,
And if, by their (actions), these limited beings should fall
   to the joyless realms,
Surely, wasn't it I who have ruined them?

(48) Based on them, my negative karmic force
Is greatly cleansed, because of my patience;
But, based on me, they fall
To the joyless realms, with long-lasting pain.

(49) Since I'm, in fact, causing harm to them,
And they're the ones who are benefiting me,
Why, unreasonable mind, do you make it the reverse
And get into a rage?

(50) If I have the advantage of wishing (to be patient),
I won't be going to a joyless realm;
But although I'm safeguarding myself (in this way),
What happens to them in this matter?

(51) And if I were to harm them back instead,
They wouldn't be safeguarded either,
While my (other bodhisattva) behavior would also decline,
And consequently, those having trials would be lost.

(52) Because of its being immaterial,
No one can destroy my mind, by any means;
But because of its obsessive involvement with my body,
It's hurt by physical suffering.

(53) Insults, cruel language,
And defaming words
Don't hurt my body,
So, why, O mind, do you become so enraged?

(54) Others' dislike for me—
   That won't devour me,
   Either in this life or in any other lifetime;
   So why do I find it undesirable?

(55) If I don't wish for it
   Because it would hinder my material gain;
   Well, though material gains in this life will have to be discarded,
   My negative karmic forces will remain secured.

(56) Death today would in fact be better for me
   Than long life through an improper livelihood;
   For even having lived a long time, there will still
   Be the suffering of death for someone like me.

(57) Someone who wakes up after having experienced
   A hundred years of happiness in a dream
   And another who wakes up after having experienced
   Just a moment of happiness:

(58) Once they've awakened, that happiness
   Doesn't return, after all, to either of the two.
   (Similarly,) it comes down to exactly the same
   For someone who's lived for long and someone who's lived
      for a short while.

(59) Though I may have obtained great material gain
   And even have enjoyed many pleasures for long,
   I shall still go forth empty-handed and naked,
   Like having been robbed by a thief.

(60) Suppose I said, "While living off my material gain,
   I'd consume my negative karmic force and do positive things."
   Well if, for the sake of material gain, I became enraged,
   Won't my positive karmic force be consumed
      and negative karmic force come about?

(61) If the very purpose for which I am living
   Should fall apart,
   What use is there with a life
   Committing only negative deeds?

(62) Well, suppose I said, "Rage for someone who maligns (me)
Is because it makes limited beings lose (their trust)."
Well then, why don't you get similarly enraged
With someone defaming someone else?

(63) If you can tolerate distrust (when it's for someone else),
Because that lack of trust depends on other things;
Then why not be patient with someone who maligns (me),
Since that's dependent on disturbing emotions arising?

(64) Even toward those who revile and destroy
Images, stupas, and the sacred Dharma,
My anger's improper,
Since there can be no harm to Buddhas and the rest.

(65) And toward those who injure my spiritual teachers,
My relatives and so on, and my friends as well,
My rage will be averted, by having seen that
This arises from conditions, as in the manner before.

(66) Since injury is inflicted on embodied beings
By both those with a mind and things having no mind,
Why single out and begrudge (only) those with a mind?
Therefore, be patient with harm!

(67) Some commit misdeeds because of naivety,
And, because of naivety, some get enraged:
Which of them can we say is without fault,
And which of them would be at fault?

(68) Why did you previously commit those impulsive actions,
Because of which others now cause me harm?
Since everything's dependent on karmic behavior,
Why do I bear a grudge against this one?

(69) Seeing it's like that, I'll put effort
Into positive things like those through which
Everybody'll become
Loving-minded toward each other.

(70) For example, when fire in a burning house
Is advancing to another home,
It's fitting to remove and throw out
Whatever it's in that would cause it to spread,
   such as straw and the like.

(71) Likewise, when the fire of anger is spreading,
Due to my mind being attached to something,
I shall throw it out at that instant,
For fear of my positive force being burned.

(72) Why would a man about to be put to death
Be unfortunate if, by having his hand chopped off, he were spared?
So why would I be unfortunate if, through human sufferings,
I were spared joyless realms?

(73) If I'm unable to bear
Even this minor suffering of the present,
Then why don't I ward off the rage
That would be the cause of hellish pain?

(74) On account of my impassioned (rage), I've experienced
   burning and the like
For thousands of times in the joyless realms;
But (through it), I haven't brought benefit to myself
Or benefit for others.

(75) But, since great benefits will be brought about
In this, which is not even a fraction of that damage,
Only delight is appropriate here
In the suffering dispelling (all) damage to wandering beings.

(76) If others obtain the pleasure of joy
From praising someone (I dislike) who possesses good qualities,
Why, O mind, don't you make yourself joyous like this,
By praising him too?

(77) That pleasure of joy of yours would be
An arising of pleasure that was not disgraceful,
Something permitted by the Ones with Good Qualities,
And superlative, as well, for gathering others.

(78) If you wouldn't like this pleasure of his,
    "Such pleasure as that would be only his!"
    Then, from stopping (as well) giving wages and the like,
    (Your) ruin will come, both seen and unseen.

(79) When your own good qualities are being extolled,
    You wish others, as well, to take pleasure;
    But when others' good qualities are being extolled,
    You don't wish yourself to take pleasure too.

(80) Having developed a bodhichitta[5] aim
    Through wishing for happiness for all limited beings,
    Then why do you become angry instead
    At the happiness that limited beings have found by themselves?

(81) (Having given your word) that you wish limited beings
    To have Buddhahood, honored throughout the three realms,
    Then why, when seeing them merely shown miserable respect,
    Do you burn up inside at it?

(82) If there were someone needing care
    Who's to be cared for by you and provided for by you,
    And that family member were to get something to live on,
    Wouldn't you be delighted, or would you be enraged in return?

(83) How could someone who doesn't want (even) that
       for wandering beings
    Be anyone who wishes for them to be Buddhas?
    Where is there bodhichitta in someone
    Who becomes enraged at others' gain?

(84) If, whether he receives it from him
    Or it remains in the benefactor's house,
    It will in no way be yours,
    So what does it matter whether or not it's given (to him)?

(85) Throw away your positive force or (others') faith (in you),
    And even your own good qualities? For what?
    Don't hold on to what could bring you gain?
    Tell me, with whom don't you get enraged?

(86) Not only do you not feel sorry
 About the negative things you've done yourself,
 You wish to compete against others
 Who've enacted positive deeds?

(87) Even if your enemy lacks any joy,
 What's there in that for you to take delight?
 The mere wish in your mind
 Won't become the cause for (any) harm to him.

(88) And even if his suffering came about through your wish,
 Still, what's there in that for you to take delight?
 If you said that you'd become gratified,
 Is there anything else more degenerate than that?

(89) This hook cast by the fishermen, the disturbing emotions,
 Is horrendously sharp. Procuring (you) from them, O mind,
 The joyless realm guards will cook me, for sure,
 In the cauldrons of hell.

(90) Praise and fame, (these) shows of respect,
 Won't bring positive force, won't bring a long life,
 Won't bring bodily strength, nor freedom from sickness;
 They won't bring physical pleasure either.

(91) If I were aware of what's in my self-interest,
 What in my self-interest would there be in them?
 If just mental happiness were what I wanted,
 I should devote myself to gambling and so on, and to alcohol too.

(92) For the sake of fame, (people) would give away wealth
 Or would get themselves killed;
 But what use is there with words (of fame)?
 Once they've died, to whom will they bring pleasure?

(93) At the collapse of his sand castle,
 A child wails in despair;
 Similarly, at the loss of praise and fame,
 My mind shows the face of a child.

(94) Because an impromptu word is something lacking a mind,
    It's impossible that it has the intention to praise me.
    But, proclaiming, "The other one (offering me praise)
        is delighted with me,"
    If I consider that a cause (also) to be delighted;

(95) Well, whether it's toward someone else or toward me,
    What use to me is another person's joy?
    That pleasure of joy is his alone;
    I won't get (even) a share of it.

(96) If I take pleasure in his pleasure (with me),
    I must do like that in all cases, in fact.
    How is it that I don't take pleasure
    When he has the pleasure of joy with another?

(97) So joy is arising in me
    (Simply due to), "Me, I'm being praised!"
    But there, in fact, because (thinking) like that is just nonsense,
    It comes down to nothing but the behavior of a child.

(98) Being praised and such things cause me distraction;
    They cause my disgust (with samsara) to disintegrate as well.
    I become jealous of those with good qualities,
    And that makes me demolish success.

(99) Therefore, aren't those who are hovering close by
    For striking down praise and the like for me
    Actually involved in protecting me from falling
    Into a worse rebirth state?

(100) For me, whose primary interest is in gaining freedom,
    Bondage to material gain and shows of respect are things I mustn't
        have.
    So how can I get enraged with those who are causing me
    To be freed from my having been bound?

(101) For me, who would enter into (a house) of suffering,
    How can I get enraged with those who've come,
    As if from Buddha's inspiration,
    In the nature of a door panel not letting me pass in.

(102) "But this one is impeding my positive practices!"
Still, it's unfitting to be enraged with him.
There isn't any trial that's equal to patience,
So shouldn't I be staying just close to that?

(103) If, in fact, it's through my own fault
That I'm not acting patiently here,
Then while a cause for positive practice is biding nearby,
It's actually me who's causing the impediment here.

(104) If there were something that wouldn't come about
    if something were absent,
But if something were present, would also be present,
That very thing would be the cause of that,
So how can it be said that it's an impediment to it?

(105) There's no impediment to giving caused by a mendicant (monk)
Gone out (for alms) at the proper time;
And it can't be said that the coming of someone conferring vows
Is an impediment for becoming a monastic.

(106) Alms-seekers are plentiful in this life,
But scarce are those who cause (me) harm,
Because no one will cause me harm
If I haven't harmed them like this (in past lives).

(107) Therefore, I shall be delighted with an enemy
Who's popped up like a treasure in my house,
Without having had to be acquired with fatigue,
Since he becomes my aide for bodhisattva behavior.

(108) It's because of its having been actualized
    through this one and me (having met)
That a fruit of patience (comes about).
(So,) let me award it first to him,
For he was, like this, the (earlier) cause of my patience.

(109) Suppose I said, "But he had no intention for (me) to actualize
     patience,
So this enemy isn't someone to be honored."
Well, how is it that the hallowed Dharma is honored
As suited to be a cause for actualizing (it)?

(110) Suppose I said, "But this enemy's intention was to cause me harm,
So he can't be honored."
Well, how could patience be actualized by me
If, like a doctor, he were intent on my benefit?

(111) Therefore, since patience arises dependently
From his vicious intention,
This one himself is fit to be honored like the hallowed Dharma,
Because he's a cause of my patience.

(112) Thus, the Sage has spoken of the field of limited beings
As well as the field of the Triumphant,
(For,) having made them happy, many have gone, thereby,
To the far-shore of excellence.

(113) When the acquisition of a Buddha's Dharma (attainments)
Is equally due to (both) limited beings and the Triumphant,
What kind of order is it that the respect shown to limited beings
Is not like that to the Triumphant?

(114) The preeminence of an intention is not from itself,
But due to its result, and by that, the preeminence
Of that which is had by limited beings is, in fact, the same;
And because of that, they are equal.

(115) Whatever is honored in having a loving intention (toward them),
That, in fact, is the greatness (coming) from limited beings;
And whatever positive force there is in confident belief in the
     Buddhas,
That, in fact, is the greatness from the Buddhas.

(116) It's the share they have in actualizing a Buddha's Dharma
      (attainments),
    And because of that, they're asserted as their equals;
    But, of course, no one can be the equal of the Buddhas
    In endless oceans of excellent qualities.

(117) If even a speck of the excellent qualities
    Of the unique syntheses of the best excellent qualities
    Were to be seen somewhere, an offering of the three planes of
      existence
    Would be inadequate for honoring it.

(118) Since a share giving rise to a Buddha's
    Foremost Dharma (attainments) exists in limited beings,
    It's fitting that limited beings be honored,
    In accordance with this very share.

(119) Further, besides making limited beings happy,
    What other repayment is there
    For those who befriend them without pretension
    And help them beyond any measure?

(120) Since it would repay them to benefit those for whose sake
    They sacrifice their bodies and plunge into joyless realms
      of unrelenting pain,
    Then even if these (limited beings) should cause great harm,
    Everything wholesome is to be done (for them).

(121) For the sake of even, in this case, my master himself,
    They disregard even their own bodies.
    So how can I, bewildered about this, act with pride
    And not act in the nature of a servant?

(122) The Sages delight in their happiness
    And enter into distress at their injury;
    And so, in (my) bringing them joy, the Sages will all have become
      delighted,
    And in bringing them harm, the Sages will have been hurt.

(123) Just as there could be no mental pleasure from desirable objects
For someone whose body were completely on fire,
Likewise, there's no way to delight the Greatly Compassionate Ones
When limited beings have, in fact, been harmed.

(124) Therefore, whatever displeasure I've brought
to all the Greatly Compassionate Ones,
By my having caused harm to limited beings,
I openly admit, today, that negative deed,
And request the Sages, please bear with that displeasure you have.

(125) From now on, for the sake of delighting the Thusly Gone (Buddhas),
I shall act, with definite restraint, as a servant to the world.
Let mobs of people kick me in the head with their feet or
even beat me to death, I shall not venture (anything back).
Let the Guardians of the World take delight!

(126) There's no doubt that Those with a Compassion Self-Nature
Have taken all wandering beings (to be the same) as themselves.
The very nature they've seen as the essential nature of limited beings
Is those Guardians' self-nature, so why don't I show (them the same)
respect?

(127) Just this, is what brings pleasure to the Thusly Gone (Buddhas);
Just this, is what perfectly accomplishes my own aims as well;
Just this, is what dispels the world's suffering too;
Therefore, let it be just this, that I always shall do.

(128) For example, even when some member of the royal court
Is harming the public,
Farsighted people do not hurt him back
Even if they're able,

(129) For that one, (acting) like this, is not alone:
On the contrary, the king's power and might are his military forces.
Likewise, some lowly person creating harm
Is not to be belittled,

(130) For his armed forces are the guards of the joyless realms
    And all the Compassionate Ones.
    So, like a commoner toward a violent king,
    I shall make all limited beings be pleased.

(131) Should even such a king be enraged (with me),
    Could he inflict the pain of a joyless realm,
    Which is what I'd be brought to experience
    By having made limited beings displeased?

(132) Should even such a king be pleased (with me),
    It's impossible that he could bestow Buddhahood,
    Which is what I'd be brought to attain
    By having made limited beings be pleased.

(133) (Leave aside) seeing that the future attainment of Buddhahood
    Arises from making limited beings be pleased,
    Don't you see that, at least in this life, great prosperity,
    Fame, and happiness come?

(134) (Moreover), with beauty and so on, freedom from sickness, and fame,
    Someone with patience, while still in samsara,
    Gains extremely long life and the abundant pleasures
    Of a universal chakra king.[6]

Notes

1. Durga—a wrathful female deity worshipped by followers of certain Hindu schools. After fasting for a certain period of time, followers of Durga engage in ritual burning, piercing, and cutting their limbs.

2. Karnata—a kingdom in South India. People of this kingdom engage in competitions of endurance of pain even to the point of losing their lives.

3. Samkhya—a school of non-Buddhist Indian philosophy that asserts twenty-five classes of phenomena: "persons" or "selves" that are equivalent to mere passive consciousness and twenty-four classes of primal matter that are made up of three universal constituents—rajas, sattva, and tamas.

4. Nyaya—a school of non-Buddhist Indian philosophy that emphasizes logic and asserts sixteen types of entities, including "persons" or "selves" that lack any quality of consciousness.

5. Bodhichitta—a mind or heart focused first on the benefit of all beings and then on one's own individual enlightenment (which has not yet happened, but which can happen on the basis of our mind's potential), with the intention to attain that enlightenment and to benefit all others by means of that attainment.

6. Universal chakra king—according to Buddhist cosmology, kings, possessing a wheel of authority, who rule over all or part of the universe during the eons when the human lifespan is steadily decreasing.

Reprinted with kind permission from www.berzinarchives.com.

CHAPTER 29

Stages on the Spiritual Path

with Alan Lokos

I have actually worked on this chapter for years and was never satisfied with it because it did not seem practical. How could a Buddhist description of a spiritual path be applied to biodynamic craniosacral therapy practice? Alan Lokos figured it out quite simply and elegantly. I am very grateful to have received permission to reprint several of Alan Lokos's Pocket Practices from his book *Pocket Peace: Effective Practices for Enlightened Living* (Lokos, 2010). I will describe the traditional meaning of the ten stages of the spiritual path in the Buddhist tradition and then give several of Alan's Pocket Practices for the reader to try out. All of the practices are meant for personal use in any life circumstance but I have found them to be excellent reminders while being with a client.

I also believe that this chapter speaks to a training for the heart. This book in general, as well as my Volume Three are about the heart at its deepest level biologically, and now in this chapter spiritually. I believe that when fear is reduced through the practices of biodynamic craniosacral therapy, happiness and equanimity replace the fear. A wonderful colleague of mine, Cator Sachoy, has drawn a beautiful lighthearted image of this experience. Figure 29.1 shows such a possibility, moving from a broken heart to a connected heart. She calls it a Buddhist heart replacement. Further development of the heart is integrated with the ten stages of the spiritual path described below.

The Buddhist tradition speaks of the lifespan of a human being as an unfolding of successive stages of spiritual development, particularly in the Mahayana traditions of India and Tibet. Buddhism itself developed in successive stages with the first phase being called the Hinayana, in which practitioners work to eliminate mental afflictions and develop a serene state of mind for themselves. Thich Nhat Hanh says that afflictions related to strong emotions are our negative mental states that disturb our peace of mind and bring about suffering and misperceptions.

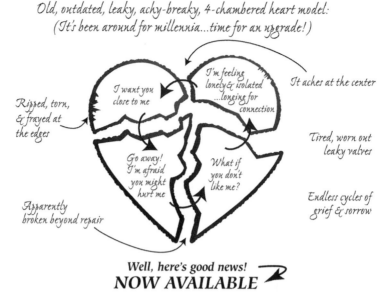

Old, outdated, leaky, achy-breaky, 4-chambered heart model:
(It's been around for millennia...time for an upgrade!)

Well, here's good news!
NOW AVAILABLE

The NEW IMPROVED Buddhist 4-Chambered Heart Model
Yours–FREE of charge! No down payment required!

To ORDER CALL 1-800-BUDDHA-Nature

WARNING: May result in loss of critical judgement, delight in change, unprecedented goodwill & generosity towards others, as well as loss of interest in material gain and worldly pursuits

Figure 29.1. Buddhist heart replacement, by Cator Sachoy
(included with permission).

Buddhism gradually evolved to eliminate cognitive obscurations or the misperceptions that come about from negative emotional states, in order to develop clear seeing. This skill or set of skills leads to more wisdom for one's self and generates compassion for others as the focus or intention of spiritual practice and life in general. This is necessary to simply see life and reality as it is presented to us through our senses and mental faculties as clearly as possible. The elimination of mental blocks and emotional blockages allows for the focus to be balanced between working on one's self and helping other people. This tradition in Buddhism is called the Mahayana or Great Vehicle.

The most basic skill for all Buddhist practice is *mindfulness,* which is the real presence of our body and mind being synchronized. Our body and mind are directed toward one point, the present moment. In addition, mindfulness includes nonjudgment of any emotional or mental blockages that one is experiencing in the present moment. Since breathing happens in the present moment unless one is dead, it is the perfect starting place for mindfulness practice. Indeed, much research has now shown the value of twenty minutes a day of mindfulness practice for alleviating a wide range of physical and emotional problems, from eating disorders to anxiety (Davidson and Begley, 2012; Siegel, 2010). The website www.mindfulexperience.org maintains a data base of all research on mindfulness. Training in mindfulness is readily available in many communities.

In the Mahayana, spiritual development is associated with becoming a Bodhisattva. Bodhisattva is the word for an enlightened being or a wise being who works tirelessly for the welfare of others with all appropriate available means. He or she is the essence of compassionate action. I imagine in the Christian tradition such a person would be a saint like Mother Teresa. In the Mahayana the spiritual developmental stages act as a roadmap, so to speak, for one's individual progress on the spiritual path. They could also be considered a series of contemplations (the previous chapter focuses on one of these stages, patience). Such a person who wishes to lead an altruistic life in service to others, and simultaneously meditates and prays on developing the perfection of wisdom for himself or herself, moves through spiritual developmental stages called the ten paramitas.

Param means "other side" or "shore," "other side of the river," while *ita* means "arrived." Thus paramita means "arriving at the other side or shore," which indicates that the activities of the bodhisattva must have the vision, the understanding that transcends the centralized notions of ego (Trungpa 1973, p. 170).

Life development in the Buddhist tradition is called a path. In the case of the Mahayana tradition it is the path of the Bodhisattva. It encompasses the ten paramitas. The Bodhisattva is one who seeks to stay awake by staying openhearted, warm, and friendly to himself or herself first and then extending that caring to others when appropriate. It is through the paramitas that one learns how and when to care for others. A central principle of the path is that providing happiness to others brings happiness to one's self. This is the central message of the Dalai Lama and has been proven to be accurate in terms of the neuroscience of empathy and compassion. (Go to www.CCARE.org for numerous research articles on compassion, available to download for free as of the writing of this chapter.)

Stanford University has started the Center for Compassion and Altruistic Research and Education (CCARE) to apply this research and make it available to school systems, especially because of the epidemic of aggression and violence in elementary schools.

The basic practices of mindfulness meditation and compassion meditations provided by Alan Lokos below naturally and gradually lead one through the path of the ten paramitas. There must be a considerable amount of life experience in each of these stages to verify if they are correct and appropriate for the practitioner. This is not a cookbook or recipe, but rather themes and practices that are experiential and must be proven to one's self in daily life.

The following ten paramitas, or Noble Virtues as they are sometimes called, begin with a brief explanation. Then I give a short list of their qualities and finally the Pocket Practices of Alan Lokos.

Generosity

The first step is *generosity*, which relates to being generous with communication first followed by material objects, spirituality, and safety. This is an attitude of giving. It means pledging non-fright to all people and living beings.

- Generosity of giving or renunciating material objects
- Generosity of giving non-fear
- Being lighthearted and vulnerable (free from co-dependency or shame, or at least able to recognize such behavior consciously)

Pocket Practices:

Greet folks with a smile.
Perform spontaneous acts of generosity.
Focus intently on what is being said by others, so as to be able to repeat accurately what they have said.

Discipline

The second step is *discipline* or *morality*, which relates to not indulging in excessive emotions or too many thoughts. It is the attitude of an ethical lifestyle.

- Not indulging in excessive emotions
- Discipline of studying and practicing sacred teachings
- Discipline of altruism—working with people wholeheartedly

Pocket Practices:

Work this sentence (or a similar one) into your conversations, especially when there is disagreement: "Let me think about that."

Contemplate often questions such as, In what situations am I most likely to stray from my values?

For a week, several times a day, as you are about to do something, anything, even the simplest act, ask yourself, What is my intention?

When you touch the phone, about to make a call or send a text message, ask yourself, What is my intention? As you are about to enter a meeting, ask yourself, What is my intention?

Each day for two weeks, sincerely praise others' words or deeds.

Take time each day, every day, to practice being the person you want to be.

Patience

The third step is *patience,* which means developing more warmth toward one's self and one's own confusion and extending that warmth to others. It is the attitude of tolerance based on the Law of Causality in which all people are equal in the common desire for happiness. If I am tolerant and giving to others, treat them ethically, then it is the cause of making me feel better.

- Patience toward one's neurosis and mental fixations

- Not being tired or impatient with various meditation practices

- Not blocking one's understanding of the nature of reality

Pocket Practices:

Find a place where you can feel completely at ease and say to yourself, Only I can destroy my peace, and I choose not to do so.

Understand and accept that in each given moment, everyone, including you, is doing the best they can.

Exertion

The fourth step is *exertion.* It takes a lot of effort to lead a spiritual life. Anyone can have spiritual experiences, but not everyone has the effort and discipline to integrate these experiences into their daily life. It is the attitude of enthusiasm for developing wisdom and compassion.

- Exertion of virtue

- Exertion of effort
- Continual exertion
- Immovable exertion
- Exertion free from pride

Pocket Practice:

Don't hold grudges—find a way to forgive.

Equanimity

The fifth step is *equanimity,* which relates to cultivating knowledge from the practice of mindfulness and extending that knowledge into compassionate action, particularly when it comes to working with others. It is an orientation to a subtle emotion inside the mind of conscious stillness called equanimity. It relates to being calm and locating a central stillness in one's mind and body.

- Sense of mental and physical calmness and ease
- Cultivating knowledge of reality
- Meditation and post-meditation experience as being equal

Pocket Practices:

Don't confuse your thoughts, feelings, and perceptions with reality. Practice seeing things as they really are.

Close your eyes and contemplate the law of impermanence: all things are changing; all things die away.

Knowledge

The sixth step is *knowledge,* which comes from conventional learning as well as transcendental learning that occurs from contemplating and meditating. Such knowledge arises from the gradual development of discriminating awareness, a side effect of meditation and concentration.

- Knowledge that comes from learning, both experiential and cognitive
- Uncommon knowledge of being interconnected to all things
- Meditation in action out in the world

Pocket Practices:

Develop listening skills.

Do not speak about anyone who is not physically present.

One day each month, every time you are about to speak, stop for a moment and consider if what you are about to say will improve upon the silence.

Skillful Means

The seventh step is called *skillful means*. This means knowing one's own method and practice of skillful means and how to use your skill for others' well-being. It is important to know your own strengths in order to help others skillfully to know happiness and the causes of happiness. The basic practice is loving kindness toward oneself and then others.

- Knowing one's own strengths and weaknesses
- Knowing how to use your skill for others compassionately

Pocket Practices:

When feeling angry, tense, or anxious, remind yourself that these feelings are grounded in fear. Stop and try to identify the cause of the fear.

Contemplate and accept that there are times when you can help and times when you cannot. Remember that just feeling bad helps no one.

Inspiration

The eighth step is called *inspiration*. This relates to the development of a joyful mind. This is the attitude of the aspiring mind or great aspiration for one's own wisdom and the attitude of infinite altruism for all others.

- Being happy and knowing the causes of happiness
- Being free from clinging and aversion to others
- Wishing others to be free from the sea of unbearable sorrow

Pocket Practices:

Spend a few quiet moments at the end of each day considering and encouraging your most positive way of thinking.

Create a personal one-hour retreat.

Strength

The ninth step is called *strength*. The Buddhist tradition speaks of the strength of fearlessness and the strength of rejoicing in taming one's mind as a significant step on the spiritual path. This is the attitude of being powerful in the sense that if I can do it then all others can do it. One can imagine oneself with the image of a king or queen sitting on a throne. It is the throne of relinquishing one's neurosis by more directly experiencing the emptiness of all phenomena.

Buddhism uses the terms emptiness or void to describe the actual reality of our existence—a concept often misunderstood, even by Buddhists. I recall Pope John Paul writing that Buddhism was a depressing religion because of such a philosophy as emptiness. Emptiness is not nothing but quite the opposite—it is the experience of everything and is known by its complete lack of fear.

It does not mean that nothing exists but rather, as Thich Nhat Hanh says, it means the absence of having an independent self. We have the shell of a personality and a family name and personal history but it does not constitute a sense of self that is different than anyone else whether it be Buddha or God. Thus from this point of view we are the same as Buddha or God, according to Thich Nhat Hanh. As a person relinquishes self, as in the actual dying process or simply letting anger die, an enormous amount of strength becomes available associated with joy, love, and compassion. These are the pre-existing conditions of our body and mind.

- Strength of emptiness—not having an independent self, no separation from others
- Strength of happiness in seeing no independent self or being separate from others

Pocket Practices:

Consider whether it's more important for you to be right or to be happy.

Consider letting someone off the hook for a deed that person committed or harsh words he or she spoke.

Wisdom

The tenth is *wisdom*. Wisdom is the culmination of one's spiritual life development and the realization of even deeper levels of emptiness or the lack of intrinsic existence of all things, especially the notion of an individual self. Emptiness further means to experience the indivisibility or interconnectedness of all things. It is sometimes called "one taste." Wisdom as discussed here has three aspects.

The first is that wisdom is a product of learning or understanding cognitively and a collection of experiences regarding the impermanence of phenomena. It is like becoming spiritually street smart.

Second, there is the aspect of wisdom that is cultivated by meditation practice and results in genuine insight into the true nature of reality. There is more and more relaxation with life and experience. It is a clear, nonthinking, panoramic awareness of the whole of life. The past is no longer compelling, as every piece of experience fits into a unified meaning. This allows one to stay in the present moment for longer periods of time.

Third, there is a wisdom in which the cultivation and collection of information falls apart. This ultimate wisdom is not a product of being wise or learned; rather, it is a product of unlearning, which leads to very direct and precise experience of remembering the origin of one's confusion or style of suffering. This type of wisdom is based on the ability to spontaneously transform the confusion of self and other into a sharp, clear wisdom. This goes back to what I mentioned at the beginning about mental afflictions and cognitive obscurations. At this stage one gives up approaching problems mechanically and seeing life as good or bad, which is aggressive. One finally sees through this and transforms both good and bad, happy and sad, into wisdom. It's a very natural process and occurs gradually. It is a deep awareness.

This is the last of the stages of opening and taming one's heart. These ten stages also replace one's heart with a higher-functioning model, as suggested in Figure 29.1. To me, they are qualities associated with the deeper intention of the dance between Primary Respiration and stillness. Thus biodynamic practice is a protocol for compassion and open-heartedness.

Pocket Practice:

Consider how your discomfort with a particular situation might be eased by accepting things as they are.

I am very grateful for permission to reprint the Pocket Practices of Alan Lokos. These ten phases of spiritual development are important measures of self-care and compassion for one's own self. They lend themselves quite well to biodynamic practice in which a great deal of time is spent waiting, watching, and wondering.

SECTION V

▪ ▪ ▪

Detoxification

CHAPTER 30

Constipation: The Whats and Whys

by Sheila Shea, MA

Viewpoint of Biological, Functional, and Naturopathic Medicine

In writing these chapters for my brother Michael's book, I draw upon the great traditions of biological, functional, and naturopathic medicine and healing. Each tradition believes that we live in harmony with ourselves and with nature. When we are out of harmony or out of balance, we return to our health through natural methods that include nutrition, detoxification, exercise, and a host of other alternative or natural ways to restore health and balance. Each tradition believes that we must get to the root cause of the problem and not just treat the symptoms.

Mark Hyman, MD, a proponent of functional medicine, writes in his foreword to *The Swiss Secret to Optimal Health* (Rau and Wyler, 2009) that the principle of biological medicine is to understand the "underlying causes of disease, ways to remove those causes and then help support and encourage the body's natural healing systems. The tools and methods of biological medicine focus on supporting the body's normal powers of regeneration, regulation and healing" (pp.xiii–xiv). Methods used in all three traditions—biological, functional, and naturopathic medicine—are detoxification, nutrition, and correcting the digestive system. All roads point to the gastrointestinal (GI) system.

Constipation is a form of imbalance and intoxication. Input does not equal output. In these chapters I review many of the naturopathic traditions for working with constipation, natural techniques that allow us to release the toxins we have taken in through our behavior and environment. The naturopathic tradition addresses the whole organism, the whole body, and places constipation in that context.

Viewpoint of a Colon Hydrotherapist

I see the world of constipation through the eyes of a colon hydrotherapist. For thirty-five years I have been seeing clients for colon hydrotherapy. During that time, I have performed more than 30,000 colon hydrotherapy sessions. First, I ask clients to fill out my health questionnaire, which I review with them. This gives me a better idea of their overall health and intestinal health. I learn about their dietary, hydration, and exercise habits.

Then we move right into the colon hydrotherapy session, which lasts about forty-five minutes. I use a "closed" system, in which the water is released when I or the client indicates and the waste flows through a closed tube or waste line through an illuminated viewing tube to the sewer system just like a toilet. While the client is relaxing on my massage table during the session and during a release or outflow, I massage his or her abdomen with my hands and a host of tools including a vibrator and hot rocks that allow for better release.

Through all of the sessions and years I have gained perspective on what helps and hinders constipation and the challenges in overcoming it. The clientele has changed over the years. Constipation is more prevalent, overweight and obesity have escalated, and sugar addiction is a major complaint. Constipation may be the reason a person comes in. Others come in to work on some condition and then say they have had constipation all their life! Is there a message here? Many of the insights I share come from my observations over years in practice and my own experience.

I also view these chapters from a personal perspective, as a lifelong sufferer of constipation. I share my story in Chapter 32. Enemas, colon hydrotherapy, nutrition, exercise, and meditation are a big part of my healing and detoxification. Constipation has a large influence on our quality of life. It can be a great source of unrecognized pain. Stay in tune as my story and others' unfold.

Constipation

Constipation is a reflection of diet, fluid intake, breathing, stressful emotions and thoughts, genes, and culture. Constipation can be lifelong, periodic, or short lived. Constipation may be the basis for seemingly unrelated illnesses. Many friends and clients with serious or chronic conditions say, coincidentally, "Oh, I've had constipation all my life!" or as long as they can remember or most of their life. The causes of constipation vary from the obvious to the more complicated or of seemingly unknown origin.

I have suffered constipation since infancy and did not even know the word constipation until I was eighteen and then I had no idea why I was constipated or what to do about it. Many are in ignorance about their condition. Many do not realize how serious constipation is. Many have such shame around constipation they cannot say the word. They use many synonyms to describe their condition but the word "constipation" is too shameful to say. Another lens through which to view constipation is how you feel about your own intestines and elimination. Constipation is a taboo subject—perhaps it just has not had the big best-seller breakthrough nor the blockbuster reality TV winner to move it into the "wow, let's talk about constipation" category.

Sylvester Yong (1999), an MD from Singapore who is overseeing a study on constipation and colon hydrotherapy, writes: "Constipation is a problem that affects almost everyone at varying periods of their lives." Dr. Yong writes that constipation affects our QOL (quality of life). For many people, constipation is the most common sign their digestive system is out of balance. One of our goals according to the naturopathic tradition is to restore balance.

So what is this balance that we are striving for? We are balancing input with output. The good old American way seems to be maximize input, very little output. At least our diets and lifestyles have lead us up this road. We are aiming for homeostasis, a balance of our intake of nutrition and our output of waste.

In these chapters, I explore all aspects of constipation. I believe constipation is a serious condition in itself. Ignoring constipation can lead to many other serious diseases and conditions. When the body is stagnating in its own waste, this toxicity in the body becomes the perfect medium for disease. Your quality of life is greatly reduced. Take the journey with me to explore and turn upside down one of my very favorite topics, constipation. Each person is unique and has an individual path in ending constipation. The path out of it is challenging, filled with trial and error, full of feedback, and rewarding.

So, what is constipation? Typically, constipation is any form of congestion and can be accompanied by dehydration. It extends to the cellular level. The major signs of constipation are less than one bowel movement a day and/or incomplete elimination. Some symptoms are overweight, bloat, gas, indigestion, lethargy, fatigue, headaches, migraines, earaches, sinus drainage, allergies, cellulite, irritability, anxiety, depression, pessimism, whining, unsatisfied hunger, poor circulation, rashes, skin conditions, anti-social behavior, attention deficit, and mental confusion and brain fog.

From the Moffitt Cancer Center and Research Institute, Susan C. McMillan (1999), a PhD and an RN, writes:

> An acceptable definition of constipation for clinical practice would be the following: a decrease in the frequency of passage of formed stools and characterized by stools that are hard and difficult to pass. This definition

suggests four characteristics that may be presented in the acronym DISH: difficult to pass, infrequent compared to normal, smaller than normal, and hard. (p. 199)

So, what is normal? Each person will define what is normal. I would say that one should hope to have formed, pliable stool more than an inch in diameter. Smaller than normal implies a change in your bowel habit. For example, many complain that their stool has become pencil-thin. That is to be avoided.

Characteristics

In the same article, McMillan quotes two additional medical studies that offer a more comprehensive list of signs of constipation. McShane and McLane (1985) and McMillan and Williams (1989) list twenty-one characteristics:

- Abdominal distention/bloating
- Abdominal growling
- Increased abdominal pressure
- Abdominal mass
- Abdominal pain
- Change in abdominal size
- Change in gas passed
- Oozing liquid stool
- Less frequent bowel movements
- Small volume of stool
- Dry, hard stool
- Straining at stool
- Inability to pass stool
- Blood with stool
- Rectal mass
- Rectal fullness or pressure
- Rectal pain at bowel movement
- Swollen rectal veins
- Indigestion

- Decreased appetite
- Headache

In addition, says Sharon McMillan, a change in mental status with confusion and increased agitation, elevated temperature, incontinence, and unexplained falls may sometimes be the only presenting symptoms of constipation in the elderly. The Stanford Study, described below and in subsequent chapters, includes fecal soiling and incontinence of feces and urine in the elderly.

Consequences

Constipation can create an accumulation of fecal matter throughout the intestines, an increase in mucus production, and be a potential feeding and breeding ground for pathogenic bacteria, fungi, yeast, virus, and parasites. These pathogens excrete toxic acids, gases, and metabolites—substances that can cause inflammation and degradation of the intestinal walls. They ultimately absorb and circulate to the cell level.

Candida, nearly epidemic, can be another consequence of constipation. Candida is an intestinal and residential yeast that grows out of healthy proportion to other residential bacteria in the presence of antibiotics, birth control pills, steroids, diabetes, nutritional deficiencies, chronic constipation, diarrhea, physical or emotional stress, and overconsumption of refined sugars.

Volumes are written on the outer manifestations of Candida. Skin conditions of all kinds, thrush in the throat and mouth, and canker sores are a few examples of Candida on the body. One client had a rash under her breasts from Candida. It was extremely uncomfortable. For some it is jock itch or athlete's foot.

As constipation continues to create enlarged intestines, organs and circulatory vessels are pressured. This pressure on the organs and circulatory system decreases their functionality. Constipation slows circulation. Uneliminated waste finds storage space throughout the body via the blood and lymph and eventually affects circulation to the organs and tissues, including the brain, feet, and hands.

Loss of our quality of life is another consequence of constipation. Socializing, studying, sleeping, and exercising while constipated are stressful because of the discomfort and muscle tension. Eating food can be painful. Our quality of life is clearly affected. As I mentioned earlier, another consequence of constipation may be the development of a far more serious and life-threatening illness such as breast cancer and IBD (inflammatory bowel disease).

Peristalsis

Peristalsis is the automatic expansion and contraction of the gut muscles that propel intestinal contents, i.e., food and fluid, from mouth to anus. This expanding and contracting muscle motion is akin to the beating of our heart to propel blood through our circulatory system. My observation of the viewing tube during colon hydrotherapy sessions shows that very few people have peristalsis.

Peristalsis and the gastrointestinal tract (gut) are governed by the enteric nervous system (ENS) and the vagus nerve of the autonomic nervous system (ANS), the tenth cranial nerve. The vagus nerve is responsible for the parasympathetic innervation of the gastrointestinal tract down to the transverse colon and contains both outgoing and incoming fibers. The outgoing parasympathetic vagal fibers enhance digestive activities by stimulating local neurons of the enteric nervous system in the gut wall. The last part of the gastrointestinal tract receives parasympathetic innervation from the pelvic nerves.

Transit Time

How long should food remain in our GI tract before we eliminate it? A wide range of possibilities exists and will reflect our uniqueness. Bowel movements are going to vary based on quantity and quality of food eaten, exercise, fluid intake (hydration), length of GI tract, and emotional and environmental states. Ideally, the colon would empty within an hour after each meal, with a total transit time of 24 to 48 hours. Some reports say that our ideal transit time is 18–24 hours; other reports say three to four days is permissible for transit time.

One pattern that I have noticed in colon hydrotherapy is that many clients present with redundant or enlarged intestines or megacolons. Redundancy means extra length of intestine with degrees of looping, coiling, and prolapsing. The enlarged bowel means an expanded wall in one or more areas of the gut. The megacolon is an exaggeratedly enlarged wall in one or more areas of the gut. The longer, wider, and more complicated the transit in the gut, the more challenging will be the ability to eliminate efficiently in 18–48 hours.

People report back to me when they had their next bowel movement after a colon hydrotherapy session. The strong intestines eliminate the next morning. However, a large group of my clients have a transit of 4–5 days. The longer the transit, the greater is the possibility of breeding pathogenic microorganisms and disease. While some reports, as mentioned above, indicate this long transit time is okay, I do not believe it is, based on my clinical experience.

Taking in food triggers the peristaltic (muscle movement of intestines) wave that goes from mouth to anus. You might not eliminate what you have immediately eaten but you will eliminate meals eaten earlier in the day or previous day. For most people, it's gravity that drives the gut. Meals build up one after the other; then we get an elimination that is one of many meals, likely eaten days ago. We think that is fine. However, we are storing days of meals inside of us. Our elimination is incomplete. Our goal of restoring an efficient transit time is dependent on restoring peristalsis.

What Is Normal?

Many clients ask how many bowel movements a day a "healthy person" has, or how many one should have normally. Personally, I am happy if people have one bowel movement a day. Chinese medicine theory would concur with once a day. Some naturopaths such as Ann Wigmore say we should eliminate after every meal. That might be 2–4 times daily. Many of my female clients report they are jealous of their husbands because after every meal they eat, they are in the bathroom evacuating their bowel. These stories inspired me to found the imaginary Constipation Club to express our jealousy toward those with such efficient elimination. Most people are lucky if they eliminate once a day.

From my experience, I am going with a once-a-day bowel movement as a norm to aim for. Then one can begin to work on the next level, two times a day. The key is to keep the intestines moving daily for health and quality of life. The bowel movement has to be substantial or otherwise we are dealing with incomplete elimination, which is what most people experience. They eliminate once a day, but it might be a small amount in the anus and rectum and not be more comprehensive or thorough. That too will create a backlog of waste that is a perfect breeding ground for disease, discomfort, distension, and dehydrated stool.

Causes

The McMillan study (1999) divides causes of constipation into three main categories: primary, secondary and iatrogenic. Primary is due to lack of fiber, exercise, fluid intake, or time and privacy for defecating. Secondary causes are due to pathologies or diseases such as Parkinson's, intestinal obstruction such as tumors, volvulus, adhesions, stroke, hypercalcemia (calcium), hypokalemia (potassium), inflammatory bowel disease (IBD) including diverticulosis, colitis, Crohn's and celiac, spinal cord compression, and rectocele. Sylvester Yong, MD (1999), in his article "Case Histories—Constipation," adds a further refinement to secondary with categories of endocrine and metabolic disorders, systemic sclerosis and other connective tissue diseases, psychological disorders (neurogenic or nervous system derived), strictures, hernias, endometriosis, surgery, and finally rectal, anal, and pelvic floor disorders such as fissure and perianal abscess.

Iatrogenic causes are pharmaceutical or substance induced constipation as a side effect of such things as antacids, anticholinergics, antidepressants, antihistamines, barium sulfate, calcium channel blockers, drugs for Parkinson's, ganglionic blockers, hypotensives, iron supplements, monoamine oxidase inhibitors, opiates, psychotherapeutic drugs, and vinca alkaloids.

Stanford Study Causes

Stanford University has prepared a primary care teaching module for constipation, which lists some of the following causes. Which of the three above categories do they relate to? For the complete study, go to:

http://www-med.stanford.edu/school/DGIM/Teaching/Modules /Constipation.html.

- Pregnancy that causes increased progesterone and decreased motility

- Slow transit of unknown origin, mainly with women, with generally 14 weeks between bowel movements, rectum usually empty, normal colonic diameter, upper GI motility disturbance, mesenteric plexus abnormal, and a higher incidence of psychological problems. The doctors indicate that dietary fiber may worsen the condition, and that stimulants are more effective and behavior modification for pelvic floor musculature may help.

- Defecatory disorder with normal transit, also mostly true with women. Characteristics include abnormal rectal evacuation, many hours on toilet, frequent digitation to aid defecation, often followed or made worse by pelvic surgery nerve damage, worsened by prolonged straining and weakening of pelvic muscles. Doctors feel that stimulants or small enemas and biofeedback may help.

- Chagas disease. The organism trypanosoma cruzi is a common cause of dilated gut in South America. It creates inflammatory changes around ganglion and severe constipation if it involves the colon. Laxatives are used initially, surgery if necessary, and treatment of the infection.

- Megarectum/megacolon affecting both sexes, usually with childhood onset

- Polypharmacy anticholinergic drugs reduce contractility, Ca++ channel blockers reduce smooth muscle motility, NSAIDs may inhibit motility via prostaglandin block, ACE inhibitors inhibit smooth muscle relaxation, diuretics reduce ability to hydrate feces in colon. And then there are aluminum antacids, anticonvulsants, and narcotics.

- Geriatric issues, including depression and dementia. The self-reported rate of constipation goes up to 60 percent of patients in some studies with 30 percent of healthy elderly using laxatives regularly ($400 million sales/year of laxatives). Depression and dementia predispose the elderly to rectal impactions.

- History of prior and current laxative use plus surreptitious use of laxatives

- History of depression

- History of physical abuse, manifesting as abdominal/bowel symptoms

My Clinical Experience of Cause

Primary

- Dehydration. A low volume of fluids can cause build-up in the intestines, weaken the immune system, and set up a breeding ground for parasites. Signs are wrinkled skin, burning eyes, sticky eyes in the morning, a heavy feeling all over, and headaches.

- Lack of exercise and insufficient breathing

- Inappropriate diet, overeating, bingeing, eating disorders

- pH and electrolyte imbalance

- Restricting intestinal muscles. Guys and girls are told to hold in their abdomens. I was told at fourteen years old that I would be popular with boys if I could hold in my stomach. Women frequently wear tight clothes around their abdomen and waist. These messages and habits can create a layer of intestinal inhibition and paralysis.

- Long-distance travel

Secondary

- Parasites obstructing passage through the intestines and obstructing ducts leading from the pancreas, liver, and gallbladder

- Dysbiosis or imbalance of intestinal microorganisms that outweigh the good flora. Some people get tested for Candida albicans, a common fungi, and other microbial irregularities.

- Adrenalization. Energy leaves our core when we are upset. Energy goes into the musculoskeletal system to mobilize for action. Major regenerative organs like the heart, intestines, and kidneys slow down or shut down. The intestines can slow down or become dysfunctional with continuous emergency, fear, threat, or abuse. It's best not to eat when angry, upset, emotionally strung out, or fatigued, until we calm down and energy returns to our heart, intestines, kidneys, and other core organs.

- Poor toilet training that was stressful. I learned to hold in my elimination and feelings during toilet training. This event can be the source of adult shame, humiliation, and constipation.

- Eating disorders such as anorexia, bulimia, bingeing and overeating, and food addiction.

- Difficult transit. Some people have extra length of intestines, twisting, looped, or coiled areas of intestines, weak muscle tone, narrowing of the intestines due to waste build-up, spasm, and genetic predisposition for disease.

- Shape of intestines. You might be a person born with extra length of intestines. I see this in many barium x-rays clients bring to me. The barium x-ray of a child or adult intestines highlights if there are any extra twists and turns and extra length. I compare the shape of the intestines in the x-ray to the ability of that person to eliminate. The incidence of the redundant bowel and enlarged intestines is increasing in my practice based on colonoscopy results and personal experience.

Tertiary

- Hemorrhoids. *The Ciba Collection,* Volume Three, by Frank Netter, MD (1962), says that an anal irritation such as hemorrhoids can cause constipation due to a "reflex spasm of the sphincters." Constipation is a double-edged sword because it can also lead to hemorrhoids!

- An anal fissure is a small tear or ulcer (open sore) in the skin around the opening of the anus. It can cause severe pain and can be caused by straining at the stool or constipation, among many causes.

- An anal fistula is an inflammatory tract between the anal canal and the skin. The fistula has many causes, but passing hard stool can be one small component.

- Carbohydrate indigestion. Inability to digest complex carbohydrates—grains, soy and other beans, starchy roots, and milk and sugar products.

Please refer to my discussion of diet called SCD/GAPS in the chapters here. In addition, I wrote extensively about it in Michael's Volume Four of this series.

- Physical, sexual, emotional, and mental abuse. Toilet training comes under this category when it is abusive. I'm sure some of Stanford's categories, in which women are the main sufferers, come from abuse somewhere in their life. Adrenalization is part of this complex. Eating disorders can generally be related to an abuse history. Abuse history is the least acknowledged aspect of constipation. It is my opinion, based on personal experience, feedback from clients, and research, that this area needs further investigation to more clearly correlate with constipation.

Iatrogenic Causes

- Radiation, chemotherapy
- Neurotoxins such as MSG, and aspartame and other artificial sweeteners
- Laxative addiction
- Metal poisoning (lead, cadmium, mercury)
- Side effects from a majority of pharmaceuticals taken by 80 percent of the population

CHAPTER 31

Constipation Exposé:
Personal Stories and My Solution

by Sheila Shea, MA

In 1978, I had a major article published in *Forum* magazine on colon hydro-therapy. Just before that article came out, my mother came clean with me on what happened during my toilet training. She rarely shared with me, so this was quite the exception. She said that she started toilet training me at six months and would scream, yell, and get angry at me when I did not eliminate. As a result, I learned the opposite of elimination. I learned to withhold.

This withholding, or constipation, has had a cascading effect on my physical and emotional health due to auto-intoxication. Numerous streptococcus infections marked my early years. Headaches began at age seven and earaches at nine. My first migraine was during my senior year in college. When I began cleansing in 1974 at age twenty-nine, I had migraines regularly for another ten years and severe headaches for ten more years. The toxins were in circulation for elimination and the pain was periodically intense.

My memories of bowel movements are few and far between: diarrhea at ages four and eleven, intestinal flu in college two times, food poisoning in Chile in 1966, after a family marriage, and then in 1970 from drinking too much. Senior year in high school, I had to pull some feces out with my fingers because the waste was so hard. My anorexia began freshman year in college as an attempt to get rid of a very distended abdomen. One friend felt it alleviated the constipation temporarily because I reduced my food intake.

During one college vacation, a friend gave me one of her tablets for elimination and I eliminated later. She gave me a word for my condition—"constipation." However, the scourge was so great I could not talk about it. I did mention it to my mother and she took me to the doctor. The doctor prescribed Senecot

383

and it quickly built a tolerance and no longer worked, plus it had a horrible taste. The issue got dropped again until 1970 when I was twenty-six.

That year, I had PID (pelvic inflammatory disease) and I feel it was exacerbated by my lifelong constipation. My intestines were a breeding ground for bacteria and fungus to reproduce, travel, and poison neighboring organs, thereby weakening them. My level of pain, gas, and intestinal toxins was so high that I would have to lie down on the floor of the bathroom at my office with the door locked. At best I would pass gas. It was a dark time.

The same year, I became bulimic in an attempt to stem the constipation and deal with an extraordinary food addiction I felt since age ten. I began to throw up my food after meals and at the same time I sought to get to the core of healing both constipation and eating disorders.

Later in 1970, I gathered up the courage to confide to a dear friend and nurse about my constipation. She exclaimed in her British accent: "My dear, if you do not eliminate regularly you will become auto-intoxicated after three or four days. You must take enemas." I thought to myself, how about twenty-five years of auto-intoxication! I took enemas as she suggested—about two of them. I forgot about enemas until I began cleansing in earnest in 1974.

I finally began to tackle my constipation following Arnold Ehret's ideas in his book *Mucusless Diet Healing System* (1976, originally published in 1922). I juice fasted every weekend for nearly two years, ate more living foods, and took regular enemas and occasional colonics. Gas pain was a constant companion. My first conscious awareness of not having regular gas pain happened after two years of cleansing. I had such a build-up of mucus secretion layers that when I started the raw juices including citrus I would get 10 to 20 feet of mucous cords out with my evening enema. This might sounds preposterous to you. It was reality for me.

At the same time, I was healing eating disorders. I began using laxatives as a break from the enemas and colonics and I became addicted. I now use enemas and/or colonics as a healthier way to recover from serious constipation rather than the use of laxatives. Constipation and eating disorders created intense irritation to my intestinal walls. My eating disorder exacerbated my constipation. A double whammy! I knew that to heal the constipation I had to heal my eating disorders and food addiction. My diet had to be stable and predictable.

I'm beginning to eliminate on my own for the first time since infancy. I am toning the tissue, regaining feeling in the intestinal muscles, and beginning to feel some peristalsis. I still take regular enemas and colonics. The colonics are most helpful in training good bowel habits and rehabilitating muscles. Enemas are convenient and useful when I feel incomplete elimination or pain. Pain is generally due to gas from eating complex sugars.

Others' Stories

The following stories about constipation come from some of the many clients I have seen over the past forty years.

BL:

I was thirty-eight years old, in my first job in a large corporation. Lots of stress and a nagging pain in the stomach. An ulcer was diagnosed followed by a then-common surgery: the cutting of the vagus nerve, which would reduce acid flow and allow the lesion to heal. To my delight my ulcer was healed but I had no idea of the lifetime cost I was destined to pay for the surgery. The severing of the vagus nerve had a side effect: decreasing the motility of my intestines, and decreasing my control over my bowel movements.

In short order a difficult pattern developed: a stubborn bout of constipation, maybe three to five days, followed by an unpredictable day of profuse elimination, with both normal and soft watery stools. During the constipation phase I was uncomfortable, with growing anxiety about the expected release days to come. On the release days the anxiety reached a maximum—I might be at work, in a meeting, in a car commuting, and constantly in worry about finding a bathroom in time if needed.

Unfortunately, while there was a pattern with some predictability it was not foolproof—there were exceptions and the dreaded release, with copious stools, could then come at unpredictable moments. The resulting anxiety turned into a serious obsession as I slowly organized my life around anticipating and planning the availability of bathrooms. Mornings were often the worst time. For a dozen years I had to commute to work for 40 miles—times of agony where I knew every bathroom on the way.

Of course, I tried to find remedies, and clung to every wisp of hope. I tried all the conventional remedies for constipation: laxatives, milk of magnesia, bulking agents, special cereals, mineral oil, suppositories, enemas, etc. I ate a healthy diet with lots of fruits and vegetables and fiber. Nothing helped in a reliable, controlled way. I consulted naturopaths and chiropractors. I even tried hypnosis and conditioning techniques. Nothing worked—my gut had a mind of its own and remained my enemy.

The psychological toll of such a condition was hurtful and hard to convey. By sheer willpower and unending cunning I managed to live a relatively normal life—job, marriage, children, hobbies—but the condition cruelly robbed me of many experiences: theatre, concerts, travel for pleasure, an abundant social life. The constant awareness of the gut issues is wearisome and feeds an anxiety that becomes an integral part of one's life.

Somehow, despite several other chronic illnesses and despite constipation, I have managed to make it to the not-so-glittering "golden years." Recently medication side effects have worsened the constipation length to over a week so I have to look for new strategies. Clearly constipation is not a minor medical issue. To me—and I am sure I am not alone—it had a powerful negative effect on my quality of life.

My life could have been much richer and sweeter if there had been a reliable answer. In this age of medical breakthroughs, MRI, CAT, genetics, etc., this basic human affliction still waits for a remedy.

(BL, now eighty, is a graduate of MIT, a computer engineer, therapist, and photographer.)

SH:

A few months ago a fabulous colon therapist I go to gave me a copy of this fantastic article. Thank you so much for writing it, for your efforts and research. I have been dealing with a constipation problem for twenty years. Over that time I've gotten much better but unexplainable hills and valleys still and consistently happen. I found that I'd done much of what you'd suggested in your article. Motivated by another downturn, I'm printing your article right now and am going to read it again.

Recently I went to a medical doctor here who is also a naturopath, a homeopath, and an Ayurvedic physician. From saliva and blood tests he found somewhat elevated blood sugar, a thyroid TSH (thyroid-stimulating hormone) reading that was too high, hormones off, so he gave me all-natural adrenal support and boost, thyroid, Sam-E, thyroid support, amongst other things. The actual thyroid pills and Sam-E [S-adenosyl methionine] I was to take for a month. The very next day I started eliminating completely! I felt like eliminating instead of feeling nothing except a discomforting fullness. For three weeks this continued, even through some stressful traveling most of that time. When I came home, the last week, with one more week of thyroid and Sam-E to go, I felt my bowel evacuation slackening. Then the thyroid and Sam-E stopped. Then my bowel evacuation went to almost nothing! I felt like I'd regressed ten years. The doctor told me to watch and see how I felt a week or two after the thyroid was up. A week and a half later I told him I was not a happy camper. He gave me more thyroid. After a week of taking the second course of thyroid my elimination is still very weak sometimes not at all. So I'm about to go back to him and add the Sam-E.

It's the big experiment. In other words, the mystery continues. Eat right, exercise, and colonics once every few weeks for right now.

G:

I am interested in trying colon hydrotherapy in an attempt to relieve constipation…. A little history: ever since I can remember I have a bowel movement once every 5 to 10 days. I take Metamucil and magnesium tablets per doctor's instruction but have not seen results as she expected so she recommended I look into this procedure. Earlier this year I had a colonoscopy that was normal. The gastroenterologist suggested taking laxatives which I try not to do because I don't want to be dependent on them. Actually the magnesium is helping after an increase to 800 mg a day but I experience pain and embarrassing gas and stomach noises; however, had a bowel movement after 3 days. Yahoo!

SA:

I have been dealing with a two-year battle with constipation. I am a twenty-six-year old female living in Manhattan and have been suffering with stomach pain, inability to concentrate, and depression for too long. I believe my constipation is due to both Candida and emotional stress. My constipation began when I started an intense internship for my masters of social work as well as after a 4-year breakup.

I have been to various doctors, wholistic practitioners, and still no longterm success going regularly. I have been following a strict Candida diet and supplements. If you can give me any advice or suggestions, I am very grateful.

Other Comments

Here are some short quotes from my clients about constipation.

I have had digestion problems ever since I could remember. I had my gallbladder removed in August due to gallstones. I continue to have problems with digestion. I mainly suffer from constipation. If I stop having a BM, after almost a week of not having one, I start to feel very sick due to the toxins. I had my gallbladder removed in August of last year due to gall stones.

I have had a constipation problem for many years, although found it more noticeable since I quit smoking 3 years ago.

I took today off work because I have been severely constipated for the past 5 days. I have done 4 enemas, Metamucil-type fiber laxative drinks, drank 60 ml of castor oil twice, lots of water and fluids, and fruits. I'm still very abnormally bloated, feel light-headed, weak, and sometimes dizzy. I have had minor problems with constipation before. The last enema I did was painful to insert and after expelling I was bleeding minorly from the rectum. I'm a little concerned about the possibility of a tumor. I'm only 32 (male), in good health, a little overweight but have had thyroid removal due to cancer at age 24.

My wife has always suffered from constipation. She is 54 years old. Please give us some ideas as to how she can kick the laxative habit.

Have had some recent surgery, 2 disks removed and fusion in my neck. Because of the surgery have been on a lot of drugs that are causing me major concerns with constipation. Have tried laxatives and even enemas, with no good results. Have been reading a lot about colonic irrigation and think it may help!

Shea Constipation Healing and Prevention Program (SCHPP)

Goals of the Shea Constipation Healing and Prevention Program (SCHPP) are to stimulate peristalsis or muscle motion of the intestinal walls, to heal the walls or lining of the intestines, to remove waste from the gut walls that inhibits assimilation, digestion, and secretion, to develop resilience with unfinished emotional and mental issues, to consciously relate to causes, and to restore a positive microbial environment.

Another goal of SCHPP is to decrease transit time of stools—the time it takes food to pass from mouth to anus. A shorter transit time lessens the effect of autointoxication and its side effects.

As this and the following chapters unfold, I will be taking the reader on a tour of my Shea Constipation Healing and Prevention Program (SCHPP). The main components of the SCHPP are:

- The Specific Carbohydrate Diet (SCD), which excludes complex carbohydrates and coincides with blood type O diet

- Raw food more than 50 percent of diet

- Eating only when hungry (that's a tough one)

- Eating foods that help elimination. (My O blood type is aligned on that one. Food such as prunes, plums, kale, spinach, pineapple, papaya, flaxseed, figs, ginger, and cayenne support elimination.)

- Drinking half one's weight in ounces daily

- Exercising daily and doing abdominal exercises

- Cleansing the GI tract using GI, liver, gallbladder, kidney, and parasite cleanses and rebuilding with right diet, plus probiotic and fermented foods

- Using enemas and colonics as needed to assure continued elimination of waste

- Meditating daily to help calm the nervous system

- Using other stress reduction techniques such as biofeedback, Heartmath biofeedback techniques, and therapy to keep the parasympathetic nervous system operational

I have spent many years cleansing and repairing my GI tract. Recently, I incorporated psyllium and bentonite cleanses which have been the most effective in removing old layers, empowering peristalsis, and reducing pain. I did my first two parasite cleanses in 1998 and eight liver flushes in the last ten years. The liver plays a role in supporting elimination.

I also work on emotional, mental, and spiritual planes to heal constipation. I use abdominal and other breathing techniques I have learned from yoga and Chi Nei Tsang classes. I practice meditation to become peaceful inside and release any unconscious tension in the abdomen. I incorporate some psychotherapy as a way to release old psychosomatic patterns and repressed emotions and thoughts. Constipation has many faces and levels and I deal with it in many different ways.

CHAPTER 32

Protocols: What to Do?

by Sheila Shea, MA

Bear with me. Now, what are you going to do about it? I will give you plenty of suggestions in this chapter and those that follow. The constipation protocols described here are the foundations of detoxification, intestinal health as well as healing constipation. I include the obvious: breathing, hydration, exercise, and diet from my Shea Constipation Healing and Prevention Program (SCHPP). I then share three other protocols developed by Stanford University, Victoria Bowmann, PhD, and Life Extension Foundation. These protocols form good guidelines for you. Give them a try and be gentle with yourself.

Breathing

The SCHPP program I have developed over many years of clinical experience involves some very basic elements. Lower abdominal breathing is essential for good elimination. Consistent, deep breathing is the key. I remember finding and perusing a book in my father's library when I was ten. It was on breathing! It planted a seed in my mind. When I was younger I would listen to others breathe. I realized I was hardly breathing at all. In the path of healing my intestines from severe and profound constipation and healing my emotional body, I have learned the importance of continuous, focused breath. The key paths I have used to learn breathing and breath focus are yoga, meditation, martial arts, rebirthing, hiking, backpacking, and Heartmath biofeedback techniques. I am currently in a therapy that uses breath and meditation as the container for the emotions. This has reinforced remembering breath in day-to-day activities like driving my car, walking across a parking lot, and working at the computer.

Each moment is an opportunity to return to the breath. The deeper it goes into the pelvic floor and abdomen, the better it is for elimination. Very often my intestinal blocks are a result of constricting my intestinal muscles and going into spasm from fright, offense, anger, or performance anxiety. I have usually reduced my breathing and restricted it to my upper lungs and neck. It never reaches my lower body and abdomen and therefore my upper body and brain are disconnected from my lower body and abdomen.

Sexual, physical, emotional, and toilet training abuse can also restrict one's breath from the lower body and put it into a state of deep freeze. The deep freeze can be reversed. Focused and continuous breath is a direct route to connect and unite the upper and lower body. The breath and water can be used very effectively during a colon hydrotherapy session to sensitize the lower body and bring it into union with the upper body. Chi Gung and Chi Lel, a variation of Chi Gung therapy, are other forms people use to learn breath practice.

Hydration

Hydration is considered more important than exercise and diet. Sufficient fluids are necessary for skin, mucosal, and immune health, not to mention efficient elimination. *Your Body's Many Cries for Water* by F. Batmanghelidj, MD (2008) is subtitled: "You are not sick, you are thirsty! Don't treat thirst with medications." We have lost our sense of thirst. I mistook it for hunger and ate instead. Steadily building up our intake of fluids restores our sense of thirst and reduces misplaced appetite. I feel that 2.5–3.5 quarts is what my body needs daily from water, herb teas, sparkling water, and raw or bottled juices. I have learned through how I feel and function how much fluid I need. I can also tell by the color of my urine. The lighter the color, the more I am hydrated.

You can calculate your fluid needs in two ways. One is to take your body weight, divide by 2, then divide by 32 to get the number of quarts you need to drink. For example, I weigh 127 pounds; 127 divided by 2 then by 32 equals 1.98 quarts, or approximately 2 quarts. However, if I am doing active outdoor exercise, as I do, like hiking or tennis, and especially in my dry desert climate, I will drink more than 3 quarts for the day. Your volume depends on your activity, too. The second way to calculate your fluid is to drink one quart for every 50 pounds of your weight. So if you are 200 pounds you would drink 4 quarts, or one gallon. See which calculation works for you.

Hydration or drinking sufficient fluids is key to healing constipation. So often constipation is accompanied by dehydration, not today's dehydration but long-standing dehydration. It takes time to rehydrate the GI tract and experience positive results from rehydration. You have to break down and dissolve with water and juices what has hardened and stagnated in your intestines from dehydration and which has contributed to your constipation.

One of the best ways to hydrate is to make raw juices from vegetables and fruits. You get a high concentration of minerals and vitamins naturally. Your intestines move well on the raw juices. Books are abundant with formulas for raw juices. For example, the fresh juices of acid fruit have the strongest ability to dissolve mucus lining the intestinal walls. The key acid fruits are lemon, lime, orange, grapefruit, tomato, and pineapple. Another helpful fluid made in a blender rather than a juicer is the green smoothie. Robin Openshaw (2009), in her book *Green Smoothies Diet* (2009), and Victoria Boutenko (2009), in *Green Smoothie Revolution,* have the premier books and recipes for green smoothies.

Exercise

Exercise is a major factor in healthy elimination. As the TV exercise guru Richard Simmons says, "If you eat every day, you work out every day!" The Stanford protocol described below promotes exercise habits, stating that immobility is a documented risk factor in constipation. The study reports that lack of movement can increase transit time from three days to three weeks! Each person has to find his or her own way with movement and especially something that person likes or loves. It can begin slow and for short periods of time, and then build up. I include testimonials of a few individuals, plus Dr. Stone's thoughts on squatting, the natural way to eliminate!

Randolph Stone, an osteopath and chiropractor, in his book *Health Building: The Conscious Art of Living Well* (1999), devotes three pages to squatting (pp.134–136). He says it is ideal for the release of gases, dealing with constipation, and getting rid of excessive abdominal fat. He notes it tones the walls of the abdomen by muscular exertion and squeezing the thighs, which also protects the muscles from excess strain in the posture. It is now possible to purchase small platforms that fit around the base of a toilet to place one's feet upon in order to mimic the squatting position. It is just as easy to build a small platform. They usually reach about halfway up toward the lip of the toilet.

How much should you exercise? How long, how often? I exercise five to six days a week. I suggest each person begin with three days a week and work up to five to six days. Start with fifteen minutes and work up to an hour. If you are the more athletic type, choose an activity that requires two to four hours of working, like cycling, tennis, or hiking. Richard Carmona, our seventeenth Surgeon General, a Tucson native and currently vice chairman of the Canyon Ranch resort and spa company, suggests that people with obesity issues should exercise seven days a week for one hour daily. Many who are obese are also constipated.

Here are some comments from my clients about exercise:

I have an abdominal workout with four variations of exercises to tone the muscles.

I am an athlete in my own way taking time daily to either hike, dance, do yoga, play tennis, practice martial arts, or swim. Occasionally, I use the weight room at my complex or do housework or gardening. I count those too. Even playing with my kids gives me great delight, not to mention a good workout. My energy is a great gift!

I'm home again after a great and strenuous backpack on the Colorado Plateau. The good news, I began eliminating on a regular basis, two times a day. I was off track eliminating before I left and taking an enema every few days. On the first and second day of the backpack, I eliminated once and very little. On the third day, generous, easy and well-formed stool kicked in. I also noticed that I lengthened my lower back as I hiked and lifted the abdominal muscles, an advance for me. I discovered I had the habit of tilting back my pelvis that cut off energy to my intestines and allowed the intestinal packet to pouch out in front. Aligning my pelvis aligned the intestines over it and allowed for better elimination.

I'm back from a two-day archeological backpack in AZ. One issue when I travel is how I will poop. My intestines are still recovering from childhood constipation. I carried in two gallons of water and was still dehydrated when we finished. I did well intestinally, meaning no major indigestion or pain. I took an enema Friday before I left and didn't poop until Monday morning; however, the backpack helped me take a break from the enemas for a few days. I go through periods of minor pain: however, I pass gas and have pooped regularly for three mornings now. I know the elimination is incomplete but I'm not bloated! I feel strenuous exercise is a big help for my intestinal health. I'm a blood type O and the big workouts are prescribed. Plus I follow a diet that promotes elimination and I am learning to drink nearly three quarts of fluids a day. I found that I was getting bad headaches after some hikes and I realized it was due to dehydration! Simply increasing my fluids alleviated my headaches.

Diet

One major factor in successfully healing constipation is your ability to manage and reduce food addiction and eating disorders. For most people, food runs them and they feel incapable of making the intelligent choices they know will resolve their constipation. Eating disorders such as anorexia, bulimia, overeating, and bingeing are some of the major hidden causes of constipation. I found that I could not heal my constipation until I healed my eating disorders. I had to be able to consistently make positive diet choices without the erratic eating behaviors I had starting at ten years old. So, if you are working on constipation, you will be working on healing any food addictions or eating disorders that you have. Food addictions are a physiological addiction or craving for highly refined substances such as sugar. That's the main food addiction. Eating disorders are a mental and emotional imbalance and require inner work to heal. Your journey has become even more challenging now!

Many ask, What is the right diet for constipation? Here is my list of diet priorities on the SCHPP:

- Eat natural
- Eat organic
- Do not eat genetically modified (GMO) foods
- Find the diet that works best for you

My sense now in terms of dealing with constipation, or any other disorder for that matter, is to first, eat natural. That means you are returning to the kitchen to prepare whole foods rather than eating out of bags, boxes, jars, cans, and plastic wrappers. You are taking more time to prepare your food from scratch. Your intestines respond well to natural foods and eliminate better on them! Say good-bye to packaged and processed foods!

My second priority for the constipated system is to eat organic. The quality of organic food is better. It is free of chemicals, additives, preservatives, and coatings. Very often, it tastes better. You want to give your GI system and body the highest quality and give it the best chance to heal from constipation.

Next, avoid genetically modified foods. The main GMO foods are corn, soy, canola oil, cotton, sugar beets, dairy, yellow squash, zucchini, aspartame, and Hawaiian papayas. Each one is a primary concern. Ninety-five percent of sugar is now genetically modified. For the best information on GMO foods, read Jeffrey Smith's *Seeds of Deception* (2003). His website is http://www.geneticroulette .com. The problem is that we do not know how deleterious they might be for our health. Some articles have said that some of the virus and bacteria used in constructing the GMO foods remain in the system after the food is consumed. The idea is to take any unnecessary burden off your system to heal from constipation. You are trying to relieve your system of anything that is unnatural and that might inhibit your best elimination.

After eating natural and organic and GMO-free, then you can split hairs on which diet works best for you. Eating, blending, and juicing vegetables seem to be the safest food category for constipation. Then you have to decide on the fruits, honey, milk-based dairy, complex sugars, proteins, and fats.

I am beginning to recognize the variety of dietary differences among my clients and friends. Some feel better with meat, some without. Some do well with grains, starchy roots, and legumes; others do not. Some need a diet high in fats; others do not metabolize fats well. Some thrive on fruit; others have so damaged their sugar metabolism they cannot even eat fruit. Some people say it's the raw food diet, the vegan diet, or the vegetarian diet; others say it's the Paleodiet, Specific Carbohydrate Diet (SCD), or the Gut and Psychology Syndrome Diet (GAPS). Many diets are helpful in healing constipation and all use natural and organic foods. You must find your own way with diet. The key is to test out, try out, and find out what works for you.

Stanford University Treatment Protocol

Here is the website link for the Stanford University treatment protocol:

http://www-med.stanford.edu/school/DGIM/Teaching/Modules/Constipation.html

The components are:

- Educate about acceptable bowel habits (twelve per week without straining)

- Discourage over-the-counter medications, discuss the possibility of positive feedback cycle

- Cultivate good toileting habits: comfort, privacy, sufficient time, taking advantage of gastrocolic reflex, elevating legs while on toilet to facilitate use of weakened pelvic and abdominal muscles

- Diet with minimum 30 grams of fiber a day

- Drink minimum 1.5 liters of fluids per day and more in the summer

- Assess the need for disimpaction, be it digital or surgical

- Use bulk laxatives such as psyllium, ispaghula husk, and methylcellulose. Bran is cheaper but bloating may be worse. Risk of impaction occurs if fluid intake is inadequate.

Victoria Bowmann's Protocol

Victoria Bowmann's protocol comes from A Plan for Constipation by Victoria Bowmann, BS, DHM—an unpublished paper she distributes to her clients. She can be reached at VBowmann@aol.com, fax 602-788-7557, or P.O. Box 31464, Phoenix AZ 85046. Here is her protocol:

- Consume 64 ounces of water or half your body weight in ounces per day. Eliminate coffee with chronic constipation; it contributes to dehydration. Water amount should also be evaluated in terms of lifestyle, weight, and environment.

- Consume healthy oils, particularly 1 tablespoon of flaxseed oil minimum daily. Use olive oil in salads and for sautées.

- Include sufficient bulk from psyllium, raw foods, fruits and vegetables and their juices.

- Appropriate reflorastation. She uses rectal implants of flora, and depending on the constipation case as often as daily for thirty days.

- Nutritional support with raw goat whey or dairy protein or fructooligosaccharides (FOS) (depending on allergies) to feed newly introduced intestinal flora. (Elaine Gottschall favors lactose over FOS. Anderson favors whey for the high concentration of naturally occurring sodium.)

Ms. Bowmann says: "I hope this helps but it will not work unless all five points are addressed simultaneously. Then the results are 85 percent or better."

Life Extension Foundation Protocol

You will find detailed information about the Life Extension Foundation at its website:

http://www.lef.org/protocols/gastrointestinal/constipation_01.htm

Life Extension has a list of suggestions for constipation. Although they include laxatives and drugs, they also have an understanding of more natural and common-sense ways to work with constipation.

The Life Extension suggestions include:

- Fiber therapy from foods and supplements
- Laxatives
- Drugs
- Supplements to aid elimination

- Supplements to relieve acute constipation
- Sufficient hydration and awareness that caffeine is dehydrating
- Eating on a regular schedule to give your body a chance to regulate elimination
- Responding to your body's signals to pass stool
- Regular exercise, including an abdominal muscle workout

CHAPTER 33

Comorbidity and Diet

by Sheila Shea, MA

Comorbidity means that a person has two or more conditions rather than presenting with one issue only. For example, clients who come in to work on their constipation might have one or more of the following: diabetes, metabolic syndrome, overweight, obesity, rheumatoid arthritis (RA), Candida, gastroesophageal reflux disease, IBS, celiac disease, interstitial cystitis, or infertility. Others come in with the listed conditions and reveal that they have had constipation all their life, or since adolescence, or for many years.

One condition that is epidemic in my practice is excessive gas. That falls under the category of a microbial overgrowth fed by complex sugars. In such cases, clients must reduce or eliminate complex sugars to heal. Sometimes, their sugar metabolism is so damaged that they cannot eat complex sugars, fruits, or honey until sufficient healing has taken place. Very often the gas itself causes the constipation or coincides with longstanding constipation. Clearly, the basis of their diet will be vegetables, proteins, and fats.

So, when choosing a diet, it's important to have a diet that works for both or all conditions. Many diets are helpful in healing constipation. The raw food diet, Specific Carbohydrate Diet, Paleodiet, instinctive eating, and blood type diet are a few that have been my personal choices for healing constipation. I have had constipation since infancy. I am a blood type O and thus need a protein-based diet with an abundance of spices, fruits, and vegetables. I sense that I have inflammatory bowel disease and that would mean eliminating complex sugars. I do react to them with gas and bloating. So, you must know yourself and make the best choices to heal.

For example, your constipation healing diet may fall on the other side of the complex carbohydrate dietary spectrum. Your dietary choices and healing may include a plant-based-only or vegan diet with fruits, vegetables, nuts, seeds, grains, beans, and starchy roots. Neil Bernard, MD, John Robbins, Richard

Anderson, Gabriel Cousens, MD, and Mishio Kushi are proponents of a purely plant-based vegan diet. As long as you are maintaining a normal body weight, constipation is helped, gas is not created, and you have a sense of fullness and satiety, then you are doing great.

One positive factor in eating natural and organic foods is that it dramatically decreases food addictions and cravings to inappropriate substances. Natural and organic foods are nutrient dense rather than calorie dense and that also helps reduce cravings, hunger, and fatigue.

Restoring the Good Bacteria

Fermented foods are a subset of raw foods and can be made inexpensively from seeds, nuts, grains, vegetables, and milk. The fermentation process allows the growth of beneficial bacteria that promote intestinal health and elimination. Victoras Kulvinskas' book *Survival into the 21st Century* (1975) is a classic work on living foods and ferments, mainly a grain-based "rejuvelac," seed and nut yogurts and cheeses, and sauerkraut. The wheat-berry-based rejuvelac has been debunked recently for containing unhealthy bacteria; however, my intestines did well with it. Robert Gray's *Colon Health Handbook* (1991) has a recipe for cabbage rejuvelac. I find his recipe easy, safe, and effective. It is rich in naturally occurring positive bacteria. Recipes for homemade yogurt are in Gottschall's *Breaking the Vicious Cycle* (1994). Donna Gates (Gates and Schatz, 2011) is well known for her vegetable and coconut ferments. Natasha Campbell-McBride MD (2010) also includes milk and vegetable ferments in her book as part of intestinal healing.

Remember, three keys in healing constipation are to clean the gut walls, restore the integrity of the gut wall, and re-establish the positive gut flora. If you are constipated and your gut wall is damaged, meaning inflamed or leaky, inappropriate substances are passing through your gut wall into your bloodstream and thus have access to your whole body. You need to choose a diet that heals the gut wall. Those key diets are Specific Carbohydrate Diet, Gut and Psychology Syndrome Diet, and the Paleodiet among others. I covered them in detail in Michael's Volume Four.

Raw Food Diet

Raw or living foods are those that are uncooked, unpasteurized, and unprocessed. They include fresh fruits and vegetables, raw nuts, seeds and sprouts, unpasteurized milk, cheese, and honey, and uncooked eggs, fish, fowl, and meat.

Most people who eat raw food are vegans—they eat no animal products. However, a group of raw foodists include raw eggs, bone marrow, organ meats, and other raw animal products in their diet. Their group is called RAF, Raw Animal Foodists.

In order to heal my constipation I went to the Hippocrates Health Institute in 1975. Ann Wigmore (1909–1994) ran this famous facility in Boston MA. After two weeks of her raw vegan diet and many classes on food preparation, I felt like a million bucks. My gut felt great, very light, clean, and happy. However, not all people can do raw food. Some who have constipation and whose gut walls are compromised cannot eat raw foods because they cannot break down the cellulose in the fruits and vegetables. Raw juices are a possibility or cooking the fruits and vegetables until further wall healing has occurred. A preferred diet for elimination and rebuilding is high in fresh fruits and vegetables and their raw fresh, unpasteurized juices because of their high water content, minerals, and enzymes.

SCD, GAPS, and Other Diets

The Specific Carbohydrate Diet (SCD) is specific for inflammatory bowel disease (IBD), irritable bowel syndrome (IBS), auto-immune conditions, Candida, and leaky gut syndrome. I wrote several chapters about this diet in Michael's Volume Four. Very often constipation is a result of these conditions or, as in my case, constipation causes the leaky gut and eating disorders further disturb the intestines. The main food group to avoid is complex carbohydrates. IBS is alternating constipation and diarrhea with stomach pain. The constipation part of this syndrome responds well to fiber or bulk that is NOT a complex carbohydrate.

A client wrote to me:

> I've suffered from irritable bowel syndrome (IBS) since I was a child. It has grown considerably worse since I moved here and entered an MFA program three years ago. My stress levels skyrocketed, paralleling my battle with constipation. I'm looking for an alternative solution. I turned twenty-five a couple months ago and I feel like I'm ninety. Can you give me further information?

Breaking the Vicious Cycle (1994) by Elaine Gottschall (1921–2005) is the bible for IBD and IBS plus Candida and other conditions such as constipation that people do not associate with intestinal inflammation. Natasha Campbell-McBride has taken over the work of Gottschall since her death and has taken the diet to the next level. Her book *Gut and Psychology Syndrome,* which I previously mentioned, has gone worldwide and she has added a cookbook and an anti-Candida version of the diet. I'm including extensive information on the GAPS, as one of my clients has recovered by using it and has provided wonderful links for us.

Here are three GAPS websites:

http://www.doctor-natasha.com

http://gapsdiet.com/introduction_diet.html

http://gaps.me

And check out my SCD/GAPS story:

http://www.blogtalkradio.com/gapsjourney/2011/05/28/gerald–healing
-digestive-disorders-on-gaps-diet

Several other GAPS stories are at this radio blog. The first guest was Dr. Natasha herself. You have to watch this interview!

Here's the address for the yahoo GAPS group I belong to:

http://health.groups.yahoo.com/group/GAPShelp/files/Personal%20
Journeys%20%26%20Reports

The Specific Carbohydrate Diet and Elaine Gottschall website is:

http://www.breakingtheviciouscycle.info

Write any time with questions. I'm happy to help. This one diet has changed my life!

Elaine Gottschall was asked many times how to deal with constipation. Her solution was first diet using homemade chicken soup with lots of pureed carrots and zucchini. She also suggested homemade applesauce. For fast action, she suggested a half cup of Welch's prune nectar and a half cup of freshly squeezed orange juice. She cautioned that one be near the bathroom for the latter as it could be quite effective.

In cases of stubborn constipation, Natasha Campbell-McBride introduces freshly pressed juices earlier in the GAPS diet, starting with carrot juice first thing in the morning and taking cod liver oil at the same time. The juice will stimulate bile production as many cases of persistent constipation are due to poor bile production. When there is not enough bile, the fats in the food do not digest well; instead, they react with salts and form soap in the gut, causing constipation. Removing dairy may also help. Check out http://www.gaps
.me/preview/?page_id=28.

Barry Sears, in his book *Enter the Zone* (1995), recommends fish oil to fix constipation, in increasing quantities until the stool floats.

Peter D'Adamo (1997) has created different diets based on blood type; these can be seen at his website: http://www.dadamo.com. Some people do well on a macrobiotic diet that is primarily cooked and based on whole grains, seaweeds, vegetables, and soups. Blood type A does well on grains. However, grains might be contraindicated with allergies, intestinal gas and bloat, inflammatory bowel disease, and Candida. The blood type O diet is a protein-based diet that includes nuts, seeds, beans, fish, and meat. Other beneficial foods for blood type O compensate for the potential constipating properties of meat with foods like prunes, plums, figs, tomatoes, cherries, pineapples, ginger, garlic, and cayenne! However, some people metabolize animal products better than others. You want to find out what you metabolize well.

Foods Known to Relieve Constipation

Magnesium is the major element in chlorophyll. Chlorophyll is the green pigment in leaves, grasses, and algaes. All chlorophyll-containing plants such as wheat and barley grass, marine and lake algaes, Essiac and culinary greens help elimination, absorption, cleansing, rebuilding, and inflammation, plus they provide a rich environment for positive flora or bacteria. You might want to see what kind of fresh and steamed greens you, your friends, and family are willing to eat! Greens can also be taken juiced, powdered, in capsules or tablets, and as teas. Essiac is an old Ojibway herbal formula containing sheep sorrel, burdock root, Indian rhubarb root, and slippery elm inner bark, used predominantly to heal cancer and taken in tea form. Chlorophyll is one of the most important foods for healing constipation.

Spinach is known to help heal constipation. It's high in oxalic acid that helps trigger peristalsis. According to Norman Walker, in his book *Raw Vegetable Juices,* the combination of spinach and carrot juice is specific for constipation. Walker said that one pint of spinach juice daily for two weeks would cure the most serious case of constipation. I never made it past seven days! Red chard, celery, and beet leaves with the carrot are high in organic sodium and help calm the nerves and stimulate peristalsis. Pineapple, grapes, apples, endive, and escarole are also specific for constipation. Powdered flax seeds are known to help elimination and flax oil is beneficial for the integrity of the intestinal walls.

Supplements

Electrolytes are the essential minerals, trace elements, and cell salts necessary to sustain all the functions of the body and mind. A high volume of quality electrolytes is consumed during a constipation program to replenish and balance your system. Diet and/or supplements are sources of electrolytes. Supplements also complement an intestinal hydrotherapy cleansing program. Raw juices, algaes, grasses, and liquid minerals are well known sources. Many people are undermineralized and toxic when they begin to make changes. They need to create a consistent and quality program to rebuild.

Daily intake of 100–150 mcg (micrograms) of iodine is recommended. Natural sources are fish, seaweed, kelp, plus water and vegetables from iodine rich soils. Iodine is required for proper thyroid gland function, is an important constituent of thyroxine and other hormones, and important for regulating energy metabolism throughout the body. A deficiency can cause hypothyroidism characterized by fatigue, weight gain, dryness of skin, headaches, and constipation.

Phosphate of iron (ferrous phosphate) is a homeopathic cell salt. Ferr phos is a component of blood and other body cells with the exception of nerve cells. An imbalance or deficiency can cause continuous diarrhea or, paradoxically, constipation.

Positive Bacteria, Flora, and Probiotics

Bacteria, flora, and probiotics are synonymous with each other. These positive microorganisms are the naturally occurring healthy and resident bacteria that live in the walls, the mural bacteria, and in the lumen, the tubes of the intestines. They provide a variety of significant functions that protect the immune system and allow proper peristalsis in the gut muscles. These resident and constructive intestinal flora are essential for healing constipation and the gut wall. One must restore intestinal flora with a variety of positive microorganisms after taking antibiotics or any other circumstance changing the flora balance. If not, constipation, lowered immunity to more infections, and general fatigue might add more insult to injury. Some use flora for related bladder infections. (See Victoria Bowmann's protocol in Chapter 33.)

I discussed the benefit of fermented food earlier. Fermented foods such as sauerkraut, kefir, 24-hour fermented yogurt, and cultured nuts and seeds provide our GI system with wonderful, healthy bacteria. We begin to feel like we are alive again when we have an abundance of the positive flora in our system.

Mucosal Health and Herbs

Very often constipation implies that the integrity or health of the intestinal wall is deficient. The purpose of the diet, supplements, and fluid is to restore this health. Many herbs are also helpful in creating this integrity via their various properties such as bitters, astringents, anti-inflammatories, and blood purifiers.

Some believe the Ayurvedic compound Triphala, three Indian fruits, is the best colon conditioner available and helps restore muscle tone to the bowels. Dashamoola, made up of ten Indian roots, is used as an implant to restore bowel function and in conjunction with Triphala in the Ayurvedic panchakarma cleansing program.

One friend reported that herbal bitters are her favorite means of stimulating peristalsis without causing dependency. Christopher Hobbs, a foremost GI herbalist, writes that bitters work in three ways. One, they activate the gastric secretion of hydrochloric acid (HCL) and other digestive enzymes such as those contained in liver bile. Two, they increase the strength and tone of the autonomic nervous system, which energizes all the digestive organs. Three, they activate the immune system. Bitters are ideal to incorporate in a constipation healing program. Hobbs lists the following herbs as bitters: angelica root, artichoke leaf, bitter orange peel, blessed thistle, cascara sagrada (laxative), gentian root, goldenseal rhizome, lemon peel, mugwort, wormwood, and devil's claw. Hobbs goes into greater depth in his book *Foundations of Health* (1994). Please feel free to research the properties of each of the bitter herbs if you wish to go into more depth.

Slippery elm bark is used to soothe the walls of the intestines. It is nutritious but contraindicated for IBD because of the polysaccharide content. Marshmallow root, comfrey leaf and root, and aloe are other demulcent herbs used to soothe the tissue of the intestinal walls. Aloe is not allowed on the Specific Carbohydrate Diet because some varieties and products have laxative effects and contain polysaccharides. Enzymes can assist in digesting foods that in turn relieve constipation. Get a good recommendation for an enzyme formula as some are more effective than others. Essential fatty acids (EFA) and vitamin A are necessary for mucosal health. L-Glutamine helps to build the bowel wall.

The Arise and Shine company (http://www.ariseandshine.com) has a new product called Intestinal Fortifier that helps rebuild the intestinal wall and is good to use after a cleanse or if the gut is compromised in any way. I had a burning sensation in my gut after one of the psyllium and bentonite cleanses. I used the Intestinal Fortifier, taking the suggested amount of the powder for thirty days. Although I continued to take the formula for the requested thirty days, the burning was gone in thirty-six hours. Ingredients are L-Glutamine, marshmallow root, white oak bark, apple pectin, chickweed leaf, goat whey, red beet root juice crystals, red raspberry leaf, slippery elm bark, ginger root, L-Glutamic acid, and L-Lysine.

Another very effective supplement for constipation is Oxy-Powder, formulated and promoted by Dr. Edward F. Group III, DC, and his Global Healing Center. It contains ozonated magnesium oxides, natural citric acid, organic germanium, and organic acacia gum. Group describes his product as an oxygen-based intestinal cleanser that releases beneficial oxygen to provide relief for symptoms of occasional constipation. He claims it melts away compacted waste. See http://www.oxypowder.com/.

Turkey rhubarb root is another very important laxative promoted by The Herb Finder online. http://theherbfinder.com/articles/colon_report01.html. The report at the link has voluminous information on its effectiveness. From personal experience, turkey rhubarb is a more gentle laxative that does not cause as much cramping as senna, aloe, and cascara.

CHAPTER 34

Detoxification Therapies

by Sheila Shea, MA

Detoxification therapies are a major component of the functional, biological, and naturopathic traditions. Detoxification is to find the balance, bring the body into homeostasis, clean the terrain, and create a healthy and vibrant body in which to live. The detoxification therapies described here are quite comprehensive. The liver, gallbladder, and pancreas are included in detoxification. Many aspects of intestinal hydrotherapies are explored. I share all the latest cleanses, products, books, and programs that my clients practice with good results. I finish by explaining a variety of other detoxing options such as laxatives, psyllium and bentonite cleanses, and castor oil packs. This chapter has something for everyone! Have at it.

Including the Liver, Gallbladder, and Pancreas in Detoxification

The liver is a major accessory organ of the GI system. Among its 500-plus functions, the liver secretes bile into the small intestines. The color of bile is generally bright yellow. Some bile is what the liver has cleansed from the bloodstream for elimination. Other bile is for the digestion of our fats and proteins.

The gallbladder is a small sack-like organ connected to the liver via the hepatic to cystic duct. The liver deposits bile into the gallbladder, which stores it until the person eats fats. Fats trigger the gallbladder to release its bile into the duodenum of the small intestine via the common duct. The bile then digests the incoming fats from the stomach. One purpose of the liver-gallbladder flushes is to cleanse the gallbladder of any stagnated or coagulated bile, or "stones" as they are called, to allow it to work more efficiently. Liver-gallbladder flushes are done routinely in cleansing.

The pancreas is another major accessory organ of the GI system. Like the liver, the pancreas has a duct leading into the small intestine. The duct from the liver and gallbladder and the duct from the pancreas meet together in the first part of the small intestine, the duodenum, at what is called the ampulla of Vater or the sphincter of Oddi. Their bile and enzymes enter the small intestine at this point. This sphincter has a ring of muscle fibers around it, which means it can spasm due to chronic constipation and interfere with digestion and especially pancreatic function.

Constipation adversely affects the health and circulation of the liver, gallbladder, and pancreas. Plus, a weak liver can lead to more constipation due to lack of digestive bile secretions. Fluids from these organs flow down the ducts. Under toxic circumstances like constipation, toxins can flow *up* the ducts to the gallbladder, liver, and pancreas. The health of these precious organs that assist digestion and other life processes may be compromised. That is why liver flushes, parasite cleanses, and coffee enemas complement any program for constipation and cleansing because they help restore the liver. Healing the pancreas is covered more fully in my chapters on sugar in Michael's Volume Four.

Intestinal Hydrotherapies

Colon hydrotherapy, colemas (also called a colema board, which is set up in the bathroom usually over the toilet), and/or enemas can be very helpful to help restore muscle tone, reposition the intestines, relax muscles, create successful bowel habits, and loosen and remove waste and gas. The therapist or individual can use abdominal massage, lymph drainage, breath techniques, and aromatherapy oils to accompany the intestinal hydrotherapies.

How often? The frequency and length of a colon hydrotherapy session depends on the condition, desire, and discipline of the person. Many options are available and I share of few of them. The idea is to get the flow going, and then keep it going, in the GI tract. For some, nothing or very little comes out in the initial sessions. The first priority then is to get the flow going. Once the person begins to eliminate, one can work on unearthing deeper layers of waste, continue rehabilitation and retraining of the gut muscles, and keep the flow going.

One has to be sensitive to the client's progress and that will help to determine the frequency and length of therapy. For anyone suffering from chronic constipation, twelve colon hydrotherapy sessions are not going to be a cure! They are a beginning. It takes months and years to cleanse and restore the GI tract, rehabilitate the muscles, and restore bacterial balance. My article, Intestinal Hydrotherapies: Colon Hydrotherapy, Colemas and Enemas, provides details on hydrotherapy procedures. (See http://sheilashea.com/faq1.html.)

High Frequency

Individuals with parasite infestations, chronic constipation, environmental illness, and various degenerative disorders might take several enemas, colemas, or colon hydrotherapies daily for a period of time or during a crisis. Some people detoxify so strongly they need up to two or three daily hydrotherapies. In the book *Cleanse and Purify Thyself,* Rich Anderson (2007) suggests one to two enemas daily when cleansing with psyllium and bentonite. Many individuals undertake an oral intestinal cleansing program when healing constipation in order to cleanse the intestines from years of built up and dehydrated waste.

Moderate Frequency

When one is fasting, detoxifying, or working with a difficult intestinal situation such as chronic constipation, then a daily or every-other-day intestinal hydrotherapy can be helpful. The use of an enema or colema every other day used in conjunction with colon hydrotherapy is also an excellent way to work with constipation. If you have severe constipation you initially might want to get more than one colon hydrotherapy session each week because it is helpful in loosening the muscles, allowing a backlog of waste to release and giving intestinal muscles a jump start. One can then graduate to once a week, once every two weeks, once a month, and then on an as-needed basis.

Low Frequency

Some individuals take the intestinal hydrotherapies weekly to cleanse and tonify the large intestinal tissue. Others use them occasionally to correct temporary constipation, reduce flu symptoms, relieve gas, undo a spasm, and before and/or after a trip, surgery, medical procedure, athletic event, or performance. People with sluggish elimination fast, cleanse, and change their diet from time to time and accompany it with colon hydrotherapy, colemas, or enemas.

In the occasional cases, people will come in and do a series of three to six hydrotherapies within close proximity. Very often receiving sessions close together will "break the log jam" and get the logs floating and moving down the river again! One women waits until her peristalsis begins to decline and she feels incomplete elimination; a session every four to six weeks keeps her muscles tonified. The point here is that people work on attaining healthy peristalsis and come in as needed—with the frequencies just described, or quarterly, annually, or even bi-annually to recharge their intestinal system.

Medical Conditions

The open-basin colon hydrotherapy equipment works especially well with spina bifida, some elderly, para- and quadriplegics, stroke patients, or other populations that have loose sphincter muscles, intense constipation, dehydration, impaction, or urgency.

Constipation resulting from irritable bowel syndrome (IBS) responds well to colon hydrotherapy using body-temperature water and accompanied by abdominal massage. One goal is to get the spasms to open up and let go and to restore a *balanced* peristalsis, according to Margaret Wright, an Australian naturopath and colon hydrotherapist (Wright, 1991).

What about parasites in the gut? Here's one testimonial: "After seeing dozens of doctors no one ever considered my constipation or colon to be an issue. After I began colonics, three times a week, almost a year later, we began seeing parasites come out. Dr. Bernard Jensen says it takes about sixty colonics to reach the layers where they live." This comment says to me that it takes time to heal the gut. If it took two years to get to the layer of parasites, we have to consider that it might take longer to heal difficult cases of constipation.

Enemas

I am giving plenty of links on how to take enemas. Kristina Amelong is an authority on the subject and her site is an excellent place to begin. Coffee implants are also discussed. The coffee implant is used for cleansing and restoring the liver. If you are healing your intestines, you definitely want to clean your liver, gallbladder, and pancreas. If you want to learn to give yourself an enema, read over the information at the sites and find a style that is personally comfortable for you. Enemas are not only excellent for self-care; they are essential for travel for those who constipate easily while traveling.

Kristina Amelong has an excellent site with an enema instruction video:

http://www.colonichealth.com

How to do a basic enema:

http://phoenixtools.org/self_healing/basic_enemas.htm

Enemas and coffee implants are explored in relation to healing cancer:

http://www.sawilsons.com/index.html

Good background material on the coffee enema:

http://www.ralphmoss.com/coff.html

Use Coffee Enemas for Detoxification, an article by Marsha Anderson:

http://www.naturalnews.com/026289_coffee_enemas_enema.html.

Here's a testimonial from a satisfied enema customer (me):

Thanks so much for posting the four articles from Monica's wonderful website! Great education. I hope to get more FAQs on my website. The need for education is tremendous. Learning how to take an enema is so important. I introduce many of my clients to the idea. It's a primary form of self-help and the most inexpensive way to go. I like that Monica states it so clearly step by step.

I brought my enema bag to Florida with me. I spent four days in Boca on the ocean, at the beach and visiting my mother who is in a nursing home. Got the bag out once a day. I tried to drink a lot of fluids and eat simply plus a two-hour workout on the beach. I still get intestinal pain almost daily and now it passes more easily. The enema will relieve the pain for me quicker than anything. I also used some H_2O_2 in the solution plus an herbal formula with propolis and other anti-bacterial herbs mainly due to a tooth infection. When I took the enema the first night, I had a large volume of liver bile—big time. So I was obviously cleansing the liver.

Retention Implants and Additives

Sometimes with constipation, it is helpful to introduce substances into the hydrotherapy water as an additive or retention implant. The constipation cause and effect as well as intention of the receiver determine which substance(s) and dosages will be useful for the condition.

Anything you can get into liquid form can be used for retention or in addition to the hydrotherapy water. Flora, chlorophyll, coffee, nystatin (for Candida), and herbs such as catnip and wheat grass are some of the more common substances that people use. Retentions and additives are also a way to get nutrition into the intestines when one's digestion, assimilation, and elimination ability are deficient or compromised. At the office, clients bring the additive or implant solution they deem best for themselves.

Retention or retention implant is for the purpose of rapid and heightened absorption in the rectum of the particular herb(s), vitamin(s), flora, and/or mineral(s) used. When doing a retention, the person first clears the colon with an enema or colonic. The implant fluid is prepared and used in a small amount, usually no more than 3 cups. The fluid is placed in a syringe or appropriate device for inflow. The fluid is then allowed to flow slowly into the rectum and is retained there. The person rests on the side, focuses on breath, relaxes, and attempts to hold the implant for twenty minutes maximum.

Although coffee retention implants can relieve constipation, Max Gerson, MD, in his book *A Cancer Therapy*, cautions: "Patients have to know that the coffee enemas are not given for the function of the intestines but for the stimulation of the liver." It is well known that healthy liver function promotes better intestinal peristalsis. Acidophilus is called for in constipation protocols.

Sometimes, substances called additives are introduced into the enema, colema, or colon hydrotherapy water during the session. Some of the additive flows in with the water each time or at decided times. This differs from a retention enema or implant because some of the substance comes out during releases and the overall volume is higher than the retention volume. In an enema or colonic, I need something that gets my peristalsis going like cayenne, H_2O_2, or lemon juice or to release spasms like valerian or catnip. I have been using a few ounces of lemon juice in my enema water and that triggers excellent peristalsis.

Electrolyte and Flora Replacement

A concern with frequent intestinal hydrotherapies is replenishing minerals and trace elements (electrolytes) and friendly bacteria or flora. Be careful to fill yourself full of high-quality minerals daily, such as through raw juices, grasses and algaes, and cultured fermented foods, or take acidophilus and bifidus cultures. Many who embark on healing their constipation already have depleted mineral reserves and imbalanced flora. So it is especially important to monitor this. Studies by the Southwest College for Naturpathic Medicine show that electrolytes and positive flora are not depleted during colon hydrotherapy.

Other Forms of Elimination, Cleansing, and Detoxifying

Dr. Thomas Rau, in his book *The Swiss Secret to Optimal Health* (Rau and Wyler, 2009), includes colon hydrotherapy cleansing in his catalog of treatments. He writes that this thorough but mild cleansing of the large intestine accompanied by a gentle abdominal massage helps stimulate the parasympathetic nervous system, cleans out toxins and bad bacteria, strengthens the immune system, and encourages the development of beneficial flora (p. 37). After the colon hydrotherapy given at his Paracelsus Clinic, the therapist administers specific intestinal flora rectally that are important for digestion and absorption of nutrients.

Another medical doctor in NYC, Alejandro Junger, is well known for his book on cleansing, *Clean* (2012):

> It's important to distinguish between a detox program (a cleanse) and the more generalized practice of slowly cleaning up our act by making gradual diet or lifestyle changes over several months. A cleanse is a distinct program, done for a concentrated period of time, that puts the body in a more intense detox mode. It has a start and an end date and a specific purpose. (p. 117)

Junger is also a proponent of using colon hydrotherapy during his Clean program to effectively boost the removal of the mucoid plaque that gets pulled out during a cleanse. He believes a detoxification program is the time when colonics are most beneficial, especially for those with a history of constipation.

Hopefully, you are already cleaning up your constipation by making a gradual diet and lifestyle change. This continues for a lifetime, not just several months. Remember, life style—you are changing the style of your life. Now that you are on that track, Junger is pointing out the marvelous choices you have today to do short, specific cleanses that move your intestinal health forward more quickly.

When you have constipation, more often than not, you have a build-up on your intestinal walls, your intestinal muscles are weak and/or leaky, and your flora is imbalanced negatively. Dysbiosis is the name given to an imbalanced floral state. The pathogenic and harmful bacteria and fungi outnumber the healthy flora. Some shorter cleanses can jump-start you to better floral balance, gut wall healing, and elimination. You have many good choices today among the various cleanses that are on the market. I am going to mention those that my clients and I have had the best success with. Each of the authors supports intestinal cleansing as part of their program. They go hand in glove.

Junger's website is http://www.cleanprogram.com/. In his twenty-one-day program, he recommends one meal in the middle of the day, two fluid meals, and a liver-gallbladder flush. Junger writes that "constipation is one of the most frequent health complaints in the Western world" (p. 71). His whole focus is to restore the intestinal flora and the integrity of the intestinal walls. He is very gut focused. The book is an excellent primer on detoxification, well worth the read. He mentions detoxifying mentally and emotionally at the same time.

Another interesting book is *21 Pounds in 21 Days: The Martha's Vineyard Diet Detox* (2009) by Roni DeLuz, RN, ND. Her recommendations are soup purees of cooked vegetables and fruits, raw juices, and supplements. DeLuz states that if you are not having at least one bowel movement a day she guarantees that you might be having some of the following problems: abdominal bloating and gas, acid reflux, stomach upset and nausea, stomach aches, body odor, and excess abdominal weight. Ring a bell? DeLuz devotes one whole chapter to understanding elimination! Her four must-have treatments for eliminating toxins are water, colonics, the kidney flush, and coffee enemas. Her program works beautifully for constipation.

The Raw Food Detox Diet by Natalia Rose (2006) is also a personal favorite. An associated web link is http://www.detoxtheworld.com/about.php. Rose, a Manhattan nutritionist, has designed a five-level diet plan to safely make the transition to eating raw foods, detoxify and achieve a perfect body no matter how you eat now. Although her program is geared to feel better and lose weight, she has a great program for the constipated! Natalia introduces us to the raw food diet, a missing piece of your education. It's an important one to know. She is a strong proponent of colon hydrotherapy and has a referral list on her site.

Next is Arise and Shine; the web link is http://www.ariseandshine.com. Rich Anderson, the principal at Arise and Shine, has formulated some of the most successful cleansing products in the world. He has seven-, fourteen-, and twenty-eight-day cleanse kits that are well tested and based on the psyllium-bentonite shakes, herbal formulas, probiotics, and a vegan diet (no animal products). According to Matt Monarch of The Raw Food World (http://www.therawfood world.com), the psyllium and bentonite shakes are the primary way to clean the intestinal walls.

Another really good detoxification program comes from Dr. Richard Schulze at http://www.herbdoc.com. Dr. Schulze has remarkable programs to cleanse the GI system, as well as the liver, gallbladder, and kidneys. A number of my clients have used his detox programs with great success. He has five-day, thirty-day, and the "incurables" programs. All are designed to clean and nourish the gut. His intestinal formulas #1 and #2 are the key to eliminating the deeper layers of waste in the gut—#1 is a laxative formula and #2 contains the psyllium as well as flax seed, apple pectin, activated willow charcoal, marshmallow root, pharmaceutical-grade bentonite clay, slippery elm bark, peppermint leaf, and cayenne pepper blend. One client has overcome a serious genetic condition, Charcot-Marie-Tooth disease, plus severe constipation using these formulas and a clean diet with juices.

I have chosen only a few of the successful, safe, reliable, and proven cleansing programs on the market. They can be used for reasons other than constipation; however, they are all aimed at healing the intestines. The idea is to try the different cleanses from time to time. They are so helpful is setting up better habits and increasing the health of your intestines.

Laxatives

Laxative sales are a multimillion-dollar industry. I'm speaking of chemical laxatives, but I'm sure the sales of both chemical and herbal laxatives are quite high as well. I was asked recently to give a talk on constipation at a local health fair. The organizer of the health fair owned the market around which the health fair booths were positioned. She told me that so many people come into the market to ask for laxatives that she decided to include the topic on the speaker's bureau! My clientele also surprises me. So many of them have worked out a daily consumption of laxatives that allows them to eliminate easily and effortlessly the next morning. More than I imagined.

Personally, I am glad that people find a way to eliminate with laxatives rather than allow their waste to remain within them. However, taking laxatives does not heal the problem—does not heal constipation. It alleviates it. Laxatives are categorized in three ways: stimulants, osmotics, and bulking agents. The major stimulant laxatives are aloe vera, senna, cascara sagrada, turkey rhubarb root, yellow dock, butternut (walnut family), and buckthorn. The osmotic laxatives are predominantly magnesium based such as magnesium sulphate (Epsom salt), magnesium oxide such as the Oxy-Powder, and magnesium citrate. They draw water into the lumen of the intestines and flush the waste out. Bulk laxatives use the power of fiber to soften the stool and stimulate a bowel movement. Psyllium, flax seed, and methylcellulose are bulk laxatives.

Christopher Hobbs, in his *Foundations of Health: Healing with Herbs and Foods,* lists all the herbal laxatives in order of potency. The strongest herbal and stimulant laxatives are aloe, senna, and cascara. Because of their stimulant nature, aloe and senna can cause cramping in the intestines and are generally mixed with another herb such as fennel or ginger to calm the cramping. Turkey rhubarb appears to be the most gentle and effective of the stimulant laxatives. Vitamin C is another common laxative used in increasing doses until elimination is achieved.

Many years ago I had a listserv on the Internet. I received a contribution from one of my subscribers on cascara sagrada. He noted that cascara helps with constipation and the peristaltic action of one's colon plus it increases bile flow and is tonic for the liver and gallbladder. The liver component is true for a number of the other stimulant laxatives. He would mix it with ginger to cut down on the gripping. However, he felt it was contraindicated with colitis or other inflammatory conditions in the bowel.

One caution with laxatives is the possibility of addiction. I can speak from personal experience as I had a laxative addiction for fifteen years. I used predominantly senna with the accompanying gripping and cramping. Some of the herbals refer to physical or psychological addiction to laxatives. In my case, it was psychological. It accompanied my eating disorder behaviors. The key thing to avoid with laxatives is electrolyte imbalance that comes from consistent overuse. For the most part, the clients who take laxatives regularly seem to have a modest pattern and use and find it highly effective for their constipation. However, they would love to eliminate naturally without the use of laxatives.

Many of the cleansing programs on the market use a mild to strong laxative depending on the company and the goal of the product. I feel that water is a healthier way to go than to take laxatives. For the most part, herbal laxatives are not harmful. They do cause melanosis coli, a black stain on the intestinal wall when viewed through a colonoscope. The condition is not harmful. The major chemical laxatives are magnesium citrate, Golytely, and ducoset. They are used as preparation for diagnostic studies such as endoscopy, pillcam, and colonoscopy.

Suppositories and Fleet enemas are two other categories of eliminators, or laxatives. The rectal suppository is small and torpedo-shaped and is placed in the anus-rectum. The glycerin or bisacodyl chemicals may generate a stool release from the rectum. One client swore by the suppositories for traveling, especially on camping trips. The Fleet phosphosoda enema is a small 2-ounce sodium phosphate solution that is infused into the rectum and may produce the desired bowel movement.

Psyllium and Bentonite

During intestinal hydrotherapies, the client enhances cleansing and rebuilding by taking orally the herb powdered psyllium seed husks and the volcanic ash bentonite to draw out old waste and clean the walls. The recommended doses range from 1 teaspoon to 5 tablespoons daily of both. Generally, the cleanses call for the smaller amounts; however, on the twenty-eight-day Arise and Shine cleanse in the final week the user has the option of taking 1 tablespoon each of psyllium and bentonite 5 times over the day!

Psyllium is not a laxative but a cleanser, bulking agent, and lubricant. The use of psyllium for the constipated person can go two ways. One, the constipated person will feel more constipated, miserable, bloated, or gaseous. Or two, the person will benefit from the lubricating properties of the psyllium and eliminate better. The lubricating quality will help matter slide through the intestines and reduce transit time.

Discomfort with the psyllium can mean that transit is compromised, or that the volume of waste build-up is extensive, or that the user is not drinking sufficient fluid. Psyllium has difficulty moving through the intestines in any case. A difficult transit might mean that the person has a redundant bowel with extra lengths, coils, spirals, and prolapses. Redundancy is quite common.

Castor Oil Packs

Palma Cristi by Edgar Cayce (1970) is the classic work to understand and practice castor oil packs. Exclusive use of castor oil packs is good for the person who is unable to use psyllium. I had two colon hydrotherapy clients in Miami who both used castor oil packs exclusively for cleansing their large intestines. One woman, a flight attendant, would use the castor oil packs for three days before her colonic session. She would pass dark flaky material that appeared to have come off her intestinal walls. Another client, the father of one of my friends, spent a week every year in Miami cleansing with castor oil packs and colonics. He did the packs and colonics daily, then flew home.

The castor oil packs are very effective for the intestines and liver. One can place the oil-saturated flannel over the intestines and liver to loosen the waste contained within. The process requires 45–60 minutes of resting on your back while you cover your abdomen with the flannel, then plastic, then a towel, and finally a heating pad. Here is a testimonial:

> I am using the castor oil packs daily plus colonics because I have a bad case of Candida and poor colon peristalsis. For me, this helps relieve constipation because it helps break down old material in the colon and promotes better releases during the colonic. It works for me to get things moving, even gas.

CHAPTER 35

Complementary and Medical Therapies

by Sheila Shea, MA

Just when you thought you had exhausted every avenue to heal constipation, I am now offering you at least seven other possibilities in this chapter. I refer to and work with natural medical doctors (NMD) in my practice of colon hydrotherapy. They can get to the root of the problem and provide coordination and resources for difficult cases. Ayurveda and traditional Chinese medicine are more than five thousand years old and have established procedures for constipation. Yes, constipation started a long time ago. Iridology gives great insight into the health of the whole body, especially how the intestines influence other organs. Some find they do very well with homeopathy. Last, I include allopathic diagnostic measures that give us a clear view of the health of the internal gut walls, mouth to anus. Read on!

Body-based modalities such as Chi Nei Tsang, craniosacral therapy, abdominal visceral manipulation, and chiropractic can be helpful in opening up the energy of the intestines. Bonnie Bainbridge Cohen, who does body-mind centering work, has developed excellent treatment for children and adults. Massage is excellent to relax the muscles.

I personally realized I had to work on planes beyond the physical to heal my constipation. This insight lead me to meditate, visualize healing, live out my life and dreams, develop and listen to my instincts and intuition, and incorporate emotional therapy and expressive arts such as dance, poetry, and cartooning. Each person finds his or her own way to healing.

Naturopathy

Naturopthic physicians work with natural means as well as viewing constipation from the greater wholistic perspective. According to one naturopathic physician: "Philosophically, naturopathic physicians believe that the human body is a self-repairing organism when given the proper circumstances. Instead of being trained to treat a symptom, NDs are trained to treat the person who has the symptoms" (Dana Myatt, ND, phone 800-376-9288). Natural Medical Doctor (NMD) appears to be the correct current title for those naturopaths or natural medical doctors who have graduated from a school accredited with the U.S. Department of Education. Previously, the name Natural Doctor or ND was used. However, now, the initials ND or "natural doctor" refer to a person who has taken an online and correspondent certification for naturopathy.

Ayurveda

Ayurveda is a 5,000-year-old system of natural healing from India. The Ayurvedic Institute, in Albuquerque NM, is run by Vasant Lad, MS (phone 505-291-9698). They offer a study program, seminars, correspondence courses, panchakarma, ayuryoga, and Ayurvedic and Western herbs and products. Panchakarma is the Ayurvedic system of cleansing. They use medicated enemas and understand cleansing very deeply. I met an employee of the panchakarma department on a backpack trip; he gave me some suggestions for my intestinal issues and suggested I come and take their program to greater benefit my clients and myself. He suggested I use Dashamoola, an Ayurvedic formula of ten roots, as a rectal implant. Another technique uses warm sesame oil enemas of one-half to one cup for chronic constipation. The book *Ayurveda: The Science of Self-Healing* by Dr. Vasant Lad (1993) has nine pages on panchakarma.

Here are some resources for Ayurvedic healing:

http://www.ayurveda.com—Ayurvedic Institute, Albuquerque NM

http://tridosha.com/contact-us—Healing Hands Massage and Ayurvedic Spa, Puerto Vallarta, Mexico

http://theraj.com/constipation/index.php—review of Ayurvedic principles for treating constipation

Homeopathy

Sujata Owens tells a touching story of a baby with Hirschsprung's disease with minimal if any elimination. He was taken to a homeopath at age seven after exhausting all medical alternatives. A prescription of a single medium-potency dose of plumbum metallicum 200c, homeopathic lead, was given and the child responded with 80 percent recovery within two weeks. You may refer to the following source for more details in this case and homeopathy in general.

> Sujata Owens, LCEH (Bom), RS Hom (NA). 1995. A Case of Severe Constipation with Colic and Congenital Deformities, Small Remedies and Interesting Cases VII, *Proceedings of the 1995 Professional Case Conference,* edited by Stephen King, ND, et al. Oegstgeest, the Netherlands: International Foundation for Homeopathy. (2366 Eastlake East, Suite 325, Seattle WA 98102, phone 206-324-8230).

Iridology

Iridology is the study of the iris of the eye, which indicates the condition of the physical, emotional, mental, and spiritual bodies, present and past. The iridologist is able to determine origins of issues whether genetic, intestinal, trauma, or accident. It is considered to be an accurate diagnostic technique. Germany is home to the most scientific treatises on it. Bernard Jensen has written most extensively on it in the United States (Jensen, 1998).

I have an iridology reading done from time to time. A reading in the early 1990s indicated that many of my organs were in acute to sub-acute condition and my intestines and heart were chronically weak, considered more serious than acute. Many organs throughout my body, including the heart, CNS (central nervous system), glands, and kidneys have been affected by the condition of my intestines, especially the effects of severe and profound constipation with an overlay of equally serious eating disorders. A recent iridology reading showed major healing of my organs, with some liver inflammation. The liver, as you remember, is a key organ in healing constipation.

Traditional Chinese Medicine

Traditional Chinese medicine (TCM) has developed systems of healing constipation via acupuncture and herbology that go back thousands of years. It is interesting to note that in China allopathic medicine is practiced side by side with TCM. I recommend finding a qualified acupuncturist where you live and explore with that person the choices he or she offers regarding your own complex of symptoms regarding constipation.

Allopathic Measures

Colonoscopy, barium x-rays, endoscopy, pillcam, sigmoidoscopy, proctoscopy, and CAT scans are various measures to view the intestines and give feedback on the condition of your gut walls. I recently asked a gastroenterologist, "How many people that you perform colonoscopy on are technically cleaned out with their bowel prep?" This particular GI doctor is excellent at performing and interpreting the diagnostic studies of the gut wall. He responded, "Technically, 70 percent are not cleaned out." That means that only 30 percent of the people receiving colonoscopy have actually cleaned out their large intestines. Personally, I believe that is a low percentage and might speak to the level of build-up as well as constipation in the 70 percent who are not cleaned out.

CHAPTER 36

Constipation and Other Conditions

by Sheila Shea, MA

Constipation comes up regularly in the context of many other conditions. Through my clients, I have found strong relationships between constipation and other conditions. Each condition described below could account for a whole book. Included are prescription drugs, Hirschsprung's disease, pregnancy, children, Hodgkin's disease, migraines and headaches, and allergies. Using case studies and a question-and-answer format, I provide jewels of information plus some surprises!

Constipation and Prescription Drugs

I do not elaborate on drugs normally, as my focus is wholistic healing and the use of natural methods to heal constipation. However, it is important to know that certain drugs slow down intestinal elimination. Some of my clients are on narcotics, muscle relaxants, or steroids and have become seriously constipated. Morphine and heroin attach to the intestine's opiate receptors and produce constipation. The cranial and intestinal brains can both be addicted to opiates. Other prescription painkillers cause a genuine slowing down or halting of peristalsis temporarily. With colon hydrotherapy, we are able to get their elimination going efficiently again. However, they need to stay on top of their elimination as long as they are on the drugs.

Antidepressants are another set of drugs influencing constipation. Prozac and its relatives prevent the uptake of serotonin by the target cells and it remains in the cranial and intestinal brains in high quantities. Higher levels in the intestines can lead to nausea, diarrhea, and constipation. Prozac increases the speed at which matter passes through the intestines and has even been used in small doses to treat chronic constipation. But it has also been shown to freeze the colon.

People who are on prescriptions and experiencing constipation should pick up a copy of *The PDR Pocket Guide to Prescription Drugs.* Find your particular prescriptions and read the common side effects. Constipation shows up quite frequently. You could then ask your doctor if alternatives exist for the prescription that do not produce constipation.

I also mentioned earlier that a number of chemical laxative formulas are used for intestinal diagnostic study preparation. Many clients complain about the taste, quantity, and resulting diarrhea from the preparatory laxatives. Doctors are using some easier alternatives such as magnesium citrate and Miralax rather that Golytely. However, colon hydrotherapy is indicated before such diagnostic intestinal studies. More clinics around the country are employing colon hydrotherapy in their centers to serve the colonoscopy population.

Constipation and Hirschsprung's Disease

This condition may also be a cause of constipation. Hirschsprung's disease occurs in one in 5,000 births; it is the absence of nerve ganglion cells in variable lengths of the intestines. One of my Internet correspondents shared her experience with a gastroenterologist on Hirschsprung's disease. The doctor felt the degree of seriousness fell on a spectrum and the most serious cases warranted surgery. Milder cases responded to regular and oil enemas. That was true of my correspondent. The doctor believed that many milder cases were misdiagnosed as something else, and conversely, that many cases of chronic, intractable constipation were likely mild forms of Hirschsprung's. Also, the use of bran for these cases made matters worse because it caused so much gas on top of an already compromised bowel!

Elaine Gottschall, author of *Breaking the Vicious Cycle,* reported a new breakthrough with Hirschsprung's using the Specific Carbohydrate Diet (SCD). She was aware of young children practicing the SCD and recovering from the Hirschsprung's. The implication is that the intestinal nerve cells are recovering, growing, and functioning through a carbohydrate-specific diet. Elaine speculated in 1995, during a visit to Tucson, that the cause could be a toxin or acid that destroys the nerves.

Hirschsprung's may also cause megacolon. The consensus is that the majority of Hirschsprung's' sufferers, even after surgery, have to rely on lifelong bowel management. Colon hydrotherapy and enemas could be very helpful for bowel management combined with appropriate diet.

Constipation during Pregnancy

During the 1990s, I had a wonderful listserv on the Internet based on intestinal health. D, a nurse, was one of the subscribers and I looked forward to her posts. I have lost touch with her but I am going to summarize the advice she wrote to an expectant mother on my listserv. Be prepared for words of wisdom.

D was excited to read an email from a young pregnant woman who was concerned about intestinal health. She congratulated her on her upcoming special event. D is a retired RN and a mother of two sons, each of whom at birth tipped the scales at more than 10 pounds. D breastfed both of her sons and did her best to eat and drink healthfully. As such, she feels she has a little inside information on potential constipation problems during pregnancy. Her position is that constipation, whether simple or chronic, will most likely become more difficult as the pregnancy advances.

D feels that any aggressive cleansing regime would not be recommended during pregnancy without constant blood monitoring and keeping electrolytes balanced. She also does not believe in laxatives, herbal or chemical. She says if one thinks that enemas can contribute to miscarriage then one should look at the probability of straining with bowel movements and the dramatic peristalsis that can accompany constipation and the stimulant laxative effects. Remember, straining of any kind is not good for a person, pregnant or not. If you do have laxatives in mind, she suggests you ask a doctor—someone you trust has you and your baby in mind—whether laxatives and/or stool softeners are recommended or wise. She doubts that a daily maintenance dose of a mild herbal laxative or stool softener product is ever warranted, and does not know whether a history of severe constipation would tip the scales in favor of such a product.

According to D, gentle is the keyword, whatever you do. She says don't let constipation make relief a major accomplishment. In other words, take care of it gently and consistently. She feels it is too bad that clear water enemas have lost their popularity with pregnancy, labor, and delivery. She believes they are a better choice than laxatives or chemical enemas. She notes that chemical enemas are in favor currently because of their convenience and the pharmaceutical influence. She asks why anyone would want to introduce more chemicals such as the Fleet enema into the body when plain water alleviates constipation with little or minimal cost.

She recommends a gentle washing with lukewarm water and raising the enema bag no higher than 24 inches above the waist. She believes an occasional small one- to two-quart plain water enema done before there is a major crisis will keep the pregnant mother more comfortable and cause no harm to mother or baby. She stresses awareness of sanitary procedures such as carefully cleansed equipment, the use of hot soapy water to wash all enema equipment, followed by a soak in 3 percent hydrogen peroxide after each use. Special care with hygiene and disinfecting is a must. Remember, the anal to urethra and/or vagina routes for possible infection warrant diligence and precaution during pregnancy.

D's protocol:

- Drink at least two quarts of pure water daily
- Eat many soluble and nonsoluble fiber foods
- Stay away from foods and drink that dehydrate you
- Do not consume salty and sugary foods or beverages
- Do not drink any soft drinks
- Read labels
- Avoid ingesting caffeine, carbonation, artificial flavors, and sugars
- Squeeze fresh lemon juice in a quart of filtered water when thirsty
- Use honey as a safe sweetener if needed
- Use moderate exercise and relaxation techniques to help the intestines

According to D: "A brisk walk followed by a warm bath may be all that is needed to improve intestinal motility, circulation, and general well-being."

D shares that she starts her day drinking a quart of unsweetened lemon water. It helps to hydrate her body, corrects her pH, strips mucus, and soothes her liver and gallbladder perhaps by softening some stored deposits. She has known for a long time that lemon juice is a healthy beverage and a great way to start the day. She provides an excellent site with a drink that helps relieve constipation and detoxifies your colon:

http://www.colonhealth.net/colon_hydrotherapy/green-drink-relieves -constipation.htm

If the mother is on an iron supplement that tends to constipate, she should either consume foods that are high in iron like apricots, grapes, and spinach, or eat foods that will counteract the problem like prunes, prune juice, and bran muffins.

Thanks, D, for your courageous words of wisdom for pregnant mothers who are experiencing constipation and want the most natural form of alleviating it. Also, encouraging gentle elimination during pregnancy will allow a more pure intestine, blood supply, and overall cleaner and thus healthier environment in which the infant and mother develop and thrive.

Constipation in Babies and Children

I realize from my own situation that constipation is a prevalent problem with babies and children. It is still a taboo topic and not on the list for acceptable discussion. It's even a blind spot for some parents, who might be in denial, or even relieved, about their offspring's discomfort. Formulas, refined food diets, insufficient fluids, birth trauma, vaccinations, and inherited situations can be origin factors. The possibility of constipation increases even more when one considers the abuse that babies and young children might receive. I include below the plaintive voices of a few concerned parents, followed by a few questions and answers.

Parents' Comments

My son has constipation. We are trying acidophilus and magnesium. I have been trying this for a few days and have seen much improvement. I am going to watch the next week and see how it goes. Then we plan to take him off the acidophilus and see if he stays regular.

My son is three and since two years old has been holding in his bowel movements. It started out to be once or twice a week and now he can hold it for two weeks. When he finally does go, he cries and complains of tummy aches. For an hour or more before elimination he finally will go into a pull-up. He verbally made it very clear he just doesn't want to let it out, afraid it will hurt. His stools are loose, never hard, and more like soft putty or clay.

I have a five-year-old who has increasing trouble with eliminating waste.… The diameter is way too big and hard for him to pass. My son sits on the stool all day, on and off, attempting to go. He knows it is going to hurt and I now believe he is trying to NOT go out of fear of pain. He is so sore after elimination I have to be extremely gentle in wiping him. The slightest pressure causes pain. Kindergarten is approaching this fall and I can't even get him to wipe himself. If this isn't solved by the fall I know he will hold it in while at school! Plus I hate to see him in so much pain!

Frequently Asked Questions

Q. What age is it healthful for children to begin colonics? Might it be helpful to children who suffer from bowel holding?

A. I have given colon hydrotherapy sessions to children as young as two to three years of age. I feel that it can be very helpful for children who hold their bowels and it is important to be accompanied by massage of the abdomen. The child needs to be fully informed about what will happen, have the treatment voluntarily, and have the parent(s) present.

Q. Is cow's milk good for babies and children?

A. I will summarize a research article on this subject in *The New England Journal of Medicine,* 1998, Volume 339:1100–1104 by G. Iacono, et al., entitled Intolerance of Cow's Milk and Chronic Constipation in Children.

The article clearly indicated that "intolerance of cow's milk can cause severe perianal lesions with pain on defecation and consequent constipation in young children."

Methods: A study was performed comparing cow's milk with soy milk in sixty-five children (age range, 11 to 72 months) with chronic constipation (defined as having one bowel movement every three to fifteen days). All of the children had been referred to a pediatric gastroenterology clinic and had previously been treated with laxatives without success. Forty-nine had anal fissures and perianal erythema or edema. After fifteen days of observation, the children received either cow's milk or soy milk for two weeks. A positive response was defined as eight or more bowel movements during a treatment period.

Results: Forty-four of the sixty-five children (68 percent) had a positive response while receiving soy milk. The anal fissures and pain with defecation issues were resolved. None of the children who received cow's milk had a positive response.

Conclusions: "In young children, chronic constipation can be a manifestation of intolerance of cow's milk."

As I read this over, I also notice a correlation between lactose and bowel inflammation. Elaine Gottschall addressed this issue through the Specific Carbohydrate Diet. For more information on this huge issue around cow's milk and constipation, see the following websites:

http://www.notmilk.com—an anti-milk site that is quite comprehensive

http://www.medicine.virginia.edu/clinical/departments/pediatrics/clinical -services/tutorials/constipation/home—University of Virginia site focusing on chronic constipation and encopresis in children

http://www.mayoclinic.com/health/constipation-in-children/DS01138 /TAB=indepth—the Mayo Clinic on constipation and encopresis in children

Constipation and Hodgkin's Disease

Q. I am twenty-eight years old and have Hodgkin's Disease, and have been constipated for a great part of my life. Are there any natural remedies I should be using to promote regularity and maximize nutrient absorption (even while on chemo)? As for eating a well-balanced, fiber-rich diet, drinking plenty of water, and exercising to the best of my daily energy supplies, I think I have all the bases covered. So is there any help or advice you can offer?

A. Thanks so much for sharing your story. I used the Hodgkin's disease juice formulas in Norman Walker's book *Raw Vegetable Juices* (2003). Since that time many more juicing books have been written and they are found in health food stores. More and more often I hear my clients who have immune-compromised diseases tell me that they have been constipated most or all of their life. I believe there is a connection between the constipation and the disease. Constipation is stagnation and a breeding ground for virus, bacteria, fungi, and other parasites, all of which can weaken the immune system. One priority would be to cleanse the GI tract and deal with the constipation.

Constipation with Migraines and Headaches

Q. Is colon hydrotherapy useful in my particular case? I suffer from bright spots, appearing continuously in my visual field for short time and disappearing soon (but on rare occasions becoming small permanent damages of the visual field). Also I feel sometimes mild headaches. Finally, I have suffered from chronic hard constipation for three years. I use laxatives continuously. The doctors do not know the cause of my visual disturbances, but do you think it is possible that they are caused by intoxication from the colon? Do you know similar cases?

A. I have had a history of headache and migraines and some of the visual patterns you describe, which I associate with migraines. I feel my head pain was and is due to initial and longstanding constipation, both emotional and physical. Plus, if my gut is full of toxins, so is my liver.

Laxatives, including herbal, are known to have some deleterious side effects, such as electrolyte imbalance, dehydration, and irritations in the intestinal mucosal wall. My headaches started to decline after improving diet, increasing my fluids to more than 3 quarts daily, receiving Rolfing, consuming wheat grass juice and raw juices, cleansing the liver, kidney, and intestines, stopping vomiting, removing or reducing trigger foods like additives, chemicals, preservatives, and wine, and doing emotional work.

Constipation and Allergies

Q. Can help for my allergies be found through colonics? I have always suffered terribly from allergies to pollen and ragweed. I thought my problem would be related to my former chronic constipation to the point of hemorrhoids.

A. The old phrase goes, "Allergies are a weakened immune system and a weakened immune system is a result of a toxic intestines." Many authorities feel that allergies are due to an overpermeability of the intestinal wall that is the beginning of an inflammatory response. The overpermeability of the wall allows substances into the blood and lymph and sets up an immune reaction. Clearly, the intestines are congested and upset with this irritated condition. Constipation can cause or be the result of this situation. Colon hydrotherapy can be part of an overall program to undermine the allergies. The Gut and Psychology Syndrome (GAPS) diet is specific for allergies.

CHAPTER 37

Constipation Resources and Glossary

by Sheila Shea, MA

Congratulations. You have made it to my final chapter on constipation—a noteworthy accomplishment. This chapter contains a comprehensive list of resources. I include information on what are called "detox spas." Sometimes it's great to reset—get away, break some old habits, and clean out! You can also explore research, websites, and a recommended reading list here. Last, I have created a glossary that takes the beginning steps in creating a vocabulary for intestinal health and constipation. The glossary is an exploration into the latest information and understanding of intestinal life. It's all here, from A to Z. Enjoy reading through your possibilities. My pleasure is to provide you with important, pressing, and needed information. Let's get on with healing ourselves.

Spa Therapy

Sometimes it seems best to find a place where we can check in and then devote full time to healing our constipation and developing new strategies and habits. I have found some wonderful spas that offer colonics, wheat grass, yoga, and mineral springs. I know a few others exist in Thailand and other countries. Do a search under colon hydrotherapy. This is what I found after a quick Internet search:

Ubud Sari Health Resort in Bali: http://www.ubudsari.com/

Hotel St. George Health Care Center, Bad Hofgastein near Salzburg Austria: http://www.stgeorg.com/engl/f-x-mayr/. This hotel is famous for its healing waters and the Mayr cure. They offer a complete healing program. The most important indications for Dr. F. X. Mayr's cure are:

- Constipation and diarrhea, flatulence, colic, gastritis, metabolism problems, heartburn, stomach and intestinal swelling
- Liver disease, obesity, anorexia
- Blood cholesterol, high or low blood pressure
- Chronic bronchial problems, migraines, chronic skin problems
- Arthritis, gout, rheumatism

We Care Health Center and Retreat, Desert Hot Springs CA: http://www.wecarespa.com. We Care is where Dr. Alejandro Junger went to heal. It's a great place. A number of my clients have spent time there.

Hippocrates Health Institute, West Palm Beach FL, Brian Clements, director: http://www.hippocratesinst.org

Optimum Health Institute in Lemon Grove CA and Austin TX: http://www.optimumhealth.org

Grace Grove Retreat Center in Sedona AZ: http://www.gracegrove.com

Tao Garden Health and Spa Resort: http://www.tao-garden.com

Research Topics

Breast Cancer and Constipation

Maruti, Lampe, Potter, et al. (2008) found limited support to the hypothesis that increased bowel motility lowers breast cancer risk. This implies the possibility of an association of breast cancer with constipation. It has to do with estrogen-uptake particles secreted by the liver. If too many are taken back into the system because of constipation, the flood of extra estrogen in the body can contribute to the creation of breast cancer.

Violence and Constipation

Carl Schultz wrote an article for *Acres, The Eco-Agricultural Journal* (in the 1970s or '80s) on a visit he made to a prison to talk to some high-security prisoners. He asked them how many had a BM daily and no one raised a hand. He kept upping the time and thought the guys were uncooperative until he got up to about two weeks. Then more men began raising their hand. Long and short, he attributed the violent behavior to internal toxicity from constipation.

Websites

These are additional websites that provide information on constipation and healing constipation:

http://www.selfhealthsystems.com/archiveletter.php?id=383—Norman Shealy, MD, PhD, on constipation

http://www.themedicalquestions.com/altmed/100954c62010.html—a home remedy for constipation

http://www.livestrong.com/constipation—a huge list of constipation healing techniques

http://www.healthandyoga.com/html/enema/enema-constipation.html—enema and constipation cure

http://chetday.com/spencedetox.html—detoxification by Ted H. Spence, DDS, ND, PhD/DSc, MPH

http://www.colonhealth.net/colon_hydrotherapy/mantell1.htm—article on colon hydrotherapy and its clinical applications, by Donald J. Mantell, MD

http://www.edgarcayce.org/are/holistic_health/data/thcolon1.html—colonics and enemas from the Cayce ARE Foundation

http://www.ability.org.uk/enemas.html—link resource for enemas, colonics, and detoxing

http://www.shirleys-wellness-cafe.com/detox.htm—the website for Shirley's Wellness Cafe, an amazing resource for detoxing and health

References and Recommended Reading

Anderson, R. 2007. *Cleanse and Purify Thyself.* Medford, OR: Christobe Publishing.

Batmanghelidj, F. 2008. *Your Body's Many Cries for Water.* Third edition. Decatur, GA: Global Health Solutions.

Bernard, [unknown], J. H. Tilden, et al. 1939, 1956. *Constipation,* three volumes. http://www.healthresearchbooks.com/pages/book_detail.php?pid=1469

Boutenko, V. 2009. *Green Smoothie Revolution: The Radical Leap toward Natural Health.* Berkeley, CA: North Atlantic Books.

Campbell-McBride, N. 2010. *Gut and Psychology Syndrome.* Revised edition. London: Medinform Publishing.

Cayce, E. 1970. *Palma Christi.* Virginia Beach, VA: Association for Research and Enlightenment.

Chia, M. 2009. *Advanced Chi Nei Tsang.* Rochester, VT: Destiny Books.

Chopra, D. 1997. *Perfect Digestion.* New York: Three Rivers Press.

Christopher, J. 1994. *Rejuvenation through Elimination.* Second edition. Springville, UT: Christopher Publications.

Clapp, L. 1998. *Prostate Health in 90 Days.* Carlsbad, CA: Hay House .

Clark, H. 1995. *A Cure for All Diseases.* Chula Vista, CA: New Century Press.

Collings, J. 1996. *The Principles of Colon Hydrotherapy.* London: Thorsons Publishing.

Cordain, L. 2010. *Paleodiet.* Revised edition. Edison, NJ: John Wiley and Sons.

D'Adamo, P., with C. Whitney. 1997. *Eat Right 4 Your Body Type: The Individualized Diet Solution to Staying Healthy, Living Longer and Achieving Your Ideal Weight.* New York: Putnam Adult.

DeLuz, R., and J. Hester. 2009. *21 Pounds in 21 Days: The Martha's Vineyard Diet Detox.* New York: HarperCollins.

Duggan, S. 1995. *Edgar Cayce's Guide to Colon Care.* Virginia Beach, VA: Inner Vision Publishing Company.

Ehret, A. 1976. *Mucusless Diet Healing System.* Paso Robles, CA: Benedict Lust Publications.

Gates, D., and L. Schatz. 2011. *The Body Ecology Diet: Recovering Your Health and Rebuilding Your Immunity.* Revised edition. Carlsbad, CA: Hay House.

Gerson, M. 1958. *A Cancer Therapy: Results of Fifty Cases and the Cure of Advanced Cancer by Diet Therapy.* Bonita, CA: Gerson Institute.

Gittleman, A. 2001. *Guess What Came to Dinner Last Night.* Revised edition. New York: Avery Trade.

Gottschall, E. 1994. *Breaking the Vicious Cycle.* Revised edition. Baltimore and Ontario, CA: Kirkton Press.

Gray, R. 1991. *Colon Health Handbook.* Twelfth revised edition. Bingley, UK: Emerald Publishing.

Hobbs, C. 1994. *Foundations of Health: Healing with Herbs and Foods.* Second edition. Loveland, CO: Interweave Press.

Jensen, B. 1998. *Doctor Jensen's Guide to Better Bowel Care.* Revised edition. New York: Avery Trade.

Jordan, L. 2001. *Detox for Life.* New York: Madison Publishing.

Junger, A. 2012. *Clean—Expanded Edition.* Second updated edition. New York: HarperOne.

Kulvinskas, V. 1975. *Survival into the 21st Century.* Fairfield, IA: 21st Century Bookstore.

Lad, V. 1993. *Ayurveda: The Science of Self-Healing.* Twin Lakes, WI: Lotus Press.

Lipski, E. 2011. *Digestive Wellness.* Fourth edition. Columbus, OH: McGraw-Hill.

Maruti, S. S., J. W. Lampe, J. D. Potter, et al. 2008. A prospective study of bowel motility and related factors on breast cancer risk. *Cancer Epidemiol Biomarkers Prev* 17:1746–1750.

Matsen, J. 1991. *Eating Alive: Prevention through Good Digestion.* Auburn, MA: Crompton Publishing.

McMillan, S. C. 1999. Assessing and managing narcotic-induced constipation in adults with cancer. *Cancer Control* 6 (2):198–204.

McShane, R. E., and A. M. McLane. 1985. Constipation: Consensual and empirical validation. *Nursing Clinics of North America* 20:801–808.

Mollison, W. 1993. *The Permaculture Book of Ferments of Human Nutrition.* Hobart, Tasmania, AU: Tagari Publications.

Moritz, A. 2007. *The Liver and Gallbladder Miracle Cleanse: An All-Natural, At-Home Flush to Purify and Rejuvenate Your Body.* Berkeley, CA: Ulysses Press.

Netter, F. H. 1962. *The Ciba Collection of Medical Illustrations.* Volume 3: A Compilation of Paintings on the Normal and Pathologic Anatomy of the Digestive System; Part II: Lower Digestive Tract. Edited by E. Oppenheimer. Summit, NJ: Ciba Pharmaceutical Company.

Oldfield, J. [No Date.] *Constipation, and How to Avoid It, and How to Cure it.* Gloucestershire, UK: Internet Bookshop UK Ltd.

Openshaw, R. 2009. *Green Smoothies Diet: The Natural Program for Extraordinary Health.* Berkeley, CA: Ulysses Press.

Owens, S. 1995. A case of severe constipation with colic and congenital deformities, small remedies and interesting cases VII. *Proceedings of the 1995 Professional Case*

Conference, edited by S. King, et al. Oegstgeest, the Netherlands: International Foundation for Homeopathy.

Page, L. 2002. *Detoxification.* Revised edition. Carmel Valley, CA: Traditional Wisdom.

The PDR Pocket Guide to Prescription Drugs. 2009. Ninth edition. New York: Pocket Books.

Rau, T., and S. Wyler. 2009. *The Swiss Secret of Optimal Health: Dr. Rau's Diet for Whole Body Healing.* Reprint edition. New York: Berkley Trade.

Rauch, E. 1993. *Diagnostics According to F. X. Mayr.* New York: Thieme Medical Publishers.

Reid, D. 2006. *The Tao of Detox.* Randolph, VT: Healing Arts.

Robinson, B. 1907. *The Abdominal and Pelvic Brain.* Chapter 29: Constipation—Its Pathologic Physiology and Its Treatment by Exercise, Diet, and "Visceral Drainage." https://play.google.com/store/books/details?id=f4dNHRg_Dg0C&rdid=book-f4dNHRg_Dg0C&rdot=1 e-book

Rogers, S. 1990. *Tired or Toxic? A Blueprint for Health.* New York: Prestige Publishing.

———. 1994. *Wellness Against All Odds.* New York: Prestige Publishing.

Rose, N. 2006. *The Raw Food Detox Diet.* New York: William Morrow Paperbacks.

Sandberg-Lewis, S. 2010. *Functional Gastroenterolgy.* Portland, OR: National College of Naturapathic Medicine Press.

Saxon, E. 1934. *Constipation.* Cambridge, UK. C. W. Daniel Company.

Schultz, C. [1970s.] Incidence of constipation in inmates. *Acres: The Eco-Agricultural Journal* [now *Acres USA*].

Sears, B., with B. Lawren. 1999. *Enter the Zone: A Dietary Roadmap.* New York: Regan-Books.

Shea, S. 1978. Colon therapy: The natural way to renewed health and sexuality. *Forum Magazine: The Journal of Human Relations.*

Smith, J. 2003. *Seeds of Deception.* Portland, ME: Yes Books.

Stone, R. 1999. *Health Building: The Conscious Art of Living Well.* Summertown, TN: Book Publishing Company.

———. 1999. *Polarity Therapy: The Complete Collected Works,* Vol. I. Summertown, TN: Book Publishing Company.

Thomson, J. 1943. *Constipation and Our Civilization.* New York: Thorsons.

Walker, N. 2003. *Raw Vegetable Juices.* Pomeroy, WA: Health Research Books.

Winters, J. 2006. *In Search of the Perfect Cleanse.* Las Vegas, NV: Tri-Sun International.

Wright, M. 1991. *Colonics.* Gympie, AU: Margaret Wright Health System.

Yong, S. 1999. Case histories—constipation. *I-ACT Quarterly,* Fall 1999:10, 24, 28.

Young, R. 2003. *The pH Miracle.* Reprint edition. New York: Wellness Central.

Zephyr. 1996. *Instinctive Eating: The Lost Knowledge of Optimum Nutrition.* Hawaii: Pan Piper Press.

Glossary

Anthraquinone. A substance found in many plants, most specifically laxatives, cathartics, and purgatives. It has a stimulant—some call it irritant—quality in the gut and causes greater elimination. The direct action of these compounds on the gut may cause cramping pains. These plants are usually used in conjunction with carminatives to relieve such symptoms. The major anthraquinone or laxative herbs are aloe, cascara sagrada, senna, yellow dock, butternut, buckthorn, frangula, and turkey rhubarb. The anthraquinones in plants are also a source of dyes. For more information, see http://herbalgyan .jimdo.com/herbal-chemistry/herbal-anthraquinones.

Anticholinergic. Blocking the effects of the neurotransmitter acetylcholine. An anticholinergic drug can cause constipation and other problematic side effects since acetylcholine is involved with learning, memory, glands, and involuntary muscles. Antidepressants and antipsychotics are two examples of anticholinergic drugs.

Atony. Referring to a muscle that has lost its strength. Atony can be a common condition among the constipated. Another name is atonic bowel.

Candida. A naturally occurring yeast in the intestines that grows in an aggressive and destructive way in the presence of overconsumption of sugars, birth control pills, steroids, or antibiotics. Overgrowth may penetrate the gastrointestinal mucosa or wall. For a photo, see http://en.wikipedia.org/ wiki/File:Candida_albicans.jpg.

Carminative. An herb or preparation that either prevents formation of gas in the gastrointestinal tract or facilitates the expulsion of gas. According to herbalist David Hoffmann, a carminative's main action is to soothe the gut wall, ease gripping pains, and reduce the production of gas in the digestive tract. The complex of volatile oils in the carminative plant have a locally anti-inflammatory, anti-spasmodic and mildly anti-microbial effect upon the lining and muscle coats of the alimentary canal. Caraway, cardamom, celery seed, chamomile, cinnamon, dill, eucalyptus, fennel, garlic, and ginger are examples of carminative herbs.

Celiac disease. A genetic and inflammatory bowel disease (IBD) that affects at least 1 in 133 Americans. Celiacs suffer damage to the villi, shortening and villous flattening, in the lamina propria and crypt regions of the small intestines. The Specific Carbohydrate Diet and Gut and Psychology Syndrome diets, with zero tolerance for complex sugars, have been the most successful in healing the condition. Symptoms of celiac disease range from diarrhea, weight loss, and malnutrition, to latent symptoms such as isolated nutrient deficiencies but no gastrointestinal symptoms. Many are asymptomatic. The premier laboratory for celiac testing is http://www.enterolab.com.

Colema. A form of intestinal cleansing similar to colonics and enemas. The colema kit includes a five-gallon bucket, the "colema board" with an oval opening and protective shield at one end, and tubing and speculum. The opening in the board sits on top of the toilet and a chair or other device supports the other end. A person rests on the board on his or her back with the buttocks positioned at the edge of the elimination opening and against the shield. The water and waste are expelled into the basin. The colema kit is an FDA Class I product. No machinery or plumbing is necessary and the person can self-administer.

Colitis. A form of inflammatory bowel disease (IBD), colitis is an inflammation of the colon or large intestine. Ulcerative colitis degrades the wall of the large intestine. Mucous colitis or "irritable colon" is a form of colitis in which the goblet cells overproduce mucus to protect the intestinal walls from further irritation or inflammation.

Colon hydrotherapy. A gentle water cleansing of the intestines with equipment that provides for temperature, pressure, and elimination. The process is a series of inflows and outflows of water. Abdominal massage may be used on the outflows of water. Equipment comes with a filtration system.

Crohn's disease. Considered the most serious of the inflammatory bowel diseases. Crohn's begins slowly, causing such symptoms as cramping abdominal pain, fever, fatigue, nausea, diarrhea, rectal bleeding, weight and/or appetite loss, and a chronic feeling of sickness. Crohn's disease tends to flare up and then subside, sometimes for months, before another episode occurs.

Over time, the disease can cause abscesses and ulcers to form, which may then deeply erode the intestinal wall. In severe cases, further complications such as fistulas and anal fissures can develop. Fistulas are abnormal passages between body organs that allow pus and fluids an avenue to drain. In Crohn's disease, fistulas form between loops of intestine, intestine and skin, or intestine and bladder.

Rarely, Crohn's disease inflammation and thickening of the small intestine is so severe that an intestinal obstruction occurs. Such an obstruction causes extreme abdominal pain with vomiting. Arthritis and skin lesions are systemic complications.

Cystocele. A form of pelvic organ prolapse, or a bladder prolapse occurring in women. A cystocele occurs when the wall of the bladder presses against and moves the wall of the vagina or rests on top of the rectum. When this occurs it may make intestinal elimination more difficult.

Diverticulum. A form of inflammatory bowel disease (IBD), a diverticulum is a small pouch or aneurysm in the colon that bulges outward through weaker areas in the intestinal walls. Multiple pouches are called diverticula, and the condition of having diverticula is called diverticulosis. When the pouches become inflamed, the condition is called diverticulitis. Diverticula are most common in the lower portion of the large intestine called the sigmoid colon.

Dysbiosis. Also called dysbacteriosis, a condition with microbial imbalances on or in the body. Dysbiosis is most prominent in the digestive tract or on the skin but can also occur on any exposed surface or mucous membrane such as the vagina, lungs, mouth, nose, sinuses, ears, nails, or eyes. It is associated with inflammatory bowel disease (IBD) as imbalances in the intestinal microbiome may be associated with bowel inflammation and chronic fatigue syndrome.

Encopresis. Also called stool holding, occurs when a child resists having bowel movements, causing impacted stool to collect in the colon and rectum. When the child's colon is full of impacted stool, liquid stool can leak around the impacted stool and out of the anus. Encopresis usually occurs after age four when the child has already learned to use a toilet. In most cases, encopresis is a symptom of chronic constipation. Less frequently, it may be the result of developmental or emotional issues. In Europe it is called paradoxical rectum because the muscles of defecation work in reverse. The urge to evacuate the bowel causes the muscles to tighten instead of relaxing. Often, the child has to heal from the encopresis to enter school.

Enlarged colon. A condition in which the large intestine or colon expands beyond what is considered a normal size. Some call it a megacolon; it is a matter of degree. An enlarged colon is somewhere between the redundant bowel and a megacolon. One could have redundancy and an enlarged colon. Causes may be constipation, poor diet, and/or excessive gas.

Enema. A form of self-care intestinal cleansing, like the colema. It is administered with a bag or bucket ranging in volume from 1.5 to 4 quarts; standard enema bag size is 2 quarts. Douche and hot water bags purchased at most drug stores and supermarkets double as an enema bag.

The bag comes with a few feet of hosing and a small 3-inch, pencil-thin speculum that is inserted a few inches into the anus. A small clasp near the speculum end of the hosing allows the recipient to regulate the water flow and pressure. The bag may be hung on a shower rod, towel rack, or hook. The higher the elevation, the greater the water pressure.

Enema positions vary. Generally, the recipient is kneeling with the upper torso and/or face resting on the floor; this is called the knee-chest position. Some individuals rest on their back with knees bent and feet on the floor. Others begin the process on their left side, moving to their back and then to their right side. Nursing training generally has the recipient lie on the left side. Gerson therapy has the recipient lie on the right side to receive the enema.

Some people feel enemas do not reach as far as the cecum, the beginning of the ascending colon. Others are highly successful in filling the entire colon. Mainly, people need to practice enemas to improve getting the water to the ascending colon and practice breathing through peristaltic waves to allow water to flow in. Learning to take a good enema is like learning any other skill. It takes time and practice.

Enemas can be combined with yoga, breathing, and abdominal massage for best effect. Using a combination of an enema, yoga postures, breathing, and abdominal massage enables the water to get all the way around to the ascending colon. The massage, breathing, and postures are also helpful in stimulating peristalsis so that the muscles work to expel all the waste and enema water.

Fissure. An anal fissure is a tear or split in the lining of the anus (anal mucosa). Symptoms include pain when passing a bowel movement and bleeding from the anus. Blood may be on the outside of the stool or on the toilet tissue (or baby wipes) following a bowel movement. Constipation may be a cause and a symptom. Healing requires an alkaline environment.

Fistula. An anal fistula is a small channel that develops between the end of the bowel known as the anal canal and the skin near the anus. Some types of fistula have one channel, while others branch out into more than one opening. The fistula ends can appear as holes on the surface of the skin around the anus. An anal fistula is painful and can cause bleeding when you go to the toilet. Some fistulae can be connected to the sphincter muscles. See http://www.nhs.uk/conditions/Anal-fistula/Pages/Introduction.aspx.

GALT. Gut-associated lymphoid tissue (GALT) is the digestive tract's immune system that works to protect the body from invasion. The digestive tract is an important component of the body's immune system and possesses the largest mass of lymphoid tissue in the human body. GALT is made up of several types of lymphoid tissue that store immune cells such as T- and B-lymphocytes that carry out attacks and defend against pathogens. GALT in the gut includes the tonsils, Peyer's patches, lamina propria, and appendix.

Dilation. Intestinal dilation is an enlargement or expansion in bulk or extent in the intestines. Causes of dilation are a build-up of fluid, feces, or gas. All cause pain of varying degree. Dilation initially increases motility and is then followed by atony or a bowel without muscle tone.

Hirschsprung's disease. Also called **aganglionic megacolon,** a congenital disorder of the colon in which ganglion nerve cells in the walls of the myenteric or Auerbach's plexus are absent. This may cause constipation. The disease has been reversed in infants and adults on the Gut and Psychology Syndrome (GAPS) diet.

Lamina propria. A constituent of the moist linings known as mucous membranes or mucosa that line various tubes in the body such as the gastrointestinal tract. It is part of the immune system and the gut-associated lymphoid tissue.

Megacolon. A dilation of the colon not caused by mechanical obstruction. Megacolon is determined by measurement of the diameter of various areas of the colon. Megacolon means that an area or many areas of the colon are very expanded. Acute, chronic, and toxic are three categories of megacolon.

Megarectum. A large rectum resulting from underlying nerve supply abnormalities or muscle dysfunction that remains after disimpaction of the rectum. The *Principles of Surgery* textbook describes any rectum that can hold more than 1500cc of fluid as a megarectum.

Mesentery. A double layer of peritoneum attached to the abdominal wall (parietal) and enclosing in its fold certain organs of the abdominal viscera (visceral). The mesentery is a fold of the peritoneum that connects the intestines to the dorsal abdominal wall, especially a fold that envelops the jejunum and ileum. The intestines are suspended from the dorsal aspect of the peritoneal cavity by a fused, double layer of parietal peritoneum called mesentery. An important feature of mesentery is that it serves as a conduit for blood vessels, nerves, and lymphatic vessels going to and from the gastrointestinal system.

Metabolic syndrome. A sugar disease characterized by any one or all of the following symptoms: large abdominal girth, abdominal visceral fat, high cholesterol LDLs and triglycerides, high blood pressure, pre-diabetes, diabetes, overweight, or obesity. Possible outcomes of metabolic syndrome are heart disease, stroke, cancer, and Alzheimer's.

Microbiome. A totality of microbes, their genetic elements (genomes), and environmental interactions in a particular environment. Joshua Lederberg coined the term "microbiome," arguing that microorganisms inhabiting the human body should be included as part of the human genome because of their influence on human physiology. The human body contains more than ten times more microbial cells than human cells. Microbiomes are in other environments as well: soil, seawater, and freshwater.

Motility. The ability of the gastrointestinal system to move food rhythmically from mouth to anus, also referred to as peristalsis. Motility means that the gut has muscle health and energy to keep a contracting-expanding motion going that successfully and efficiently allows contents to move through the system and the waste on out.

Parasympathetic nervous system. The PNS is the branch of the autonomic nervous system (ANS) responsible for the body's ability to recuperate and return to a balanced state known as homeostasis. While the sympathetic system is also known as the "fight-or-flight" response, the parasympathetic is often called "relax-and-renew." The primary parasympathetic nerve is the vagus nerve, also known as cranial nerve X. When active, the parasympathetic system slows down heart rate, dilates blood vessels, activates digestion, facilitates peristalsis, and stores energy.

Peristalsis. A propagating contraction in the gastrointestinal system of successive sections of circular smooth muscle preceded by a dilation. The dilated intestinal wall is drawn over its content in this reflex mechanism that transports the content aborally, meaning opposite to or away from the mouth.

Peritoneum. Thin membrane that lines the abdominal and pelvic cavities (parietal) and covers most abdominal viscera (visceral). The intestines are suspended from the dorsal aspect of the peritoneal cavity by a fused, double layer of parietal peritoneum called mesentery.

Rectal prolapse. Downward displacement of the rectum, when the tissue that lines the rectum falls down into or sticks through the anal opening. It occurs most often in children under six years and in the elderly. It is associated with constipation, cystic fibrosis, malnutrition, and malabsorption such as with celiac disease among other conditions.

Rectocele. Also called protocele, occurring in women. Happens when the thin wall of fibrous tissue fascia, separating the rectum from the vagina, becomes weakened allowing the front wall of the rectum to bulge into the vagina. Very often the rectocele inhibits bowel movements and may contribute to constipation.

Redundant bowel. Occurs when extra loops form in the intestines, resulting in a longer than normal organ. Rarely volvulus occurs, resulting in obstruction and requiring immediate medical attention. A colonoscopy is difficult and in some cases impossible when a redundant colon is present because of too many twists and turns.

SBBOS. Small bowel bacterial overgrowth syndrome (SBBOS), or small intestinal bacterial overgrowth (SIBO), also termed bacterial overgrowth, is a disorder of excessive bacterial growth in the small intestine. Generally, the small intestine has a low number of bacteria, whereas the colon has a large number. In this condition, the small intestine has a very high count of pathogenic bacteria and fungi that interfere with digestion and absorption.

Steatorrhea. The presence of excess fat in the feces. Stools may also float due to excess lipid, have an oily appearance, and be foul smelling. The liver and pancreas may be compromised with steatorrhea.

Volvulus. A major bowel obstruction with an abnormal and complete twisting of a loop of intestine around its mesenteric attachment site or around itself. A volvulus is a rotation of part of the intestine around an axis resulting in partial or complete obstruction of the lumen. If not relieved, the condition can lead to ischemia of the bowel wall, gangrene, and perforation, often with significant mortality. In general, volvulus is responsible for 1–7 percent of large bowel obstructions. In a researched series of large bowel volvulus cases, the sigmoid was involved in 76 percent, the cecum in 22 percent, and the transverse colon in 2 percent. Volvulus of the splenic flexure accounts for 1 percent of cases. See http://www.medscape.org/viewarticle/737667_2.

Appendixes

Client Brochure: Practicing Biodynamic Craniosacral Therapy

Biodynamic craniosacral therapy is an empathy-based practice focused on the felt sense of wholeness. Slowness and stillness are key in the method used to recover physical wholeness.

From the time of conception until now, we are always one whole body. The billions of cells in our body know where each other is located. All the fluids in the body are connected in the same way as all the cells. The practitioner senses fluid flows, currents, and tidal movements in your body as it swells and recedes.

Why is this important?

The fluids provide nutrition and waste removal. They are in a delicate balance and are easily stressed, causing disease. A biodynamic practitioner can sense imbalances in the fluid movement with his or her hands. He or she will use several different hand positions to assist your body in having a uniform, whole movement that is slow and still.

How does he or she do this?

First, the biodynamic practitioner begins by slowing down and settling his or her own body through the practice of mindfulness. Mindfulness means paying attention to any experience that is occurring, without judgment. Research shows that this produces a state of balance between the body and the brain. Thus the client's health can be restored more deeply when the practitioner is personally mindful while working.

Second, the biodynamic practitioner is regularly mindful of his or her own breathing and heart rate, to build empathy. This reduces fear and repairs the brain and heart regions that control love, happiness, and compassion. This allows the biodynamic practitioner to become sensitive to you and your unique challenges.

You are considered an equal partner in this therapeutic process. How do you become an equal partner in the session? The mindfulness techniques being used by the practitioner are gradually taught to you. This allows you to self-regulate your own mind and body with the practitioner during the session and between sessions. Together, you and your practitioner can feel whole and healthy in body, mind, and heart.

What can you expect from a session or series of sessions?

Very deep relaxation is the first effect of a biodynamic session. It balances the brain. Second, since the practitioner is focused on the whole body, you may be able to let go of your symptoms slowly and, in many cases, actually feel the health in your body as happiness or joy. Third, you get more mental and physical clarity from the session. This allows you to make better choices about how to live and how to heal yourself.

Biodynamic Practitioner Competencies

with Carol Agneessens, MS

1. Orienting

Be still and know

    a. Sit still in a comfortable and aligned position

    b. Sense the support of the chair, the floor and the air around you

    c. Sense and imagine your body shape three dimensionally (3D)

    d. Relax and breathe gently 3D into the whole surface of your skin

    e. Settle into Stillness in and around your mind and fluid body

2. Synchronizing

Breathing with the Wholeness

    a. Relax and welcome Primary Respiration (PR) in and around your soma

    b. Sense the back of your body relaxing and opening to the space behind you

    c. Open the front of your soma and go to the horizon and back with PR

3. Attuning

Building coherency and self-regulation

    a. Relax, breathe, and negotiate contact with the client from your heart

    b. Touch like "a feather on the breath of God"

    c. Reorient and resynchronize to your 3D body after contact

    d. Practice cycles of attunement through the zones with each window

4. Therapeutic Gates

There are many; wait for one to open
Your touch remains on the surface of the client
Your hands float and eventually disappear

    I. Disengagement
        a. Periodically rest attention on the back of your hands
        b. Wait for the autonomic nervous system in your soma and client's to settle
        c. Sense zone B to zone B whenever possible

    II. Buoyancy
        a. Find an alive, playful, lifting shape with your fluid body
        b. Balance the fluid fields of the face, neck, brain, trunk, pelvis and extremities of the client sequentially and slowly over time

    III. Ignition
        a. Reverently establish a sense and image of the client being a 3D fluid body
        b. Deepen into PR in the 3D fluid body of yourself and the client
        c. Deepen into Stillness in the Midline of yourself, client and the natural world

    IV. Heart
        a. Allow your hands to become an extension of your heart pulsation
        b. Attend to the heart and vascular system in yourself and client as a unified circulatory system
        c. Visualize the zones as embryonic fluid globes held by a loving mother and father

5. Healing

Primary Respiration is the origin story of love
Stillness is the story of being

        a. A therapeutic process may begin after disengagement of the autonomic nervous systems of both the practitioner and client
        b. A healing process in the client may be initiated by the natural world
        c. PR-Stillness may become more clear through the zones at session's end
        d. Life makes sense when there is a breathing whole oriented to a still Midline

e. You cannot know your client's spiritual path

f. Create a profoundly gentle container and be the organizing center

6. Session Reminders

Biodynamic practice is a protocol for compassion

a. Perception of your whole soma and fluid body is crucial

b. Open all your sense doors through the zones

c. Hands and arms are like an umbilical cord, your body like an embryo, placenta, or uterus

d. Periodically take a deep breath in synch with PR

e. Teach the client 3D and PR very slowly and with great kindness

f. Practice with humility; bow

g. Patience is a priority

The Cranial Sutures

Sutures are named after the bones they connect.

The sutures in the cranial vault can all be palpated in the course of the examination of the skull. The other sutures lie in the depth of the orbital cavity, the mouth cavity, the nasal fossae, and at the base of the skull.

The Cranial Vault

The **metopic suture** separates the frontal into two frontal halves, right and left.

The **coronal suture** separates the frontal from the two parietals and from the greater wings of the sphenoid.

The **sagittal suture** separates the occipital squama from the two parietals and from the two mastoids.

The **lambdoid suture** separates the occipital squama from the two parietals and the two mastoids.

The **parietosquamosal suture** (right and left) separates the parietal from the temporal squama.

The **sphenofrontal suture** (right and left) separates the lower and external part of each side of the coronal suture from the upper half of the anterior border of the greater wing of the sphenoid.

The **frontonasal suture** (right and left) separates the nasal spine (external part) from the upper border of the nasal process of the upper maxilla.

The **sphenoparietal suture** (right and left) separates the posterior-external (or lower posterior) angle of the parietal from the base of the mastoid.

The **sphenosquamosal suture** (right and left) separates the greater wing of the sphenoid (posterior border) from the anterior part of the temporal squama.

The **occipitoparietal suture** (right and left) separates the posterior border of the parietal from the occipital squama.

The **occipitomastoid suture** (right and left) separates the lower external border of the occipital squama from the posterior border of the mastoid.

The **frontomalar suture** (right and left) separates the external angular process of the frontal from the frontal process of the malar.

The **temporomalar suture** (right and left) separates the temporal (zygomatic process) from the malar.

The **nasomaxillary suture** (right and left) separates the anterior border of the nasal process of the upper maxilla from the posterior border of the nasal bone.

The **maxillomalar suture** (right and left) separates the malar from the upper maxilla.

The **intermaxillary suture** (maxillamaxillary) separates the two upper maxillaries at their anterior border and at the nasal crest.

The **internasal suture** separates the two nasal bones.

Orbital Cavity

The **frontolacrimal suture** (right and left), between the frontal and the lacrimal. Situated behind the nasal process of the upper maxilla (behind the internal angular process of the frontal), it separates the orbital arch from the upper border of the lacrimal, over a distance of approximately 1 centimeter.

The **frontoethmoidal suture** (right and left). Situated behind the suture of the frontal and the lacrimal, it separates the remainder of the internal border of the orbital arch from the upper border of the os planum of the ethmoid.

The **sphenofrontal suture** (lesser wing, right and left) separates the orbital arch of the frontal (posterior border) from the anterior border of the lesser wing of the sphenoid.

The **sphenofrontal suture** (greater wing, right and left) separates the external border of the orbital arch from the upper anterior border of the greater wing of the sphenoid.

The **lacrimoethmoidal suture** (right and left) separates the posterior border of the lacrimal from the anterior border of the os planum.

The **ethmoidomaxillary suture** (right and left) separates the lower border of the os planum from the internal border of the orbital surface of the upper maxilla.

The **palatoethmoidal suture** (right and left) separates the posterior border of the os planum from the lesser wing of the sphenoid.

The **sphenoethmoid suture** (right and left) separates the antero-external border of the greater wing from the internal border of the orbital process of the malar.

The **frontomalar suture** (right and left) separates the external part of the orbital arch from the upper border of the orbital surface of the malar.

The **malomaxillary suture** (right and left) separates the external border of the orbital process of the upper maxillar from the lower border of the orbital process of the malar.

The **palatomaxillary suture** (right and left) separates the orbital process of the palatine from the internal border of the orbital process of the upper maxilla.

The **lacrimomaxillary suture** (right and left) separates the lower border of the lacrimal from the antero-internal border of the orbital process of the upper maxilla (formation of the lacrimal canal).

Sutures in the Mouth Cavity, Intracranial Cavities, and Nasal Fossae

The **frontoethmoidal suture** separates the ethmoid notch of the frontal from the upper part of the alteral bodies, right and left, of the ethmoid. (The cribriform plate of the ethmoid fits into the center of this notch.)

The **sphenovomeric suture** separates the lower surface of the body of the sphenoid from the alae of the vomer.

The **vomerothmoid suture** separates the lower posterior border of the perpendicular border of the ethmoid from the upper and anterior border of the vomer.

The **vomeropalatine suture** connects the lower border of the vomer with the interpalatine suture of the palatines and the intermaxillary suture.

The **sphenopalatine suture** (right and left) separates the body of the sphenoid at the side from the upper and lower processes of the sphenopalatine notch of the upper posterior angle of the palatine (vertical plate), and thus marks off the sphenopalatine foramina, right and left.

The **pterygopalatine suture** (right and left) connects the anterior border of the pterygoids with the posterior border (vertical plate) of the palatine.

The **palatomaxillary suture** (right and left) is between the anterior border of the horizontal plate of the palatine and the posterior border of the palatine processes of the upper maxilla.

The **interpalatine suture** is between the two internal edges of the horizontal plates of the palatines.

The **intermaxillary suture** separates the internal edges of the palatine processes of the upper maxilla.

The **ethmoidonasal suture** separates the upper anterior border of the perpendicular plate of the ethmoid from the two nasal bones.

The **sphenopetrosal suture** (right and left). Between the anterior extremity of the petrous portion of the temporal and the posterior external part of the body of the sphenoid, it marks off the foramen lacerum.

The **petrobasilar suture** (right and left). Between the lower and internal border of the petrous portion of the temporal and the external border of the basilar part of the occiput, it marks off the opening of the jugular foramen.

The **palatomaxillary suture** (right and left) connects the external surface of the vertical plate of the palatine with the internal surface of the upper maxilla.

The **lower turbinate bone suture** connects:

- At the front with the nasal process of the upper maxilla, its internal surface with the turbinated crest

- Just at the rear with the lower border of the lacrimal (closing the circumference of the lacrimal canal)

- With the ethmoid through the uniform process

- With the palatine on the turbinated crest of the internal surface of the vertical plate

- With the internal surface of the upper maxilla, obstructing with its vertical plate the lower part of the opening of the upper maxillary sinus (Antrum of Highmore).

RESOURCES

Michael J. Shea, PhD
13878 Oleander Ave.
Juno Beach, FL 33408-1626
561.775.9912
www.michaelsheateaching.com
info@michaelsheateaching.com

Sheila Shea, MA
Colon hydrotherapy instructor and
practitioner, raw food counselor
4427 East 5th St.
Tucson, AZ 85711
520.325.9686
www.sheilashea.com
intestines@sheilashea.com

Carol Agneessens, MS
Pacific School of Biodynamic Integration
Santa Cruz, CA
831.662.3057
www.holographictouch.com
carolagneessens@mac.com

Wendy Anne McCarty, PhD, RN
Prenatal and perinatal psychology practice for all ages, supporting families and
professionals; publications and information for individual support available at
www.wondrousbeginnings.com
315 Meigs Road, A306
Santa Barbara, CA 93109
wmccarty@wondrousbeginnings.com

Sarajo Berman, MFA, CMT, LMT, RCST
Body therapist
2615 Cone Ave.
Durham, NC 27704
919.688.6428
www.bodyrevitalizations.com
sjberman@me.com

"What Babies Want"
Hana Peace Works
DVDs and books on birthing
P.O. Box 681
Los Olivos, CA 93441
www.whatbabieswant.com

Sara Dochterman, LCSW
Psychotherapist
521 Lake Avenue, Suite 5
Lake Worth, FL 33460
561.533.0948
www.saradochterman.com
sara@saradochterman.com

Ann Diamond Weinstein, PhD
Preconception, Prenatal and Early
Parenting Specialist
Offering consultation, coaching and
education to individuals and professionals on issues related to fertility,
pregnancy, birth and the early parenting period and their impacts over the
lifespan
347.878.8031
www.anndiamondweinstein.com
adw@anndiamondweinstein.com

Castellino Prenatal and Birth Training
Contact: Sandra Castellino, MEd
1105 N. Ontare Rd.
Santa Barbara, CA 93105
805.687.2897
castellinotraining.com
sandra@castellinotraining.com

Tim Shafer, MS
Biodynamic craniosacral therapy
instructor
3500 JFK Parkway, Suite 209
Ft. Collins, CO 80525
970.229.1925
www.indianpeaks.biz
Rolfer email: rolfer@indianpeaks.biz

Valerie A. Gora, LMT, BCST, NSCA-CPT
Excellent Bodywork, Inc.
Biodynamic craniosacral therapy instructor; continuing education in pre- and
perinatal massage, infant massage, and
myofascial therapies
North Palm Beach, FL 33408
561.283.3404
excellent-bodywork.com
Valerie@excellent-bodywork.com

Pacific Distributing—Books and Bones
An extensive catalog in the fields of
osteopathy, craniosacral therapy, embryology, anatomy, pre-and perinatal,
neuroanatomy, physiology, somatic and
trauma resolution, and movement therapies. The catalog also carries some of the
finest anatomical models in the world.
Contact:
Christopher or Mary Louise Muller
39582 Via Temprano
Murrieta, CA 92563
951.677.0652
www.BooksandBones.com
booksandbones@verizon.net

BIBLIOGRAPHY

Abram, D. 1996. *The Spell of the Sensuous.* New York: Vintage Books.

Agneessens, C. 2001. *The Fabric of Wholeness: Biological Intelligence and Relational Gravity.* Santa Cruz, CA: Quantum Institute Press.

Ainsworth, M. D. S. 1985. I. Patterns of infant-mother attachment: Antecedents and effects on development, and II. Attachments across the life span. *Bulletin of New York Academy of Medicine* 61:771–791, 791–812.

Als, H., F. H. Duffy, G. B. McAnulty, M. J. Rivkin, and R. V. Vajapeyam. 2004. Early experience alters brain function and structure. *Pediatrics* 113 (4):846–857.

Amiel-Tison, C., D. Cabrol, R. Denver, P.-H. Jarreau, E. Papiernik, and P. V. Piazza. 2004. Fetal adaptation to stress, part II: Evolutionary aspects, stress-induced hippocampal damage, long-term effects on behavior, consequences on adult health. *Early Human Development* 78:81–94.

Anand, K. J. S. 1986. Hormonal metabolic functions of neonates and infants undergoing surgery. *Current Opinion in Cardiology* 7:681–689.

———. 2005. A scientific appraisal of fetal pain and conscious sensory perception. Written testimony offered to the Constitution Subcommittee of the House of Representatives U.S. House Committee on the Judiciary 109th United States Congress.

Anand, K. J. S., and A. Aynsley-Green. 1985. Metabolic and endocrine effects of surgical ligation of patent ductus arteriosus in the human preterm neonate: Are there implications for further improvement of postoperative outcome? *Modern Problems in Paediatrics* 23:143–157.

Anand, K. J. S., and P. R. Hickey. 1987. Pain and its effect on the developing fetus. *New England Journal of Medicine* 377 (21):1321–1329.

Anand, K. J. S., and F. M. Scalzo. 2000. Can adverse neonatal experiences alter brain development and subsequent behavior? *Biology of the Neonate* 77 (2):69–82.

Association for Prenatal and Perinatal Psychology and Health. 2009. *Birth Psychology.* http://www.birthpsychology.com/apppah/introducing_APPPAH.htm.

Bailey, B. A. 2010. Partner violence during pregnancy: Prevalence, effects, screening, and management. *International Journal of Women's Health* 2:183–197.

Bailey, B. A., and R. A. Daugherty. 2007. Intimate partner violence during pregnancy: Incidence and associated health behaviors in a rural population. *Maternal and Child Health Journal* 11:495–503.

Barral, J., and A. Croibier. 2011. *Visceral Vascular Manipulations.* London: Churchill Livingstone.

Beebe, B., and F. Lachmann. 2002. *Infant Research and Adult Treatment: Co-Constructing Interactions.* Hillsdale, NJ: The Analytic Press.

Behnke, E. A. 2003. Embodiment work for the victims of violation: In solidarity with the community of the shaken. In *Essays in Celebration of the Founding of the Organization of Phenomenological Organizations,* edited by C. Cheung, I. Chvatik, I. Copoeru, L. Embree, J. Iribarne, and H. R. Sepp. http://www.o-p-o.net/prague essaylist.html.

Bergman, K., P. Sarkar, V. Glover, and T. G. O'Connor. 2008. Quality of child-parent attachment moderates the impact of antenatal stress on child fearfulness. *Journal of Child Psychology and Psychiatry* 49:1089–1098.

Bergner, S., C. Monk, and E. W. Werner. 2008. Dyadic intervention during pregnancy? Treating pregnant women and possibly reaching the future baby. *Infant Mental Health Journal* 29 (5):399–419.

Blechschmidt, E. 2004. *The Ontogenetic Basis of Human Anatomy: A Biodynamic Approach to Development from Conception to Birth.* Translated by B. Freeman. Berkeley, CA: North Atlantic Books.

Blechschmidt, E., and R. Gasser. 1978. *Biokinetics and Biodynamics of Human Differentiation: Principles and Applications.* Springfield, IL: Charles C. Thomas.

———. 2012. *Biokinetics and Biodynamics of Human Differentiation: Principles and Applications.* Revised edition. Berkeley, CA: North Atlantic Books.

Boivin, J., and L. Schmidt. 2005. Infertility-related stress in men and women predicts treatment outcome 1 year later. *Fertility and Sterility* 83 (6):1745–1752.

Bowlby, J. 1988. *A Secure Base: Parent-Child Attachment and Healthy Human Development.* New York: Basic Books.

Briere, J., and D. M. Elliot. 2003. Prevalence and psychological sequelae of self-reported childhood physical and sexual abuse in a general population sample of men and women. *Child Abuse and Neglect* 27 (10):1205–1222.

Bromberg, P. 1998. *Standing in the Spaces.* Hillsdale, NJ: The Analytic Press.

———. 2006. *Awakening the Dreamer.* Mahwah, NJ: The Analytic Press.

Campbell-McBride, N. 2010. *Gut and Psychology Syndrome.* Revised edition. London: Medinform Publishing.

Castellino, R. 1995. *The Polarity Therapy Paradigm Regarding Pre-Conception, Prenatal and Birth Imprinting.* Santa Barbara, CA: Castellino Prenatal and Birth Therapy Training.

———. 2000. *The Stress Matrix: Implications for Prenatal and Birth Therapy.* Santa Barbara, CA: Castellino Prenatal and Birth Therapy Training.

Chamberlain, D. 1990. The expanding boundaries of memory. *Journal of Prenatal and Perinatal Psychology and Health* 4 (3):171–189.

———. 1998. *The Mind of Your Newborn Baby.* Berkeley, CA: North Atlantic Books.

———. 1999. Babies don't feel pain: A century of denial in medicine. *Journal of Prenatal and Perinatal Psychology and Health* 14 (1):145–168.

Cheek, D. B. 1986. Prenatal and perinatal imprints: Apparent prenatal consciousness as revealed by hypnosis. *Journal of Prenatal and Perinatal Psychology and Health* 1 (2):97–110.

———. 1992. Are telepathy, clairvoyance and "hearing" possible in utero? Suggestive evidence as revealed during hypnotic age-regression studies of prenatal memory. *Journal of Prenatal and Perinatal Psychology and Health* 7 (2):125–137.

Coalson, R. E., and J. J. Tomasek. 1992. *Embryology.* Second edition. New York: Springer-Verlag.

Cwikel, J., Y. Gidron, and E. Sheiner. 2004. Psychological interactions with infertility among women. *European Journal of Obstetrics and Gynecology and Reproductive Biology* 117:126–131.

Davidson, R. J., and S. Begley. 2012. *The Emotional Life of Your Brain: How Its Unique Patterns Affect the Way You Think, Feel, and Live—and How You Can Change.* London: Hudson Street Press.

Davis, E. P., L. M. Glynn, F. Waffarn, and C. A. Sandman. 2011. Prenatal maternal stress programs infant stress regulation. *Journal of Child Psychology and Psychiatry* 52 (2):119–129.

Davis, E. P., and C. A. Sandman. 2010. The timing of prenatal exposure to maternal cortisol and psychosocial stress associated with infant cognitive development. *Child Development* 81 (1):131–148.

DiPietro, J. A., M. H. Bornstein, K. A. Costigan, E. K. Pressman, C. Hahn, K. Painter, et al. 2002. What does fetal movement predict about behavior during the first two years of life? *Developmental Psychobiology* 40:358–371.

DiPietro, J. A., K. A. Costigan, P. Nelson, E. D. Gurewitsch, and M. L. Laudenslager. 2008. Fetal responses to induced maternal relaxation during pregnancy. *Biological Psychiatry* 77:11–19.

DiPietro, J. A., K. A. Costigan, and E. K. Pressman. 2002. Fetal state concordance predicts infant state regulation. *Early Human Development* 68:1–13.

DiPietro, J. A., K. A. Costigan, E. K. Pressman, and J. Doussard-Roosevelt. 2000. Antenatal origins of individual differences in heart rate. *Developmental Psychobiology* 37:221–228.

Dobson, H., S. Ghuman, S. Prabhakar, and R. Smith. 2003. A conceptual model of the influence of stress on female reproduction. *Reproduction* 125 (2):151–163.

Elliot, D. M., D. S. Mok, and J. Briere. 2004. Adult sexual assault: Prevalence, symptomology, and sex differences in the general population. *Journal of Traumatic Stress* 17 (3):203–211.

Elliot, L. 1999. *What's Going On in There? How the Brain and Mind Develop in the First Year of Life.* New York: Bantam Books.

Emerson, W. R. 1997. *Birth Trauma: The Psychological Effects of Obstetrical Interventions.* Petaluma, CA: Emerson Training Seminars.

———. 2000. *Collected Works II: The Pre- and Perinatal Treatment of Children and Adults.* Petaluma, CA: Emerson Training Seminars.

Entringer, S., E. S. Epel, R. Kumsta, J. Lin, D. H. Heilhammer, et al. 2011. Stress exposure in intrauterine life is associated with shorter telomere length in young adulthood. *Proceedings of the National Academy of Sciences* 108 (33):13377–13378.

Eugster, A., A. J. J. M. Vingerhoets, G. L. van Heck, and J. M. W. M. Merkus. 2004. The effect of episodic anxiety on an in vitro fertilization and intracytoplasmic sperm injection treatment outcome: A pilot study. *Journal of Psychosomatic Obstetrics and Gynecology* 25:57–65.

Feinstein, D. 2010. Rapid treatment for PTSD: Why psychological exposure with acupoint tapping may be effective. *Psychotherapy: Theory, Research, Practice, Training* 47 (3):385–402.

Ferin, M. 1990. Stress and the reproductive cycle. *Journal of Clinical Endocrinology and Metabolism* 84 (6):1768–1774.

Field, T., M. Diego, and M. Hernandez-Reif. 2010. Prenatal depression effects and interventions: A review. *Infant Behavior and Development* 33 (4):409–418.

Field, T., B. Figueiredo, M. Hernandez-Reif, M. Diego, O. Deeds, and A. Ascencio. 2008. Massage therapy reduces pain in pregnant women, alleviates prenatal depression in both parents and improves their relationships. *Journal of Bodywork and Movement Therapies* 12:146–150.

Figueiredo, B., T. Field, M. Diego, M. Hernandez-Reif, O. Deeds, and A. Ascencio. 2008. Partner relationships during the transition to parenthood. *Journal of Reproductive and Infant Psychology* 23:99–107.

Findeisen, B. 2001. *The Psychology of Birth* (DVD). Geyserville, CA: STAR Foundation.

Flynn, H. A., F. C. Blow, and S. M. Marcus. 2006. Rates and predictors of depression treatment among pregnant women in hospital-affiliated obstetrics practices. *General Hospital Psychiatry* 28:289–295.

Fogel, A. 2009. *The Psychophysiology of Self-Awareness: Rediscovering the Lost Art of Body Sense.* New York: W. W. Norton.

Fonagy, P., G. Gergely, E. Jurist, and M. Target. 2002. *Affect Regulation, Mentalization and the Development of the Self.* New York: Other Press.

Foster, S. M., and T. R. Verny. 2007. The development of sensory systems during the prenatal period. *Journal of Prenatal and Perinatal Psychology and Health* 21 (3):271–280.

Freeman, B. 2010. *Biodynamic Embryology.* Bath, England: www.biodoc.uk.

Gallinelli, A., R. Roncaglia, M. LuciaMatteo, I. Ciaccio, A. Volep, and F. Facchinetti. 2001. Immunological changes and stress are associated with different implantation rates in patients undergoing in vitro fertilization-embryo transfer. *Fertility and Sterility* 76 (1):85–91.

Gasser, R. F. 1975. *Atlas of Human Embryos.* New York: Harper and Row.

Gill, J. M., S. L. Szanton, and G. G. Page. 2005. Biological underpinnings of health alterations in women with PTSD: A sex disparity. *Biological Research for Nursing* 7 (1):44–54.

Gitau, R., A. Cameron, N. M. Fisk, and V. Glover. 1998. Fetal exposure to maternal cortisol. *The Lancet* 352 (9129):707–708.

Glover, V., K. Bergman, P. Sarkar, and T. G. O'Connor. 2009. Association between maternal and amniotic fluid cortisol is moderated by anxiety. *Psychoneuroendocrinology* 34 (3):430–435.

Grimstad, J., and B. Schei. 1999. Pregnancy and delivery for women with a history of child sexual abuse. *Child Abuse and Neglect* 23 (1):81–90.

Grof, S. 1975. *Realms of the Human Unconscious.* New York: Viking.

———. 1985. *Beyond the Brain: Birth, Death and Transcendence in Psychotherapy.* Albany, NY: State University of New York Press.

Hayes, B. 2007. Stress, prenatal imprinting and childhood development disorders. Presentation at the Institute for Functional Medicine 14th International Symposium, Tuscon, AZ.

Hesse, E., M. Main, K. Y. Abrams, and A. Rifkin. 2003. Unresolved states regarding loss or abuse can have "second-generation" effects: Disorganization, role inversion and frightening ideation in the offspring of traumatized, non-maltreating parents. In *Healing Trauma: Attachment, Mind, Body and Brain,* edited by M. F. Solomon and D. J. Siegel. New York: W. W. Norton.

Hilden, M., K. Sidenhuis, J. Langoff-Roos, B. Wijma, and B. Shei. 2003. Women's experiences of the gynecologic examination: Factors associated with discomfort. *Acta Obstetricia and Gynecologica Scandinavica* 82 (11):1030.

Hill, S., M. DeBellis, M. Keshavan, L. Lowers, S. Shen, et al. 2001. Right amygdala volume in adolescent adult offspring from families at high risk for developing alcoholism. *Biological Psychiatry* 49:894–905.

Huizink, A. C., E. J. H. Mulder, and J. K. Buitelaar. 2004. Prenatal stress and risk for psychopathology: Specific effects or induction of general susceptibility. *Psychological Bulletin of New York Academy of Medicine* 130 (1):115–142.

Ingber, D. 2006. Mechanical control of tissue morphogenesis during embryological development. *International Journal of Developmental Biology* 50:255–266.

Issokson, D. 2004. Effects of childhood abuse on childbearing and perinatal health. In *Health Consequences of Abuse in the Family; A Clinical Guide for Evidence-Based Practice* (Chap. 11, pp. 1–25), edited by Kathleen A. Kendall-Tackett. Washington, D.C.: American Psychological Association.

Kaplan, L. A., L. Evans, and C. Monk. 2007. Effects of mothers' prenatal psychiatric status and postnatal caregiving on infant biobehavioral regulation: Can prenatal programming be modified? *Early Human Development* 84 (4):249–256.

Karr-Morse, R., and M. S. Wiley. 2012. *Scared Sick: The Role of Childhood in Adult Disease.* New York: Basic Books.

Khashan, A. S., R. McNamee, K. M. Abel, P. B. Mortensen, L. C. Kenny, M. G. Pedersen, et al. 2009. Rates of preterm birth following antenatal maternal exposure to severe life events: A population-based cohort study. *Human Reproduction* 1 (1):1–9.

Kilpatrick, D. G., C. N. Edmunds, and A. Seymour. 1992. *Rape in America: A Report to the Nation.* Charleston, SC: National Victims Center and Crime Victims Research and Treatment Center.

Kilpatrick, D. G., B. E. Saunders, A. Amick-McMullan, C. L. Best, L. J. Veronen, and H. S. Resnick. 1989. Victim and crime factors associated with the development of crime-related post-traumatic stress disorder. *Behavior Therapy* 20:199–214.

Kinsella, M. T., and C. Monk. 2009. Impact of maternal stress, depression and anxiety on fetal neurobehavioral development. *Clinical Obstetrics and Gynecology* 52 (3):425–440.

Kirby, M. 2007. *Cardiac Development.* Oxford: Oxford University Press.

Kirkengen, A. L. 2001. *Inscribed Bodies: Health Impact of Childhood Sexual Abuse.* Dordecht, The Netherlands: Kluwer Academic Publishers.

———. 2008. Inscriptions of violence: Societal and medical neglect of child abuse—impact on life and health. *Medicine, Health Care and Philosophy* 11:99–110.

———. 2010. *The Lived Experienced of Violation: How Abused Children Become Unhealthy Adults.* Translated by E. S. Shaw. Bucharest: Zeta Books.

Kloneff-Cohen, H., E. Chu, L. Natarajan, and W. Sieber. 2001. A prospective study of stress among women undergoing in vitro fertilization or gamete intrafallopian transfer. *Fertility and Sterility* 76 (4):675–687.

Larsen, W. 2001. *Human Embryology.* Third edition. New York: Churchill Livingstone.

Levine, P. A., and M. Kline. 2007. *Trauma through a Child's Eyes: Infancy through Adolescence.* Berkeley, CA: North Atlantic Books.

Lipton, B. H. 2005. *The Biology of Belief: Unleashing the Power of Consciousness, Matter and Miracles.* Santa Rosa, CA: Mountain of Love/Elite Books.

Llinas, R. 2001. *i of the vortex: From Neurons to Self.* Cambridge, MA: MIT Press.

Loewy, J., C. Hallan, E. Friedman, and C. Martinez. 2005. Sleep/sedation in children undergoing EEG testing: A comparison of chloral hydrate and music therapy. *Journal of Peranesthesia Nursing* 20 (5):323–331.

Lokos, A. 2010. *Pocket Peace: Effective Practices for Enlightened Living.* New York: Jeremy P Tarcher/Penguin.

Lupien, S. J., B. S. McEwen, M. R. Gunnar, and C. Heim. 2009. Effects of stress throughout the lifespan on the brain, behavior and cognition. *Nature Reviews* 10:434–445.

Lyman, B. J. 2007. *Prenatal and Birth Memories: Working with Your Earliest Memories to Help Your Life Today.* Santa Barbara, CA: Santa Barbara Graduate Institute Publishing.

Lyons-Ruth, K., and D. Jacobovitz. 1999. Attachment disorganization: Unresolved loss, relational violence, and lapses in behavioral and attentional strategies. In *Handbook of Attachment,* edited by J. Cassidy and P. Shaver. New York: The Guilford Press.

Marcus, S. M., H. A. Flynn, F. C. Blow, and K. L. Barry. 2003. Depressive symptoms among pregnant women screened in obstetrics settings. *Journal of Women's Health* 12:373–380.

McCarty, W. A. 2000. *Being with Babies: What Babies Are Teaching Us.* Revised edition. Vol. 2: Supporting Babies' Innate Wisdom. Goleta, CA: Wondrous Beginnings.

———. 2002. The power of beliefs: What babies are teaching us. *Journal of Prenatal and Perinatal Psychology and Health* 16 (4):341–360.

———. 2004. *Welcoming Consciousness: Supporting Babies' Wholeness from the Beginning of Life, An Integrated Model of Early Development.* W. B. Publishing (ebook available from www.wondrousbeginnings.org).

———. 2008. EFT for mom, baby and dad from the beginning of life. In *Fifteen Ways to Health, Happiness and Abundance* (ebook available from http://www.thetapping-solution.com/free_ebook.shtml).

———. 2011. Consciousness at the beginning of life. *Bridges Magazine* 21 (1):12–15.

Meaney, M. J. 2010. Epigenetics and the biological definition of gene-environment interactions. *Child Development* 81 (1):41–79.

Merleau-Ponty, M. 1958. *Phenomenology of Perception.* Translated by C. Smith. London: Routledge Classics. Original edition published in 1945.

Miranda, L., S. Schick, C. Dobson, L. Hogan, and B. D. Perry. 1999. Positive developmental effects of a brief music and movement program at a public preschool: A pilot project [Abstract]. www.childtrauma.org/etaServices/neigh_arts, www.childtrauma.org/etaServices/neigh_arts.

Monahan, K., and C. Forgash. 2000. Enhancing the health care experiences of adult female survivors of childhood sexual abuse. *Women and Health* 30 (4):27–41.

Monk, C., W. Fifer, M. Myers, R. Sloan, L. Trien, and A. Hurtado. 2000. Maternal stress responses and anxiety during pregnancy: Effects on fetal heart rate. *Developmental Psychobiology* 36:67–77.

Myowa-Yamakoshi, M., and H. Takeshita. 2006. Do human fetuses anticipate self-oriented actions? A study by four-dimensional (4D) ultrasonography. *Infancy* 10 (3):289–301.

Nathanielsz, P. W. 1999. *Life in the Womb: The Origin of Health and Disease.* Ithaca, NY: Promethean Press.

Netter, F. H. 1962. *The Ciba Collection of Medical Illustrations.* Volume 3: A Compilation of Paintings on the Normal and Pathologic Anatomy of the Digestive System; Part II Lower Digestive Tract. Edited by E. Oppenheimer. Summit, NJ: Ciba Pharmaceutical Company.

Ng, P. C. 2000. The fetal and neonatal hypothalamic-pituitary-adrenal axis. *Archives of Disease in Childhood* 82:F250–F254.

Noble, E. 1993. *Primal Connections.* New York: Simon and Schuster.

Norwitz, E. R., D. J. Schust, and S. Fisher. 2001. Implantation and the survival of early pregnancy. *New England Journal of Medicine* 35 (19):1400–1408.

O'Connor, T. G., Y. Ben-Shlomo, J. Heron, J. Golding, D. Adams, and V. Glover. 2005. Prenatal anxiety predicts individual differences in cortisol in pre-adolescent children. *Biological Psychiatry* 58 (3):211–217.

O'Connor, T. G., J. Heron, J. Golding, V. Glover, and ALSPAC study team. 2003. Maternal antenatal anxiety and behavioural/emotional problems in children: A test of a programming hypothesis. *Journal of Child Psychology and Psychiatry* 44 (7):1025–1036.

O'Rahilly, R., and F. Muller. 1987. *Developmental Stages in Human Embryos.* Washington, DC: Carnegie Institution of Washington.

———. 2001. *Human Embryology and Teratology.* Third edition. New York: Wiley-Liss.

Odent, M. 2002. *Primal Health.* East Sussex, England: Clairview Books.

———. 1984. *Birth Reborn.* New York: Pantheon Books.

Ogden, P., K. Minton, and C. Paine. 2006. *Trauma and the Body: A Sensorimotor Approach to Psychotherapy.* New York: W. W. Norton.

Perry, B. D. 1999. The memories of states: How the brain stores and retrieves traumatic experience. In *Splintered Reflections: Images of the Body in Trauma,* edited by J. M. Goodwin and R. Attias. New York: Basic Books.

———. 2002. Childhood experience and the expression of genetic potential: What childhood neglect tells us about nature and nurture. *Brain and Mind* 3:79–100.

———. 2006. Applying principles of neurodevelopment to clinical work with maltreated and traumatized children. In *Working with Traumatized Youth in Child Welfare,* edited by N. B. Webb. New York: Guilford Press.

Pert, C. 1997. *Molecules of Emotion.* New York: Random House.

Peterson, G. 1994. Chains of grief: The impact of prenatal loss on subsequent pregnancy. *Pre- and Perinatal Psychology Journal* 9 (2):149–158.

Piontelli, A. 1992. *From Fetus to Child: An Observational and Psychoanalytic Study.* New York: Brunner-Routledge.

Plichta, S. B., and M. Falik. 2001. Prevalence of violence and its implications for women's health. *Women's Health Issues* 11 (3):244–258.

Porges, S. 2001. The polyvagal theory: Phylogenetic substrates of a social nervous system. *International Journal of Psychophysiology* 42:123–146.

———. 2004. Neuroception: A subconscious system for detecting threats and safety. *Zero to Three* May 2004:19–24.

———. 2011. *The Polyvagal Theory: Neurophysiological Foundations of Emotions, Attachment, Communication, and Self-regulation.* New York: W.W. Norton.

Putnam, F. 1992. Discussion: Are alter personalities fragments or figments? *Psychoanalytic Inquiry* 25:95–111.

Reida, C. R., T. Lattya, A. Dussutourc, and M. Beekmana. 2012. Slime mold uses an externalized spatial "memory" to navigate in complex environments. *Proceeding in the National Academy of Sciences* October 23, 109 (43):17490–17494.

Resnick, H. S., D. G. Kilpatrick, B. S. Dansky, B. E. Saunders, and C. L. Best. 1993. Prevalence of civilian trauma and post-traumatic stress disorder in a representative national sample of women. *Journal of Consulting and Clinical Psychology* 61 (6):984–991.

Robohm, J. S., and M. Buttenheim. 1996. The gynecological care experience of adult survivors of childhood sexual abuse: A preliminary investigation. *Women and Health* 24 (3):59–75.

Rossi, E. L., and D. B. Cheek. 1988. *Mind-Body Therapy: Methods of Ideodynamic Healing in Hypnosis.* New York: W. W. Norton.

Rothschild, B. 2000. *The Body Remembers: The Psychophysiology of Trauma and Trauma Treatment.* New York: W.W. Norton.

Sandman, C. A., and Davis, E. P. 2012. Neurobehavioral risk is associated with gestational exposure to stress hormones. *Expert Review of Endocrinology & Metabolism* 7 (4):445–459.

SART. 2008. Assisted Reproductive Technologies: A Guide for Patients. http://www .asrm.org/Patients/patientbooklets/ART.pdf.

Schachter, C., C. Stalker, and E. Teram. 2001. *Handbook on Sensitive Practice for Health Professionals: Lessons from Women Survivors of Childhood Sexual Abuse.* National Clearinghouse on Family Violence, Public Health Agency of Canada. Available from http://www.phac-aspc.gc.ca/ncfv-cnivf/familyviolence/html.

Schore, A. 1994. *Affect Regulation and the Origin of the Self: The Neurobiology of Emotional Development.* Hillsdale, NJ: Lawrence Erlbaum Associates.

———. 2001. The effects of early relational trauma on right brain development, affect regulation, and infant mental health. *Infant Mental Health Journal* 22 (1–2):201–269.

———. 2002. The neurobiology of attachment and early personality organization. *Journal of Prenatal and Perinatal Psychology and Health* 16 (3):249–263.

———. 2003. *Affect Dysregulation and Disorders of the Self.* New York: W. W. Norton.

———. 2003. *Affect Regulation and the Repair of the Self.* New York: W. W. Norton.

———. 2012. *The Science of the Art of Psychotherapy.* New York: W. W. Norton.

Schultz, P., and R. Feitis. 1996. *The Endless Web: Fascial Anatomy and Physical Reality.* Berkeley, CA: North Atlantic Books.

Schweiger, A. P., L. Pellerin, C. Hubold, K. M. Oltmanns, M. Conrad, B. Shultes, et. al. 2004. The selfish brain: Competition for energy resources. *Neuroscience and Biobehavioral Reviews* 28:143–180.

Seckl, J. R. 2008. Glucocorticoids, developmental "programming" and the risk of affective dysfunction. *Progress in Brain Research* 167:17–34.

Selver, C. 1995. Coming to our senses. Interview with Charlotte Selver (John Schick). In *Bone, Breath and Gesture: Practices of Embodiment,* edited by D. H. Johnson. Berkeley, CA: North Atlantic Books.

Seng, J. S., S. A. Rauch, H. Resnick, C. D. Reed, A. King, L. K. Low, et al. 2010. Exploring post-traumatic stress disorder symptom profile among pregnant women. *Journal of Psychosomatic Obstetrics and Gynecology* 31 (3):176–187.

Seng, J. S., D. J. Oakley, C. M. Sampselle, C. Killion, S. Graham-Bermann, and I. Liberzon. 2001. Post-traumatic stress disorder and pregnancy complications. *Obstetrics and Gynecology* 97 (1):17–22.

Seng, J. S., K. J. H. Sparbel, K. K. Low, and C. Killion. 2002. Abuse related post-traumatic stress and desired maternity care practices: Women's perspectives. *Journal of Nurse Midwifery and Women's Health* 47 (5):360–370.

Shea, M. 2010. *Biodynamic Craniosacral Therapy.* Volume Three. Berkeley, CA: North Atlantic Books.

Shonkoff, J. P., W. T. Boyce, and B. S. McEwen. 2009. Neuroscience, molecular biology and the childhood roots of health disparities. *Journal of the American Medical Association* 301 (21):2252–2259.

Shumake, J., N. Conejo-Jiminez, H. Gonzalez-Pardo, and F. Gonzalez-Lima. 2004. Brain differences in newborn rats predisposed to helpless and depressive behavior. *Brain Research* 1030:267–276.

Siegel, D. 1999. *The Developing Mind: Toward a Neurobiology of Interpersonal Experience.* New York: Guilford Press.

———. 2010. *Mindsight: The New Science of Personal Transformation.* New York: Bantam Books.

———. 2012a. *The Developing Mind, Second Edition: How Relationships and the Brain Interact to Shape Who We Are.* New York: Guilford Press.

———. 2012b. *Pocket Guide to Interpersonal Neurobiology.* New York: W. W. Norton.

Simkin, P., and P. Klaus. 2004. *When Survivors Give Birth: Understanding and Healing the Effects of Early Sexual Abuse on Childbearing Women.* Seattle, WA: Classic Day Publishing.

Sonne, J. C. 2004. On tyrants as abortion survivors. *Journal of Prenatal and Perinatal Psychology and Health* 19 (2):149–167.

Stern, D. 2004. *The Present Moment: In Psychotherapy and Everyday Life.* New York: W. W. Norton.

Stough, C. 1981. *Dr. Breath: The Story of Breathing Coordination.* New York: The Stough Institute.

Sutherland, W. G. 1998. *Contributions of Thought: The Collective Writings of William Garner Sutherland, D.O.* Second edition. Portland, OR: Rudra Press.

Szejer, M. 2005. *Talking to Babies: Healing with Words on a Maternity Ward.* Boston, MA: Beacon Press.

Talge, N. M., C. Neal, and V. Glover. 2007. The early stress translational research and prevention science network: Fetal and neonatal experience on child and adolescent mental health. *Journal of Child Psychology and Psychiatry* 48 (3/4):245–261.

Thomson, P. 2004. The impact of trauma on the embryo and fetus: An application of the diathesis-stress model and the neurovulnerability-neurotoxicity model. *Journal of Prenatal and Perinatal Psychology and Health* 19 (1):9–63.

———. 2007. "Down will come baby": Prenatal stress, primitive defenses and gestational dysregulation. *Journal of Trauma and Dissociation* 8 (3):85–113.

Tjaden, P., and N. Thoennes. 1998. Prevalence, incidence, and consequences of violence against women: Findings from the National Violence Against Women Survey. In *National Institute of Justice Centers for Disease Control and Prevention, Research in Brief.* Washington, DC: U.S. Department of Justice, National Institute of Justice.

———. 2000. Prevalence and consequences of male-to-female and female-to-male intimate partner violence as measures by the National Violence Against Women Survey. *Violence Against Women* 62 (2):142–161.

Tollenaar, M. S., R. Beijers, J. Jansen, M. A. Riksen-Walraven, and C. De Weerth. 2011. Maternal prenatal stress and cortisol reactivity to stressors in human infants. *Stress* 14 (1):53–65.

Tronick, E. 2007. *The Neurobehavioral and Social-Emotional Development of Infants and Children.* New York: W. W. Norton.

Trungpa, C. 1973. *Cutting through Spiritual Materialism.* Boston: Shambhala Press.

Tsiaris, A. 2002. *From Conception to Birth: A Life Unfolds.* New York: Doubleday.

Tucker, D. M. 2001. Motivated anatomy: A core-and-shell model of corticolimbic architecture. In *Handbook of Neuropsychology* (second edition), edited by F. Boller and J. Grafman. New York: Elsevier Science.

Uvnäs-Moberg, K. U. 2003. *The Oxytocin Factor: Tapping the Hormone of Calm, Love and Healing.* Cambridge, MA: Da Capo Press.

Van den Bergh, B. R. H., and A. Marcoen. 2004. High antenatal maternal anxiety is related to ADHD symptoms, externalizing problems, and anxiety in 8- and 9-year olds. *Child Development* 75 (4):1085–1097.

Van den Bergh, B. R. H., E. J. H. Mulder, M. Mennes, and V. Glover. 2005. Antenatal maternal anxiety and stress and the neurobehavioral development of the fetus and child: Links and possible mechanisms. A review. *Neuroscience and Biobehavioral Reviews* 29:237–258.

Van den Bergh, B. R. H., H. Van Calster, T. Smits, S. Van Huffel, and L. Lagae. 2008. Antenatal maternal anxiety is related to HPA-axis dysregulation and self-reported depressive symptoms in adolescence: A prospective study on the fetal origins of depressed mood. *Neuropsychopharmacology* 33 (3):536–545.

Van der Kolk, B. 2012. How Trauma Traps Survivors in the Past—A Look at Trauma Therapy. Webinar presentation June 6, 2012 from The National Institute for the Clinical Application of Behavioral Medicine, www.nicabm.com.

Verny, T. R., and K. Kelly. 1981. *The Secret Life of the Unborn Child.* New York: Summit Books.

Verny, T. R., and P. Weintraub. 2002. *Tomorrow's Baby: The Art and Science of Parenting from Conception through Infancy.* New York: Simon and Schuster.

Vieten, C., and J. Astin. 2008. Effects of a mindfulness-based intervention during pregnancy on prenatal stress and mood: Results of a pilot study. *Archives of Women's Mental Health* 11 (1):67–74.

Wade, J. 1998. Physically transcendent awareness: A comparison of the phenomenology of consciousness before birth and after death. *Journal of Near Death Studies* 16 (4):249–275.

———. 1998. Two voices from the womb: Evidence for physically transcendent and a cellular source of fetal consciousness. *Journal of Prenatal and Perinatal Psychology and Health* 13 (2).

Wadhwa, P. D. 2005. Psychoneuroendocrine processes in human pregnancy influence fetal development and health. *Psychoneuroendocrinology* 30:724–743.

Wadhwa, P. D., L. Glynn, C. J. Hobel, T. J. Garite, M. Porto, A. Chicz-DeMet, A. K. Wiglesworth, and C. A. Sandman. 2002. Behavioral perinatology: Biobehavioral processes in human fetal development. *Regulatory Peptides* 108:149–157.

Wambach, H. 1981. *Life before Life.* New York: Bantam.

Weinstein, A. D. 2010. The Experiences of Women Who Received Reproductive Endocrinology Treatment for Infertility. Dissertation. Santa Barbara, CA: Santa Barbara Graduate Institute.

Weinstock, M. 1997. Does prenatal stress impair coping and regulation of hypothalamic-pituitary-adrenal axis? *Neuroscience and Biobehavioral Reviews* 21 (1):1–10.

Weitensteiner, J. 2005. Key Factors in Sensory Development [unpublished course handout]. Santa Barbara, CA.

Weitlauf, J. C., J. W. Finney, J. I. Ruzek, T. T. Lee, M. Thraikill, and S. Jones. 2008. Distress and pain during pelvic examinations: Effect of sexual violence. *Obstetrics and Gynecology* 112 (6):1343–1350.

Williamson, G., and M. Anzalone. 2001. *Sensory Integration and Self-Regulation in Infants and Toddlers: Helping Very Young Children Interact with Their Environment.* Washington: Zero to Three.

Yehuda, R., editor. 2002. *Treating Trauma Survivors with PTSD.* Washington, DC: American Psychiatric Publishing.

Yehuda, R., S. M. Engel, S. R. Brand, J. Seckl, and S. M. Marcus. 2005. Transgenerational effects of post-traumatic stress disorder in babies of mothers exposed to the World Trade Center attacks during pregnancy. *Journal of Clinical Endocrinology and Metabolism* 90 (7):4115–4118.

CLOSING THOUGHT

Unlimited compassion
Infinite compassion
Unbiased compassion
The seed is there from conception.

ABOUT THE AUTHOR

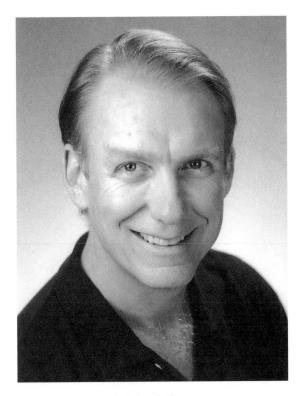

Michael Shea

One of the Upledger Institute's first certified full instructors of craniosacral therapy in 1986, Michael Shea, PhD, has taught somatic psychology, myofascial release, visceral manipulation, and craniosacral therapy worldwide for more than thirty years. He is co-founder of the International Affiliation of Biodynamic Trainings, a founding board member of the Biodynamic Craniosacral Therapy Association of North America, and a student of His Holiness the Dalai Lama. Dr. Shea has also taught in the somatic psychology and pre-and perinatal doctoral programs at the Santa Barbara Graduate Institute and has served on several pre- and perinatal doctoral committees. He lives in Juno Beach, Florida, with his wife Cathy. For more information on his courses and trainings, visit www .michaelsheateaching.com.